Serum free light chain analysis

4th Edition

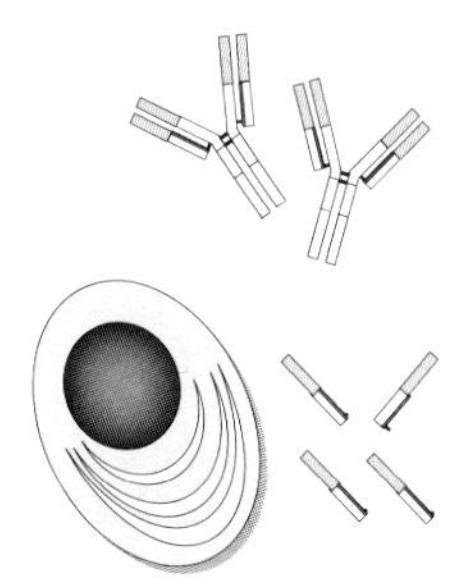

Distributors:
The Binding Site Ltd., PO Box 11712, Birmingham, B14 4ZB, UK.
U.S.A.: Binding Site Inc: San Diego, Ca 92121

Published by The Binding Site Ltd., PO Box 11712, Birmingham, B14 4ZB, UK
Printed in the UK by HSWprint., Rhondda, Wales, UK
This book was produced using QuarkXpress 5.0 and Powerpoint 97
A CIP record for this book is available from the British Library.

ISBN: 0704425297

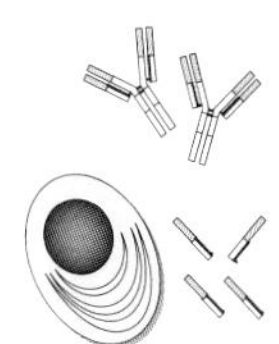

Serum free light chain analysis

4th Edition

AR Bradwell MB ChB, FRCP, FRCPath.

Professor of Immunology, The Medical School, University of Birmingham, B15 2TT, UK and The Binding Site Ltd., PO Box 11712, B14 4ZB, UK.

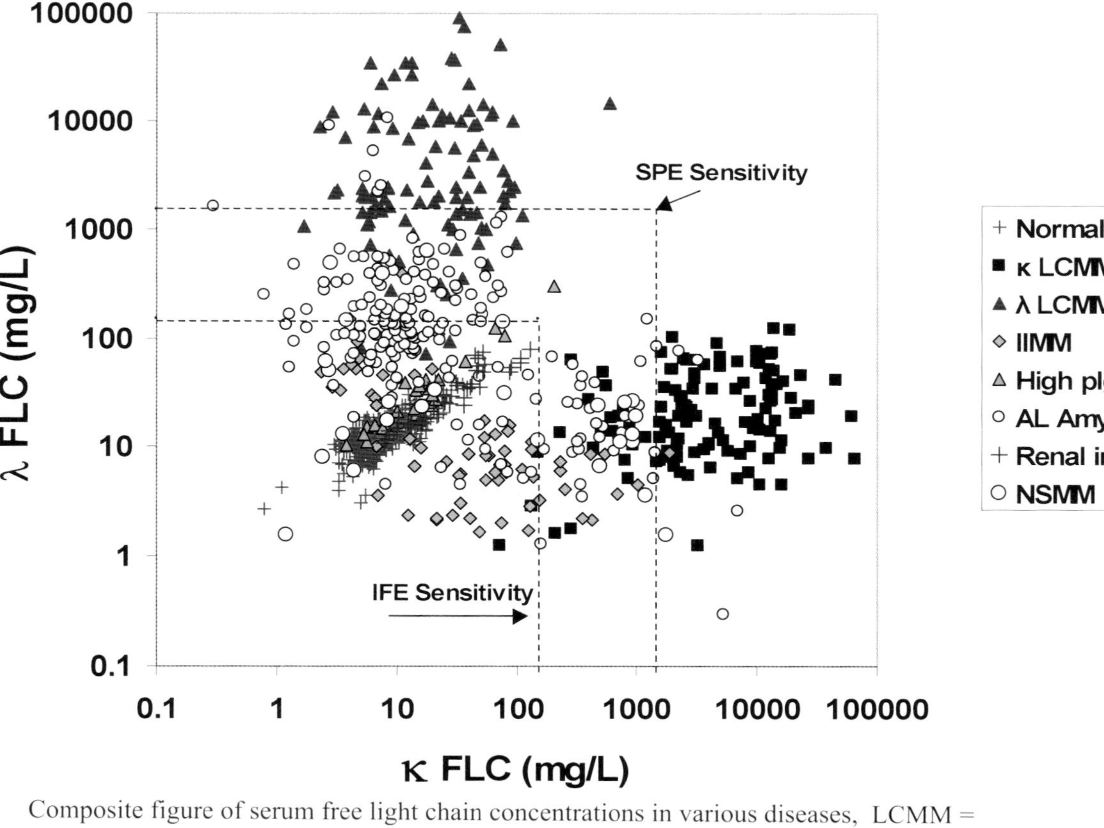

Composite figure of serum free light chain concentrations in various diseases, LCMM = light chain multiple myeloma; IIMM = intact immunoglobulin multiple myeloma; High pIgG = polyclonal hypergammaglobulinaemia; NSMM = nonsecretory multiple myeloma.

Contents

SECTION 1

Immunoglobulin free light chains and their analysis

SECTION 2

Diseases with monoclonal free light chains

SECTION 2A. Multiple myeloma

SECTION 2C. Other diseases with monoclonal free light chains

SECTION 3

Diseases with increased polyclonal free light chains

SECTION 4

General applications of free light chain assays

SECTION 5

Practical aspects of serum free light chain testing

SECTION 6

Appendices

Preface to fourth edition 2006

The first edition of this book was published only three years ago. Since then the subject has evolved enormously. The stumbling infant has grown through childhood into a young adult and has developed stature, presence and impact. Now the rate of change is slowing, fewer new concepts are being discovered and horizons are being defined.

An important recent development has been the use of free light chain measurements in patients with monoclonal gammopathies of undetermined significance. In combination with M-spike concentrations and immunoglobulin class, risk stratification for progression is now possible. This should allow many patients to be confidently reassured about the benign nature of their cancer marker. Others, at high risk, might enter prophylactic trials in an attempt to prevent disease progression.

There is great interest in using serum free light chain measurements alongside serum protein electrophoresis to screen symptomatic patients for monoclonal gammopathies. The strategy is more sensitive than testing for Bence Jones proteinuria; both simpler and clinically more accurate. Many centres are now using the test in this manner, leading to improvements in patient diagnosis and management. Support for this approach is seen in the emerging International Guidelines for treating patients with multiple myeloma and AL amyloidosis. Uniform Response criteria have been defined, and patients previously thought to have nonsecretory disease can now enter clinical trials.

The full impact of free light chains as fast response markers to therapy is yet to be realised. But, in some centres, failure of serum free light chain concentrations to fall rapidly following treatment alterations is interpreted as therapeutic failure. Drug doses or regimens are altered accordingly and ineffective chemotherapy terminated.

Of emerging importance is knowledge of the relationship between serum free light chain concentrations and nephrotoxicity. Many patients with multiple myeloma develop acute and chronic renal failure because of free light chain damage. Identifying patients at risk allows early drug treatment and may prevent progression of renal disease. In addition, serum free light chains can be quickly removed by novel 'protein leaking' dialysis membranes. This may impact on patients with renal failure from light chain multiple myeloma and AL amyloidosis.

The purpose of this fourth edition is to ensure that the new data on serum free light chain tests is readily available to all those who are interested. Modernisation from the use of urine to serum analysis is underway as free light chain tests gather momentum. The impact is considerable, but.........

Change is not made without inconvenience, even from worse to better.

Samuel Johnson: 1755 in the preface to
'A dictionary of the English Language'.

AR Bradwell March 2006

Preface to first edition 2003

Imagine the scene in a darkened room of an immunology laboratory. Four people, a professor, a junior doctor, a medical student and a technician were reviewing gels over a light-box. They were struggling to ascertain which of the serum electrophoresis tests were normal and which would need immunofixation:

Slightly irritated, the elderly, white-haired professor studied the gels again.
"Can you see that small band in the gamma region?" asked the junior doctor.
"Pass me my other glasses," the professor demanded of the technician.
Carefully adjusting his bifocals, he set the line between the two lenses onto the gamma region of the gel, and guessed at the location of the band. In his youth he could see bands as well as anyone - even better.
"Yes, I can clearly see the band now," he stated emphatically.
The young medical student was not so certain and enjoyed provoking the professor.
"I think there might be two bands," she suggested, in a teasing manner, but received a warning elbow nudge from the junior doctor.
He was looking for promotion. He liked the old man and was trying to impress him. Furthermore, he had already seen the results of the serum free light chain tests that showed 625mg/L of free kappa and 5 mg/L of free lambda with a free kappa/lambda ratio of 125.
"We could test for serum free light chains" he suggested cautiously.
"I'm not using those new-fangled methods. A urine test will be fine. What was good enough for Henry Bence Jones is good enough for me," the professor resolutely replied.

The opportunity to develop and evaluate important, new clinical assays rarely occurs. Over a five-year period, we gradually realised that serum assays for immunoglobulin free light chains were both technically feasible and clinically important. Initial results from Birmingham showed that the assays could detect free light chains in serum from patients with light chain multiple myeloma, nonsecretory multiple myeloma and AL amyloidosis that hitherto had no detectable serum abnormalities. These results were confirmed in studies from the Mayo Clinic in Rochester, the National Amyloidosis Centre at the Royal Free Hospital in London, and elsewhere.

It has since been shown that serum free light chain measurements can be used to detect and monitor over 95% of all types of patients with myeloma and AL amyloidosis. Furthermore, serum concentrations provide a more accurate marker of variations in disease than urine measurements. The convenience of serum and the enhanced sensitivity and precision of the free light chain immunoassays suggest that urinalysis may rarely be required. Further studies should also allow a re-evaluation of the existing guidelines for assessment of myeloma. Many questions however, remain unanswered:

- Are serum free light chain assays useful for assessing early responses to chemotherapy?
- Are they an early marker of relapse?
- How sensitive are they for assessing minimal residual disease?
- Are they a prognostic marker in MGUS?

Present observations also need to be checked and confirmed by other laboratories. Until such time as their full clinical role is determined, it seemed opportune to review historical, analytical and clinical aspects of free light chain assays to both stimulate and substantiate this evolving subject.

AR Bradwell. Serum Free Light Chain Assays. January 2003

Dedication

This book is dedicated to my wife Barbara and my children, Edward, Annie and Susie. They have given me the indulgence of time, discovery and innovation. This has allowed faster entry of serum free light chain assays into clinical practice. I much appreciate their love and patience.

Acknowledgements

Many people have been involved in the research, development and application of free light chain immunoassays. They include the following at The Binding Site Ltd:- Graham Mead, Hugh Carr-Smith, Paul Showell, Steven Reid, Richard Hampton and Laura Smith. The clinical data were obtained in collaboration with the following:- Mark Drayson, University of Birmingham, UK; Jerry Katzmann, Robert Kyle, Roshini Abraham, Vincent Rajkumar and Raynell Clark, The Mayo Clinic, USA; David Keren, University of Michigan Medical School, USA; Philip Hawkins and Helen Lachmann, UK Amyloidosis Centre, Royal Free Hospital, London; Peter Hill and Julia Forsyth, Derby NHS Trust, UK; G Pratt, Heartlands Hospital, Birmingham; M Chappell and N Evans, University of Warwick; S Abdalla, St Mary's Hospital, London; Timothy Harvey and Gary Galvin, Walsall Manor Hospital, UK; Mohammad Nowrousian, Essen University, Germany; and numerous other physicians who have sent samples to the laboratory. I am also indebted to Margaret Richards for the setting and presentation of this book and the numerous other jobs she has performed that have made the project possible. My grateful thanks go to them all.

The initial stages of the project were supported by a grant from the Department of Trade and Industry (No. WMR/26799/SP).

Abbreviations

ABCM	adriamycin (doxorubicin), busulphan, cyclophosphamide, melphalan
ASMM	asymptomatic multiple myeloma
B-CLL	B cell chronic lymphocytic leukaemia
CZE	capillary zone electrophoresis
CSF	cerebrospinal fluid
C-VAMP	cyclophosphamide and VAMP
Dex	dexamethasone
FcBr	Brambell Fc receptor
FLC	free light chain
FLCs	free light chains
HDM	high dose melphalan
IFE	immunofixation electrophoresis
IgG	immunoglobulin G
IIMM	intact immunoglobulin multiple myeloma
κ	kappa
κ/λ	kappa/lambda (ratio)
λ	lambda
LCDD	light chain deposition disease
LCMM	light chain multiple myeloma
MGUS	monoclonal gammopathy of undetermined significance
MM	multiple myeloma
NR	normal range
NSMM	nonsecretory multiple myeloma
NT-proBNP	amino-terminal fragment of naturetic peptide type B
PBSCT	peripheral blood stem cell transplant
PIgs	polyclonal immunoglobulins
SAP	serum amyloid P (scans)
sFLC	serum free light chain
sIFE	serum IFE
SLE	systemic lupus erythematosus
SPE	serum protein electrophoresis
TSP	total serum protein (in IFE tests)
uFLC	urine free light chain
uIFE	urine IFE
UPE	urine protein electrophoresis
VAD	vincristine, adriamycin (doxorubicin), dexamethasone
VED	vincristine, epirubicin, dexamethasone
VAMP	vincristine, adriamycin, melphalan, methyl-prednisolone

Overview - The importance of serum free light chain analysis

For 150 years, the presence of Bence Jones protein (immunoglobulin free light chains - FLCs) in the urine has been an important diagnostic marker for multiple myeloma. Indeed, it was the first cancer test and a century before any others.[1] Over the last few years, however, interest in FLCs has undergone a renaissance. Development of serum tests for free kappa (κ) and free lambda (λ) has opened the door to new applications and increased their clinical importance.[2] By way of comparison, the management of diabetes mellitus was hugely improved when blood replaced urine for glucose analysis.

From a physiological viewpoint, blood tests for small molecular weight proteins have clear advantages over urine tests. Serum FLCs are rapidly cleared through the renal glomeruli with a serum half-life of 2-6 hours and are then metabolised in the proximal tubules of the nephrons. Under normal circumstances, little protein escapes to the urine so serum FLC concentrations have to increase many-fold before the absorption mechanisms are overwhelmed.[3] This makes urinalysis a fickle witness to changing FLC production. Conversion to a serum test provides clarity in assessing disease processes that were previously hidden from view.

Serum concentrations of FLCs are dependent upon the balance between production by plasma cells and their progenitors, and renal clearance. When there is increased polyclonal immunoglobulin production and/or renal impairment, both κ and λ FLC concentrations can increase 30-40 fold. However, the relative concentration of κ to λ, i.e. the κ/λ ratio, remains unchanged. In contrast, tumors produce a monoclonal excess of only one of the light chains, often with bone marrow suppression of the alternate light chain, so that κ/λ ratios become highly abnormal. Accurate measurement of κ/λ ratios underpins the utility of the serum FLC immunoassays and provides a numerical indicator of clonality.[4] Urine κ/λ ratios are not as dependable because the non-tumor light chain production is too low to pass consistently through the nephrons. Electrophoretic tests are used only to quantify the monoclonal light chain peak because they are not sensitive enough to identify the non-tumor FLC concentrations.

Early clinical studies with serum FLC tests were in patients with Bence Jones (light chain) multiple myeloma. In two studies, on 270 sera taken at the time of clinical presentation, highly abnormal serum FLC concentrations were found in every case.[5,6] Furthermore, during chemotherapy, urine tests frequently normalised while serum tests remained abnormal, indicating their increased sensitivity for residual disease. In this patient group, urinalysis can now be replaced by serum FLC tests. This is particularly helpful for frail, elderly patients because 24-hour urine samples are difficult to collect and results may be unreliable.[7]

3-4% of patients with multiple myeloma have so called nonsecretory disease. By definition, these patients have no monoclonal proteins by serum and urine electrophoretic tests. Nevertheless, in a study by Drayson et al.,[8] serum FLC tests identified monoclonal proteins in 70% of 28 patients. A study by Katzmann et al.,[9] found that all of 5 patients with nonsecretory myeloma had abnormal FLC concentrations. It is apparent that these patients' tumor cells produce small amounts of monoclonal protein. Their serum FLC concentrations are below the sensitivity of serum electrophoretic tests and below the threshold for clearance into the urine. Importantly, these patients can now be closely monitored by serum FLC tests rather than repeated bone marrow biopsies or whole body scans.

Approximately 20% of all patients with myeloma have light chain or nonsecretory myeloma. Among the remaining patients, those who produce intact monoclonal immunoglobulins, FLCs are abnormal in 95% at disease presentation.[10] Interestingly, the serum concentrations of FLCs and intact monoclonal immunoglobulins are not correlated ($R = <0.02$). Monoclonal serum FLCs are, therefore, independent markers of the disease process. This is of potential clinical use when the tumor produces large amounts of FLCs and small amounts of intact monoclonal immunoglobulins. Patients who are in apparent remission, as judged by study of their intact monoclonal immunoglobulins, may still have monoclonal FLCs indicating residual disease. Using a similar argument, when these patients relapse, FLC concentrations may increase first. Free light chain, "breakthrough", is thought to occur in 2-5% of patients who relapse after modern, intensive treatment.

An additional feature of serum FLCs is that, in contrast to intact immunoglobulin molecules, they are potentially nephrotoxic. In many patients with intact monoclonal immunoglobulins the serum FLC concentrations are >1,000mg/L (50-100 times normal). This is characteristic of patients with IgD multiple myeloma but is also apparent in 10-15% of IgG and IgA producing patients. The assays now allow assessment of the pre-renal load of monoclonal light chains. There is early evidence that in some patients, treatment should be aimed at normalising serum FLC concentrations in order to prevent renal damage.[11]

One particularly interesting aspect of serum FLCs is their short half-life in the blood (κ 2-4 hours: λ 3-6 hours). This is approximately 100-200 times shorter than the 21-day half-life of IgG molecules. Hence, responses to treatment are seen in "real time". This is apparent from the good correlation between bone marrow assessment of disease status and FLC concentrations but a poor correlation with IgG concentrations.[12] Thus, FLC concentrations allow more rapid assessment of the effects of chemotherapy than does monoclonal IgG. The impact of this is likely to be considerable. For instance, the resistance of patients to particular drugs or drug combinations can be observed quickly and alternative treatments chosen. The short half-life of FLCs also allows distinction between partial and complete tumor responses after one or two cycles of chemotherapy and before stem cell transplantation. The 21-day half-life of IgG hides complete responses whereas FLC analysis allows more accurate assessments.[13,14]

Serum FLC tests are also having considerable impact in AL (primary) amyloidosis. Characteristically, light chain fibrils are deposited in various organs and tissues and directly lead to disease. The origin of the fibrils is monoclonal FLCs produced by a slowly growing clone of plasma cells. Concentrations are usually insufficient for measurement by serum electrophoretic tests. However, serum FLC assays provide quantification of the circulating fibril precursors in 90-95% of patients.[15,16] Furthermore, the tests allow assessment of treatment responses and disease relapses that, in turn, correlate with survival. As recently stated by Dispenzieri et al., "*The introduction of the serum immunoglobulin free light chain assay has revolutionised our ability to assess hematological responses in patients with low tumor burden*".[17]

Further support for the role of serum FLCs in AL amyloidosis is given by Katzmann et al.[9] The combination of serum FLC and serum immunofixation electrophoretic tests identified 109 of 110 patients at diagnosis. The FLC analysis alone identified 91% of the patients while immunofixation electrophoresis identified only 69%, and urinalysis failed to identify the sole patient that was normal by both serum tests. A similar high sensitivity for the FLC assays has been found in light chain deposition disease.[4,9]

The new UK and international guidelines for the management of AL amyloidosis and multiple myeloma include use of serum FLC measurements.[18,19] Reduction of the κ/λ ratio to normal, alongside the intact monoclonal immunoglobulins, will become the benchmark for complete serological responses to therapy in these and other diseases.

An emerging role of serum FLC analysis is for assessing the risk of progression in individuals with monoclonal gammopathies of undetermined significance (MGUS). These are pre-cancer markers and patients progress to multiple myeloma, AL amyloidosis or other plasma cell dyscrasias at a rate of approximately 1% per year. Rajkumar et al.[20] have recently shown that the presence of an abnormal serum FLC κ/λ ratio is a major independent risk factor for progression. In particular, the 40% of MGUS patients with low levels of IgG M-spike $<$15g/L and normal κ/λ ratios had a 21-fold lower risk of progression than patients with an M-spike of $>$15g/L, abnormal κ/λ ratios and non-IgG immunoglobulin class. It seems that the low risk patients can be reassured about their disease and may not need to be monitored on a long-term basis.

The high sensitivity of serum FLC immunoassays for tumor detection suggests they have a role in screening for plasma cell dyscrasias. Currently, symptomatic patients are assessed using serum and urine protein electrophoretic tests. Since urine is frequently unavailable, it is logical to add serum FLC analysis to current test protocols. In a study of 1,003 consecutive unknown samples by Bakshi et al.,[21] serum FLC analysis identified an additional 16 patients with monoclonal proteins above the 39 detected by serum capillary zone electrophoresis. B-cell/plasma cell tumours were present in 9 of the 16, including 3 with light chain multiple myeloma. These early results indicate that the combination of serum protein electrophoresis and FLC analysis is a clinically sensitive strategy for identifying patients with monoclonal gammopathies and will be widely adopted. Adding serum immunofixation electrophoresis is of modest extra clinical consequence. Katzmann et al.,[9] showed that there was an additional AL detection rate of 9%. However, this is a rare disease. If the choice is between serum FLCs and serum or urine immunofixation electrophoresis, then FLC tests are more useful.

FLC concentrations have been assessed in cerebrospinal fluid (CSF). In a study by Fischer et al.,[22] kappa concentrations provided information comparable with oligoclonal band measurements. They concluded that CSF kappa FLC measurements may be a useful diagnostic procedure for detecting and potentially monitoring, intrathecal immunoglobulin synthesis.

Is there a remaining role for urine FLC analysis? The answer is a qualified yes. When both serum and urine tests are available, it is always clinically reassuring when different tests provide similar results. Also, samples do occasionally get incorrectly analysed, mislabelled or misplaced, so additional evidence for making a diagnosis or changing treatment is always helpful. And, there are rare patients who have normal serum FLCs but low-level monoclonal proteins in the urine, although the clinical relevance of the urinary findings is doubtful.

In summary, serum FLC tests are assuming an increasing role in the detection and monitoring of monoclonal gammopathies. This new approach is bringing benefits to the many patients with plasma cell dyscrasias.

*This overview is largely based upon an article originally published in Clinical Chemistry (2005; **51**(5): 805-807), and is reprinted here with their permission.*

References

1. **Jones HB.** Papers on Chemical Pathology, Lecture III. Lancet 1847; **II**: 88-92.
2. **Bradwell AR, Carr-Smith HD, Mead GP, Tang LX, Showell PJ, Drayson MT, Drew R.** Highly sensitive automated immunoassay for immunoglobulin free light chains in serum and urine. Clin Chem 2001; **47**: 673-680.
3. **Bradwell AR.** Serum Free Light Chain Analysis (**4th Edition**). Pub: The Binding Site Ltd., 2006; ISBN: 0704425297.
4. **Katzmann JA, Clark RJ, Abraham RS, Bryant S, Lymp JF, Bradwell AR, Kyle RA.** Serum Reference Intervals and Diagnostic Ranges for Free κ and Free λ Immunoglobulin Light Chains: Relative Sensitivity for Detection of Monoclonal Light Chains. Clin Chem 2002; **48**: 1437-1444.
5. **Bradwell AR, Carr-Smith HD, Mead GP, Harvey TC, Drayson MT.** Serum test for assessment of patients with Bence Jones myeloma. Lancet 2003; **361**: 489-491.
6. **Abraham RS, Clark RJ, Bryant SC, Lymp JF, Larson T, Kyle RA, Katzmann JA.** Correlation of serum immunoglobulin free light chain quantitation with urine Bence Jones protein in Light Chain Myeloma. Clin Chem 2002; **48**: 655-657.
7. **Alyanakian MA, Abbas A, Delarue R, Arnulf B, Aucouturier P.** Free Immunoglobulin Light-chain Serum Levels in the Follow-up of Patients With Monoclonal Gammopathies: Correlation with 24-hr Urinary Light-chain Excretion. Am J Hematology 2004; **75**: 246-248.
8. **Drayson MT, Tang LX, Drew R, Mead GP, Carr-Smith HD, Bradwell AR.** Serum free light-chain measurements for identifying and monitoring patients with nonsecretory multiple myeloma. Blood 2001; **97**: 2900-2902.
9. **Katzmann J, Abraham RS, Dispenzieri A, Lust JA, Kyle RA.** Diagnostic performance of Quantitative Kappa and Lambda Free Light Chain Assays in Clinical Practice. Clin Chem 2005; **51**: 878-881.
10. **Mead GP, Carr-Smith HD, Drayson MT, Morgan GJ, Child JA, Bradwell AR.** Serum Free Light Chains for Monitoring Multiple Myeloma. Br J Haem 2004; **126**: 348-354.
11. **Nowrousian MR, Brandhorst D, Sammet C, Kellert M, Daniels R, Schuett P, Poser M, Mueller S, Ebeling P, Welt A, Bradwell AR, Buttkereit U, Opalka B, Flasshove M, Moritz T, Seeber S.** Serum Free Light Chain Analysis and Urine Immunofixation Electrophoresis in Patients with Multiple Myeloma. Clin Cancer Res 2005; **11** (24): 8706-8714.
12. **Mead GP, Reid S, Augustson B, Drayson MT, Bradwell AR, Child JA.** Correlation of Serum Free Light Chains and Bone Marrow Plasma Cell Infiltration in Multiple Myeloma. Blood 2004; **104**: 4865, p299b.
13. **Cavallo F, Rasmussen E, Zangari M, Tricot G, Fender B, Fox M, Burns M, Barlogie B.** Serum

Free-Lite Chain (sFLC) Assay in Multiple Myeloma (MM): Clinical Correlates and Prognostic Implications in Newly Diagnosed MM Patients Treated with Total Therapy 2 or 3 (TT2/3). Blood 2005; **106** (11): 3490, p974a.

14. Hassoun H, Reich L, Klimek VM, Dhodapkar M, Cohen A, Kewalramani T, Zimman R, Drake L, Riedel ER, Hedvat CV, Teruya-Feldstein J, Filippa DA, Fleisher M, Nimer SD, Comenzo RL. Doxorubicin and dexamethosone followed by thalidomide and dexamethasone is an effective well tolerated initial therapy for multiple myeloma. Br J Haem 2006; **132**: 155-161.

15. Lachmann HJ, Gallimore R, Gillmore JD, Carr-Smith HD, Bradwell AR, Pepys MB, Hawkins PN. Outcome in systemic AL amyloidosis in relation to changes in concentration of circulating free immunoglobulin light chains following chemotherapy. Br J Haematol 2003; **122**: 78-84.

16. Abraham RS, Katzmann JA, Clark RJ, Bradwell AR, Kyle RA, Gertz MA. Quantitative analysis of serum free light chains. A new marker for the diagnostic evaluation of primary systemic amyloidosis. Am J Clin Pathol 2003; **119**: 274-278.

17. Dispenzieri A, Gertz MA, Kyle RA. Determining appropriate treatment options for patients with primary systemic amyloidosis. Blood 2004; **104**: 2992.

18. Bird JM, Cavenagh J, Samson D, Mehta A, Hawkins P, Lachmann H. Guidelines on the diagnosis and management of AL amyloidosis. Br J Haematol 2004; **125**: 681-700.

19. Kumar S, Gertz MA, Hayman SR, Lacy MQ, Dispenzieri A, Zeldenrust AR, Lust JA, Greipp PR, Kyle RA, Fonseca R, Rajkumar SV. Use of the Serum Free Light Chain Assay in Assessment of Response to Therapy in Multiple Myeloma: Validation of Recently Proposed Response Criteria in a Prospective Clinical Trial of Lenalidomide Plus Dexamethasone for Newly Diagnosed Multiple Myeloma. Blood 2005: **106** (11): 3479, p971a.

20. Rajkumar SV, Kyle RA, Therneau TM, Melton LJ III, Bradwell AR, Clark RJ, Larson DR, Plevak MF, Dispenzieri A, Katzmann JA. Serum free light chain ratio is an independent risk factor for progression in monoclonal gammopathy of undetermined significance. Blood 2005; **106**: 812-817.

21. Bakshi NA, Guilbranson R, Garstka D, Bradwell AR, Keren DF. Serum Free Light Chain (FLC) Measurement Can Aid Capillary Zone Electrophoresis (CZE) In Detecting Subtle FLC M-Proteins. Am J Clin Path 2005;**124**: 214-218.

22. Fischer C, Arneth B, Koehler J, Lotz J, Lackner K. Kappa Free Light-chains in Cerebrospinal Fluid as Markers of Intrathecal Immunoglobulin Synthesis. Clin Chem 2004; **50**: 1809-1813.

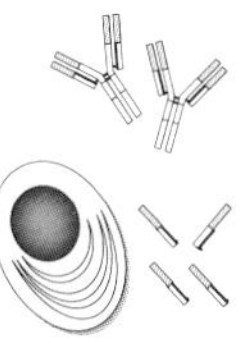

Section 1

Immunoglobulin free light chains and their analysis

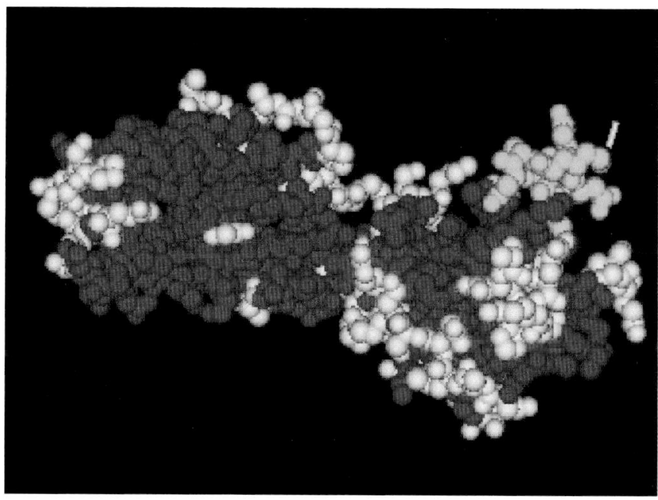

Figure 1.0. Three-dimensional structure of a κ light chain molecule.

Tumour type	Cancer deaths	Tumour markers	Specificity	Sensitivity	Tumour Detection	Clinical Utility
Lung + bronchus	28%	Neuron specific enolase	Poor	Poor	Late	Poor
Colon + rectum	10%	Carcinoembryonic antigen	Poor	Modest	Late	Modest
Breast	8%	CA 15-3; CEA	Poor	Modest	Late	Modest
Pancreas	5%	CA 19-9; CEA	Poor	Poor	Late	Poor
Prostate	5%	Prostate-specific antigen	Good	Good	Intermediate	Good
Stomach	3%	CEA; CA 19-9	Modest	Modest	Late	Poor
Ovary	2.5%	CA 125; PLAP	Modest	Modest	Intermediate	Good
Liver	1%	Alpha feto-protein (αFP)	Good	Good	Intermediate	Good
Myeloma	**1.5%**	**Monoclonal protein/FLC**	**Good**	**Good**	**Early**	**Very good**
AL amyloidosis	**0.3%**	**Monoclonal protein/FLC**	**Good**	**Good**	**Early**	**Very good**
Germ cell	~0.1%	αFP; hCG	Good	Good	Early	Very good
Choriocarcinoma	<0.1%	Chorionic gonadotrophin	Good	Good	Early	Very good
Neuroendocrine	<0.1%	Chromogranin A	Good	Good	Early	Very good

Table 1. Some common serum tumour markers and their clinical utility. All these analytes are measured using highly sensitive immunoassays apart from monoclonal proteins. FLC = free light chains

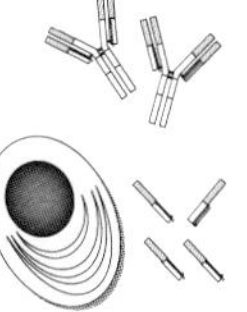

Chapter 1

Introduction

Multiple myeloma is a disease with many faces. It usually presents in old age but may occur in youth; bone pain and fractures are characteristic yet there are soft tissue plasmacytomas; patients may die within weeks of presentation while others 'smoulder' for years. Patients may have renal failure, acute and chronic infections or amyloidosis and will need stem cell transplantations, intensive chemotherapy, etc. Consequently, many specialists become involved in disease management such as haematologists, nephrologists, immunologists, orthopaedic surgeons and chemical pathologists. Furthermore, the prevalence of MM is increasing with a slowly rising incidence and a longer life expectancy.[1-4]

Despite the complexity of this disease one feature has been a great lighthouse in the fog, alerting the unwary to the diagnosis and guiding the hand of management; the presence of monoclonal immunoglobulins. Produced in excess, and in a variety of shapes and sizes, these molecules have been linked to MM since they were first identified by Henry Bence Jones, FRS., over 150 years ago.[5] Notwithstanding their substantial history and great utility, measurement of these tumour markers, particularly FLCs, has remained imperfect. Techniques used for their measurement have failed to keep pace with analytical developments in other fields.

Most serum cancer tests are now based on state-of-the-art immunoassays and are highly automated. (*A selection of the more common serum markers is shown in Table 1*). In contrast, tests for MM and AL amyloidosis are based on old-fashioned, electrophoretic techniques. These are rather insensitive, require considerable experience for interpretation and are labour-intensive.[6-8] How ironic that the first tumour marker to be identified should be the last to benefit from modern technology.

Perhaps it is not surprising that errors occur in FLC measurements.[9] And, why measure FLCs in urine? It is difficult to imagine a less attractive fluid in which to evaluate these molecules. The prime function of the kidneys is to ***prevent*** the loss of FLCs and other small protein molecules into the urine. Furthermore, urine samples are voluminous, difficult to obtain, awkward to transport and need concentration prior to analysis.

An alternative strategy is to measure FLCs in serum. In 1981, it was shown that serum concentrations were elevated when Bence Jones proteinuria occurred (*Chapter 2*) and serum was diagnostically more accurate than urine in patients with renal failure.[10,11] Why, therefore, have serum immunoassays not been used before?

It appears that the over-riding problem had been the difficulty in developing satisfactory antibodies. To function correctly, they must not only be of high affinity to allow measurement of the low concentrations of FLCs in serum, but they must also be highly specific. Serum FLC concentrations are several orders of magnitude lower than serum light chains bound to intact immunoglobulins, so even minor antibody cross-reactivity produces unacceptable results. Only recently have suitable antibodies been developed that bind exclusively to the hidden epitopes of FLC molecules. Serum FLC assays are now specific, sensitive and quantitative.[12,13]

Serum FLC immunoassays offer the following benefits:

- Better sensitivity and precision than current electrophoretic assays.
- Numerical results for disease monitoring.
- Convenience of serum as a test medium.
- Identification of AL amyloidosis and NSMM patients who have no detectable monoclonal proteins by conventional tests.
- More accurate marker of complete disease remission than existing assays.
- Short half-life marker for rapid assessment of treatment responses.
- Identification of progression risk in individuals with MGUS.
- Better screening of symptomatic patients.

General statements have been formulated on the clinical applications of cancer markers.[14] Most of these have now been determined for FLC immunoassays:-

1. Differential diagnosis in symptomatic patients. Serum FLC analysis is most helpful in the differential diagnosis of patients with bone pain, fractures, equivocal bone marrow biopsy results, unexplained renal impairment and other features of MM and AL amyloidosis *(Sections 2 and 4)*.

2. Clinical staging of disease. Serum FLC concentrations show a relationship with the staging of monoclonal diseases and are helpful in assessing residual disease after treatment *(Chapters 10 and 12)*.

3. Estimating tumour burden. Serum FLC concentrations correlate poorly with tumour volume at the time of diagnosis but changing concentrations correlate well with changing tumour burden during treatment *(Section 2)*.

4. Prognostic indicator for disease progression. There is evidence that sFLC concentrations are helpful. Patients who are in remission, but have elevated FLC levels in the absence of other abnormalities are at risk of early relapse. Of particular interest is the use of the assays for predicting progression of MGUS. Recent studies from the Mayo Clinic indicate that elevated monoclonal FLCs are the most sensitive risk factor for progression to plasma cell dyscrasias *(Section 2)*.

5. Evaluating the success of treatment. FLC analysis is particularly helpful in assessing treatment responses in patients with AL amyloidosis, LCMM and NSMM. There are also indications that the short half-life of FLCs can be used to assess early treatment responses in nearly all patients with monoclonal proteins. Many studies are currently underway *(Section 2)*.

6. Detecting the recurrence of cancer. Serum FLCs are useful for detecting disease recurrence and are more sensitive than other tests in patients with AL amyloidosis, LCMM and NSMM. They are useful in a proportion of patients with IIMM and some other monoclonal gammopathies *(Section 2)*.

7. Screening symptomatic patients. At present, patients with symptoms of MM or related disorders are screened for monoclonal proteins by serum and urine electrophoretic tests. Several recent studies have shown that serum FLC analysis identifies more patients and can replace urine tests *(Chapters 23 and 24)*.

8. Screening the general population. There is evidence that sFLC measurements identify a new set of MGUS patients in otherwise healthy people *(Chapter 19)*. The importance of this is not clear. Since one of the criteria for a successful screening test includes a beneficial outcome for the population screened, it will be many years before it is clear whether serum FLCs are useful in this context.

In addition, the assays are allowing new guidelines to be written for the diagnosis and monitoring of patients with MM, AL amyloidosis and other diseases producing excess FLCs.

This book describes the discovery of Bence Jones protein, the structure and synthesis of light chain molecules and assays for sFLC quantitation. A detailed account is given of the current use of the assays in clinical and laboratory practice together with some potential applications in other situations. Finally, there are appendices for guidance in their clinical and laboratory use.

References

1. **Alexanian R, Weber D, Liu F.** Differential Diagnosis of Monoclonal Gammopathies. Arch Pathol Lab Med 1999; **123**: 108-113.

2. **Kyle RA.** Multiple Myeloma and Other Plasma Cell Disorders. Haematology: Basic Principles & Practice 1995, 2nd edition New York: Churchill Livingstone: 1354-1374.

3. **Merlini G.** Monoclonal Gammopathies. Cancer J 1995; **8**: 173-180.

4. **Rajkumar SV, Greipp PR.** Prognostic Factors in Multiple Myeloma. In Hematology/Oncology Clinics of North America: Monoclonal Gammopathies & related disorders. Eds. RA Kyle & M A Gertz; Pub: W B Saunders Co. Philadelphia; 1999; **13** (6): 1295-1314.

5. **Jones HB.** Papers on Chemical Pathology, Lecture III. Lancet 1847; **II**: 88-92.

6. **Levinson SS, Keren DF.** Free Light Chains of Immunoglobulins: Clinical Laboratory Analysis. Clin Chem 1994; **40**: 1869-1878.

7. **Merlini G, Aguzzi F, Whicher J.** Monoclonal Gammopathies. J Int Fed Clin Chem 1997; **9**: 171-177.

8. **Attaelmannan M, Levinson SS.** Understanding and Identifying Monoclonal Gammopathies. Clin Chem 2000; **46**: 1230-1238.

9. **Ward AM, White PAE, Beetham R.** UK NEQAS Monoclonal Protein Identification Distribution 986. UK NEQAS Sheffield, 1998.

10. **Sölling K.** Free light chains of immunoglobulins: studies of radioimmunoassay of normal values, polymerisation, mechanisms of renal handling and clinical significance. Scand J Clin Lab Invest 1981; **41** (Suppl 157): 15-83.

11. **Sinclair D, Dagg JH, Smith JG, Stott DI.** The incidence and possible relevance of Bence Jones protein in the sera of patients with multiple myeloma. Br J Haematol 1986; **62**: 689-694.

12. Bradwell AR, Carr-Smith HD, Mead GP, Tang LX, Showell PJ, Drayson MT, Drew R. Highly sensitive automated immunoassay for immunoglobulin free light chains in serum and urine. Clin Chem 2001; **47**: 673-680.

13. Katzmann J, Abraham RS, Dispenzieri A, Lust JA, Kyle RA. Diagnostic performance of Quantitative Kappa and Lambda Free Light Chain Assays in Clinical Practice. Clin Chem 2005; **51** (5): 878-881

14. Chan DW, Schwartz MK. Tumor Markers: Introduction and General Principles. In: Tumor Markers Physiology, Pathology, Technology and Clinical Applications. Eds. EP Diamandis, HA Fritsche, H Lilja, DW Chan, MH Schwartz.Pub: AACC Press, Washington, DC, 2002: Chapt 2: 9-17.

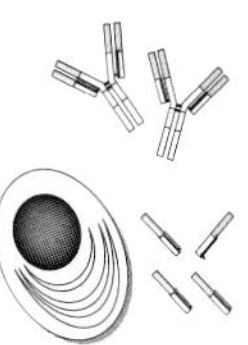

Chapter 2

Dr Bence Jones and the history of free light chains

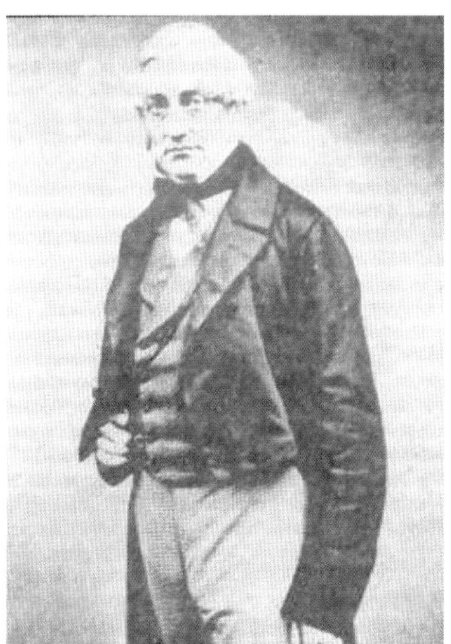
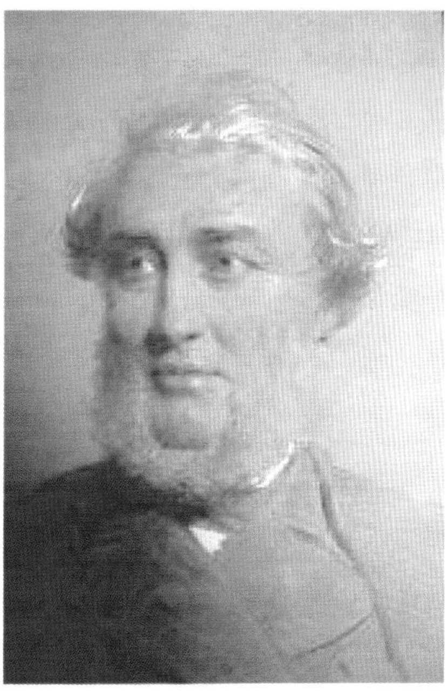

Figure 2.1. Henry Bence Jones (Courtesy of RA Kyle and The British Journal of Haematology).

Although immunoglobulin FLCs are synonymous with Bence Jones proteins, history might have been more generous to others involved in their discovery.[1-4]

On Friday, October 30th 1845, the 53 year old Dr William MacIntyre, physician to the Western General Dispensary, St. Marylebone, London, left his rooms in Harley Street. He had been called to see Mr Thomas Alexander McBean, a 45 year-old, highly respectable grocer, who had severe bone pain and fractures. He had been under the care of his general practitioner, Dr Thomas Watson, for several months. Upon examination of the patient, William MacIntyre noted the presence of oedema. Considering the possibility of nephrosis, he tested the urine for albumin. To his consternation, the albuminous protein precipitate found on warming the urine, uncharacteristically, re-dissolved when heated to 75°C.

Both Dr MacIntyre and Dr Watson then sent urine samples to the chemical pathologist at St.George's Hospital. A note accompanying the urine sent by Dr Watson read as follows:-

"Dear Dr Bence Jones,
The tube contains urine of very high specific gravity. When boiled it becomes highly opaque. On the addition of nitric acid, it effervesces, assumes a reddish hue, and becomes quite clear; but as it cools assumes the consistence and appearance which you see. Heat reliquifies it. What is it?"

Over the next two months, the patient deteriorated, became emaciated, weak, and was racked with pain. He eventually died on January 1st 1846, in full possession of his mental faculties. Dr MacIntyre subsequently published the post-mortem examination and the description of the peculiar urine in 1850.[5] Unfortunately for him, Henry Bence Jones had already described the patient's urinary findings in two, single author articles, one of which was published in *The Lancet*, in 1847.[6,7] He considered the protein to be an "*hydrated deutoxide of albumen*". He wisely commented:

"I need hardly remark on the importance of seeking for this oxide of albumen in other cases of mollities ossium".

Bence Jones's reputation was assured, while the contributions of his colleagues were consigned to the footnotes of history.

For all the apparent injustice to his colleague, William MacIntyre, Henry Bence Jones achieved much else in his career. He published over 40 papers and became rich and famous based on his clinical practice, lecturing and original observations and was elected to fellowship of The Royal Society at the tender age of 33. Florence Nightingale once described him as 'the best chemical doctor in London.' Surprisingly, there was no mention of Bence Jones protein in his obituary and the eponym (and the hyphen in his name) was not used until after his death.[2]

By 1909, over 40 cases of Bence Jones proteinuria had been reported,[8] and the protein was thought to originate in bone marrow plasma cells which were first identified by Waldeyer in 1875.[9] In 1922, Bayne-Jones and Wilson characterised two types of Bence Jones protein by observing precipitation reactions using antisera made by immunising rabbits with the urine of several patients.[10] The proteins were classified as group I and group II types. However, it was not until 1956 that Korngold and Lapiri,[11] using the Ouchterlony technique,[12] showed that antisera raised against the different groups also reacted with myeloma proteins. As a tribute to their observations the two types of Bence Jones protein were designated kappa and lambda (κ and λ). Edelman and Gally, in 1962,[13] subsequently showed that FLCs prepared from IgG monoclonal proteins were the same as Bence Jones protein. It had taken 117 years from the original observation for the function of Bence Jones protein to be finally determined. Remarkably, the format of the urine test had remained unchanged for a similar period. The following is a protocol from Levinson and MacFate's "Clinical Laboratory Diagnosis," a standard textbook published in 1946.[14]

Bence-Jones* Protein Test

Principle. Bence-Jones protein is soluble in urine at room and body temperature. When the urine is heated to 40°C, a white cloud appears and at 60°C, a distinct precipitate forms. The precipitate disappears on boiling but reappears on cooling. Excessive amounts of acid or salt will prevent the appearance of the precipitate.
Reagent. Acetic Acid, approximately 10% aqueous solution.
Procedure. Add urine to a 6-inch test tube until it is about two-thirds full. Place in a water bath and heat slowly. Do not allow the bottom of the test tube to touch the bottom of the beaker, as it may become hotter than the rest of the water. Suspend a thermometer in the water bath. Note the temperature and the appearance of the urine every few minutes, especially between the temperatures of 40°C - 60°C. If a slight cloud appears when the urine is heated to the boiling point, 100°C, add a few drops of acetic acid. This will dissolve any phosphates that have separated out. If a precipitate forms at the boiling point, it is due to albumin. Boil the urine with a few drops of dilute acetic acid, filter rapidly, and repeat the test on the cooled filtrate.
Interpretation. Bence-Jones protein is found in urine in many cases of multiple myeloma, osteogenic sarcoma, osteomalacia, carcinomatosis.

**(The hyphen was only added after his death)*

In parallel with the clinical and scientific observations of the role of Bence Jones protein, electrophoretic techniques for protein separation were entering clinical laboratories. Longsworth et al., in 1939,[15] recognised tall, narrow-based, "church spire" peaks in the sera of patients with MM, using moving boundary protein electrophoresis. Electrophoresis was subsequently improved by using paper as a substrate followed by cellulose acetate then agarose in the 1950's and 1960's. Finally, immunofixation electrophoresis became established in the 1980's.[16]

Clear identification of κ and λ molecules was possible with the use of antibodies specific for each type of protein. Immunodiffusion was initially used,[12] followed by immunoelectrophoresis in 1953,[17] radial immunodiffusion and ultimately nephelometry and turbidimetry. However, serum assays for Bence Jones protein or "FLCs" remained unattainable because the antibodies could not distinguish between FLCs and the overwhelming amounts of light chains bound in intact immunoglobulin molecules.

The first successful attempt to measure FLCs in serum was in 1975. Size-separation column chromatography,[18-20] was used to isolate them from intact immunoglobulins, prior to analysis. Although the results were accurate and showed the potential use of serum analyses, these assays were clearly impractical for routine use. Subsequent assays focussed on the use of antibodies directed against "hidden" epitopes on FLC molecules. These are located at the interface between the light and heavy chains of intact immunoglobulins and become detectable when the FLCs are unbound. Radio-immunoassays and enzyme immunoassays using polyclonal antisera against FLCs were used to analyse urine samples but specificity remained inadequate for serum measurements,[21,22] and variations in FLC polymerisation caused measurement errors.[18,23]

The use of monoclonal antibodies was an obvious approach to improving specificity but satisfactory reagents were difficult to develop,[24-27] and their use was restricted to radio-immunoassays and enzyme immunoassays. Attempts were made to develop turbidimetric,[28,29] and latex-enhanced nephelometric assays,[30] using polyclonal antibodies but they could not detect normal sFLC concentrations, and cross-reactions with intact immunoglobulins were unacceptable. In 2001, immunoassays, based on polyclonal antibodies, were finally developed that could measure FLCs at normal serum concentrations.[31] Their utility was quickly made apparent when monoclonal FLCs were detected in the sera of most patients classified as having "nonsecretory myeloma".[32] Furthermore, as described in *The Lancet*, all of 224 patients with LCMM who had Bence Jones proteinuria, also had elevated sFLC concentrations.[33] The serum tests were also better at detecting residual disease than urinalysis. Further studies have recently shown that sFLC assays can be used for screening symptomatic patients (*Chapter 23)*, are more sensitive than urine tests *(Chapter 24)* and are markers for progression in MGUS (*Chapter 19)*.

These results and many others, herald the widespread use of sFLC immunoassays. The enduring story of Bence Jones protein and Bence Jones proteinuria may be entering its final act, 160 years after it began.

References

1. Clamp JR. Some Aspects of the First Recorded Case of Multiple Myeloma. Lancet 1967; **II** 1354-1356.

2. Rosenfeld L. Henry Bence Jones (1813-1873): the best 'chemical doctor' in London. Clin Chem 1987; **33**: 1687-1692.

3. Kyle RA. Multiple myeloma: an odyssey of discovery. Brit J Haem 2000; **111**: 1035-1044.

4. Kyle RA. Henry Bence Jones - Physician, Chemist, Scientist and Biographer: A man for all seasons. Brit J Haem 2001; **115**: 13-18.

5. MacIntyre W. Case of Mollities and Fragilitas Ossium. Med Chir Tran; 1850: 211-232.

6. Jones HB. Papers on Chemical Pathology, Lecture III. Lancet 1847; **II:** 88-92.

7. Jones HB. On the new substance occurring in the urine of a patient with mollities ossium. Philosophical Transactions of the Royal Society of London. Series B: Biological Sciences 1848; **138**: 55-62.

8. Weber FP, Ledington JCG. A note on the history of a case of myelomatosis (multiple myeloma) with Bence-Jones protein in the urine (myelopathic albumosuria). Proceedings of the Royal Society of Medicine 1909; **2**: 193-206.

9. Waldeyer W. Ueber Bindegewebszellen. Archiv fur Microbiologie und Anatomie 1875; **11**: 176-194.

10. Bayne-Jones S, Wilson DW. Immunological reactions of Bence-Jones proteins. II. Differences between Bence-Jones proteins from various sources. Bulletin of the John Hopkins Hospital 1922; **33**: 119-125.

11. Korngold L, Lapiri R. Multiple Myeloma proteins. II. The antigenic relationship of Bence-Jones proteins to normal gamma-globulin and cancer multiple myeloma serum proteins. Cancer 1956; **9**: 262-272.

12. Ouchterlony O. Antigen-antibody reactions in gels. IV. Types of reactions in coordinated systems of diffusion. Acta path et microbiol Scand 1953; **32**: 231-240.

13. Edelman GM, Gally JA. The nature of Bence-Jones proteins: chemical similarities to polypeptide chains of myeloma globulins and normal g-globulins. J Exp Med 1962; **116**: 207-227.

14. Levinson SA, MacFate RP. Bence-Jones Proteins, pp 374-375. In: Clinical Laboratory Diagnosis, 3rd Edition, 1946. Publishers: Lea and Febiger, Philadelphia.

15. Longsworth LG, Shedlovsky T, MacInnes DA. Electrophoretic patterns of normal and pathological human blood serum and plasma. J Exp Med 1939; **70**: 399-413.

16. Whicher JT, Hawkins L, Higginson J. Clinical applications of immunofixation: a more sensitive technique for the detection of Bence Jones protein. J Clin Pathol 1980; **33**: 779-780.

17. Grabar P, Williams CA. Methode permettant l'etude conjugee des proprietes electrophoretiques et immunochimiques d'un melange de proteines. Allication au serum sanguin. Biochimica et Biophysica Acta 1953; **10**: 193-194.

18. Sölling K. Free Light Chains of Immunoglobulins in Normal Serum and Urine Determined by Radioimmunoassay. Scand J Clin Lab Invest 1975; **35**: 407-412.

19. Sölling K. Normal values of free light chains in serum in different age groups. Scand J clin Lab Invest 1977; **37**: 21-25.

20. Cole PW, Durie BGM, Salmon SE. Immunoquantitation of free light chain immunoglobulins: applications in multiple myeloma. J Imm Methods 1978; **19**: 341-349.

21. Robinson EL, Gowland E, Ward ID, Scarffe JH. Radioimmunoassay of Free Light Chains of Immunoglobulins in Urine. Clin Chem 1982; **28**/11: 2254-2258.

22. Brouwer J, Otting-van de Ruit M, Busking-van der Lely H. Estimation of free light chains of immunoglobulins by enzyme immunoassay. Clin Chim Acta 1985; **150**: 257-274.

23. Heino J, Rajamaki A, Irjala K. Turbidimetric measurement of Bence-Jones proteins using antibodies against free light chains of immunoglobulins. An artifact caused by different polymeric forms of light chains. Scand J Clin Lab Invest 1984; **44**: 173-176.

24. Ling NR, Lowe J, Hardie D, Evans S, Jefferis R. Detection of free κ chains in human serum and urine using pairs of monoclonal antibodies reacting with Cκ epitopes not available on whole immunoglobulins. Clin Exp Immunol 1983; **52**: 234-240.

25. Axiak SM, Krishnamoorthy L, Guinan J, Raison RL. Quantitation of free κ light chains in serum and urine using a monoclonal antibody based inhibition enzyme-linked immunoassay. J Imm Methods 1987; **99**: 141-147.

26. Nelson M, Brown RD, Gibson J, Joshua DE. Measurement of free kappa and lambda chains in serum and the significance of their ratio in patients with multiple myeloma. Br J Haemat 1992; **81**: 223-230.

27. Abe M, Goto T, Kosaka M, Wolfenbarger D, Weiss DT, Solomon A. Differences in kappa and lambda (κ:λ) ratios of serum and urinary free light chains. Clin Exp Imm 1998; **111**: 457-462.

28. Hemmingsen L, Skaarup P. Urinary Excretion of Ten Plasma Proteins in Patients with Febrile Diseases. Acta Med Scand 1977; **201**: 359-364.

29. Tillyer CR, Iqbal J, Raymond J, Gore M, McIlwain TJ. Immunoturbidimetric assay for estimating free light chains of immunoglobulins in urine and serum. J Clin Pathol 1991; **44**: 466-471.

30. Wakasugi K, Suzuki H, Imai A, Konishi S, Kishioka H. Immunoglobulin free light chain assay using latex agglutination. Int J Clin Lab Res 1995; **25**: 211-215.

31. Bradwell AR, Carr-Smith HD, Mead GP, Tang LX, Showell PJ, Drayson MT, Drew R. Highly sensitive automated immunoassay for immunoglobulin free light chains in serum and urine. Clin Chem 2001; **47**: 673-680.

32. Drayson MT, Tang LX, Drew R, Mead GP, Carr-Smith HD, Bradwell AR. Serum free light-chain measurements for identifying and monitoring patients with nonsecretory multiple myeloma. Blood 2001; **97**: 9; 2900-2902.

33. Bradwell AR, Carr-Smith HD, Mead GP, Harvey TC, Drayson MT. Serum test for assessment of patients with Bence Jones myeloma. Lancet 2003; **361**: 489-491.

Test questions

1. Who was the first person to observe 'Bence Jones proteinuria'?
2. What is the origin of the names, kappa and lambda?

Answers

1. Dr William MacIntyre in 1845 (page 7).
2. The first letters of Korngold and Lapiri who showed that light chains were located on immunoglobulin molecules in 1956 (page 8).

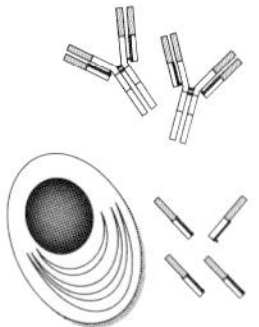

Chapter 3

Biology of immunoglobulin light chains

3.1. Structure

Antibody molecules have a two-fold symmetry and are composed of two identical heavy chains and two identical light chains, each containing variable and constant domains. The variable domains of each light chain, heavy chain pair combine to form an antigen-binding site, so that both chains contribute to the antigen-binding specificity of the antibody molecule. Light chains are of two types, κ and λ and any given antibody molecule has either light chain but never both. There are approximately twice as many κ as λ molecules produced in humans but this is quite different in some mammals. Each FLC molecule contains approximately 220 amino acids in a single polypeptide chain that is folded to form the constant and variable region domains (*Figure 3.1*).

Domains are constructed from two β sheets, which are elements of protein structure made up of strands of the polypeptide chain (β strands) packed together in a particular

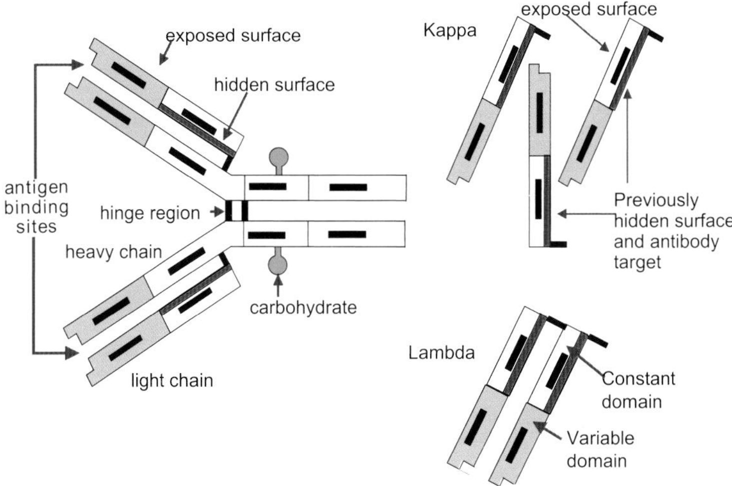

Figure 3.1. An antibody molecule showing the heavy and light chain structure, together with free κ and λ FLCs.

shape. The sheets are linked by a disulfide bridge and together form a roughly barrel-shaped structure known as a β barrel (*Figure 3.2*).

The constant (C) domains of the FLCs show little variation except for the amino acid substitutions found in the Km allotypes on κ molecules and the Oz and Kern isotypes on λ molecules. In contrast, the variable (V) domain has huge structural diversity, particularly in association with the antigen binding amino acids. In addition, the first 23 amino acids of the 1st variable domain framework region have a limited number of variations known as subgroups. Using monoclonal antibodies, 4 kappa (Vκ1 - Vκ4) and 6 lambda subgroups (Vλ1 - Vλ6) can be identified.[1] The specific subgroup structures influence the potential of the FLCs to polymerise such that AL amyloidosis is associated with Vλ6 and LCDD with Vκ1 and Vκ4.

3.2. Synthesis

κ FLC molecules (chromosome 2) are constructed from approximately 40 functional Vκ gene segments, five Jκ gene segments and a single Cκ gene. λ molecules (chromosome 22) are constructed from about 30 Vλ gene segments and four pairs of functional Jλ gene segments and a Cλ gene *(Figure 3.3)*.

FLCs are incorporated into immunoglobulin molecules during B lymphocyte development and are expressed initially on the surface of immature B-cells. Production of FLCs occurs throughout the rest of B-cell development and in plasma cells, where secretion is highest. Tumours associated with the different stages of B-cell maturation will secrete monoclonal FLCs into the serum where they may be detected by FLC immunoassays (*Figures 3.4 and Chapter 18*).

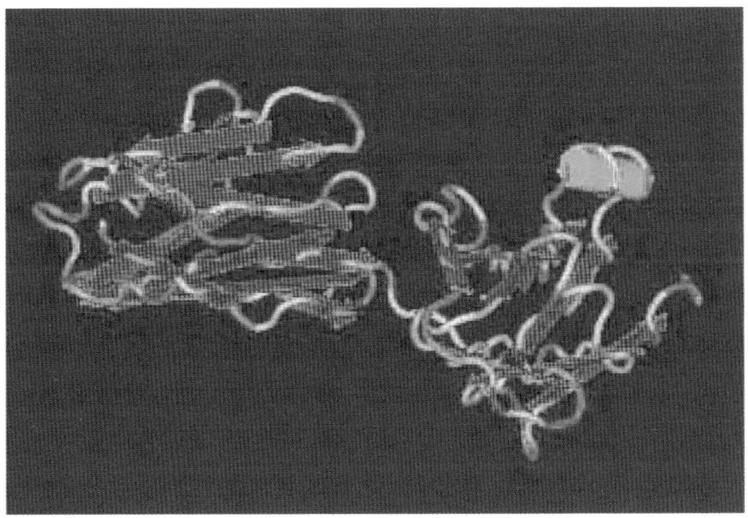

Figure 3.2. A κ FLC molecule showing the constant region (left), and the variable region (right) with its alpha helix (green).

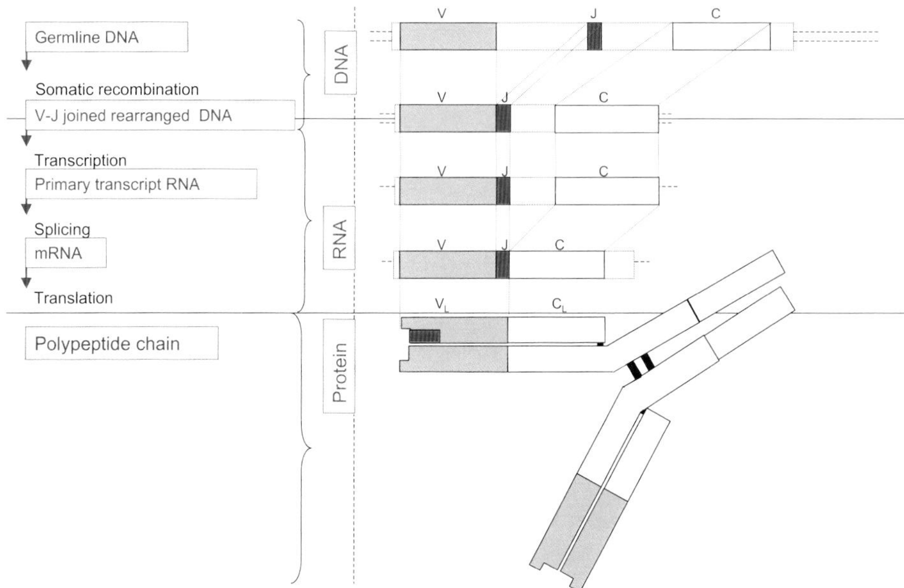

Figure 3.3. Construction of light chains.

3.3. Production

Production of FLCs in normal individuals is approximately 500mg/day from bone marrow and lymph node cells.[1,2] The molecules enter the blood and are rapidly partitioned between the intra-vascular and extra-vascular compartments. The normal plasma cell content of the bone marrow is about 1% while in MM the plasma cell content can rise to over 90%. The bone marrow may contain 5-10% plasma cells in chronic infections and autoimmmune diseases and this is associated with hypergammaglobulinaemia and corresponding increases in polyclonal sFLC concentrations. Bone marrow identification of monoclonal plasma cells by histology is an essential part of MM diagnosis and is frequently based on identifying intracellular κ and λ by direct immunofluorescence techniques (*Figure 3.5*).

Plasma cells produce one of five heavy chain types together with κ or λ molecules. There is approximately 40% excess FLC production over heavy chain synthesis to allow proper conformation of the intact immunoglobulin molecules. As already indicated, there are twice as many κ producing plasma cells as λ, and κ FLCs are normally monomeric, while λ FLCs tends to be dimeric, joined by disulphide bonds but higher polymeric forms of both FLCs can occur (*Figure 3.6*).

3.4. Clearance and metabolism

In normal individuals, sFLCs are rapidly cleared and metabolised by the kidneys depending upon their molecular size. Monomeric FLCs, characteristically κ, are cleared

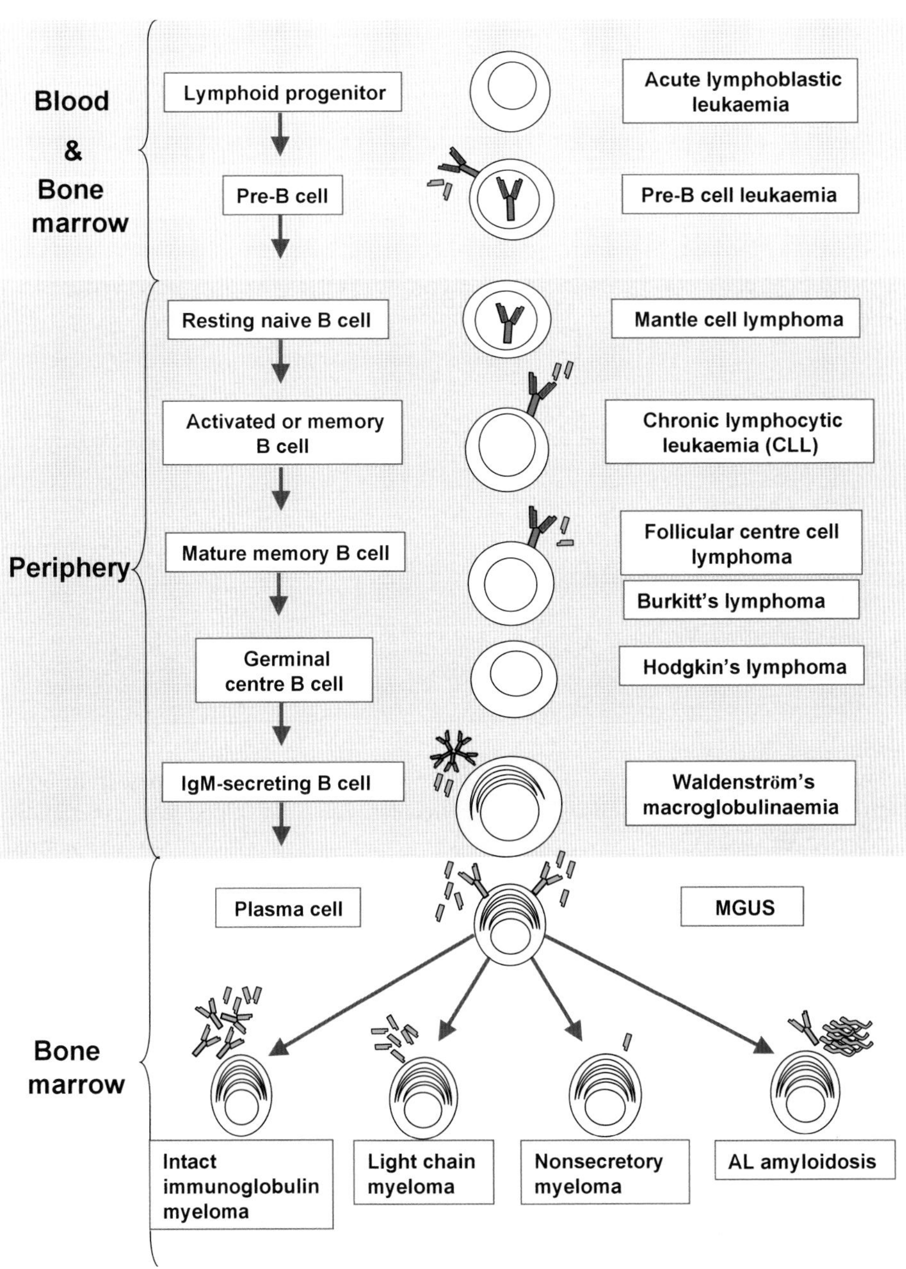

Figure 3.4. Development of the B-cell lineage and associated diseases.

in 2-4 hours at 40% of the glomerular filtration rate. Dimeric FLCs, typically λ, are cleared in 3-6 hours at 20% of the glomerular filtration rate, while larger polymers are cleared more slowly. Removal may be prolonged to 2-3 days in MM patients in complete renal failure *(Chapter 14)*.[1-3] In contrast, IgG has a half-life of 21 days.

Figure 3.7 shows a nephron, of which there are approximately one million in both

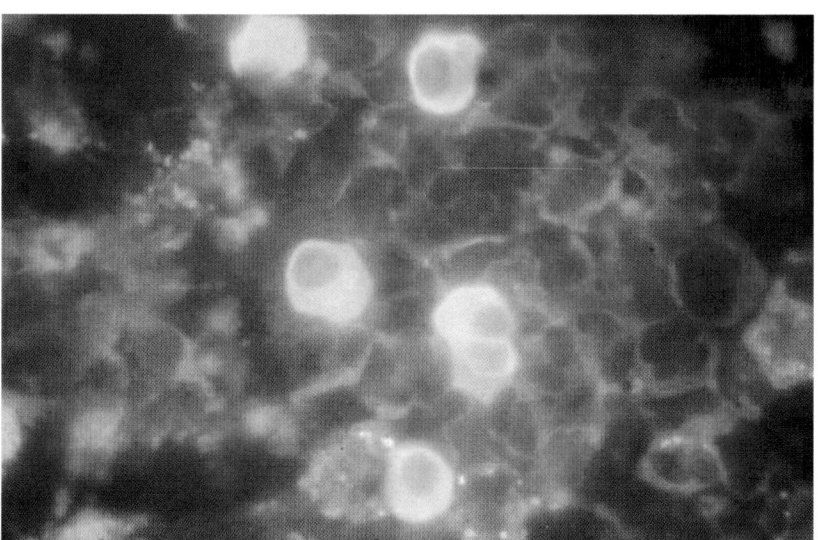

Figure 3.5. Immunohistochemical staining of κ producing bone marrow plasma cells from a patient with MM using fluorescein-conjugated, anti-κ antiserum. 5 plasma cells can be seen.

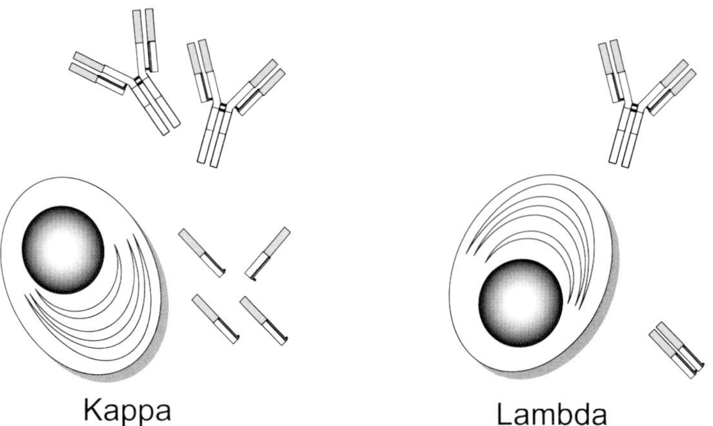

Figure 3.6. Diagrammatic representation of plasma cells producing intact immunoglobulins and FLC molecules.

kidneys. Each contains a glomerulus with basement membrane fenestrations, that allows filtration of serum molecules into the proximal tubules. The pore sizes are variable with a restriction in filtration commencing at about 20-40kDa and being complete by 60kDa. Protein molecules that pass the glomerular pores are then either absorbed unchanged (such as albumin) or degraded in the proximal tubular cells and absorbed or excreted as fragments.[4] This is an essential mechanism that is designed to prevent loss of large amounts of proteins and peptides into the urine, and is very efficient. The exact pathway for FLC metabolism is unknown but between 10-30g of small molecular weight proteins can be processed by the kidneys per day, so under normal conditions, none passes beyond the proximal tubules.[5-7]

The distal tubule secretes large amounts of uromucoid (Tamm-Horsfall protein). This is the dominant protein in normal urine and is thought to be important in preventing ascending urinary infections. It is a relatively small glycoprotein (80kDa) that aggregates into polymers of 20-30 molecules. Interestingly, it contains a short peptide motif that specifically binds FLCs.[8] Together they form waxy casts that are characteristically found in acute renal failure associated with LCMM (*Figures 3.8, 3.9 and Chapter 14)*.[9,10]

In normal individuals, 1-10mg of FLCs is excreted per day into the urine. Its exact origin is unclear but it probably enters the urine via the mucosal surfaces of the distal part of the nephrons and the urethra, alongside secretory IgA. This secretion is part of a

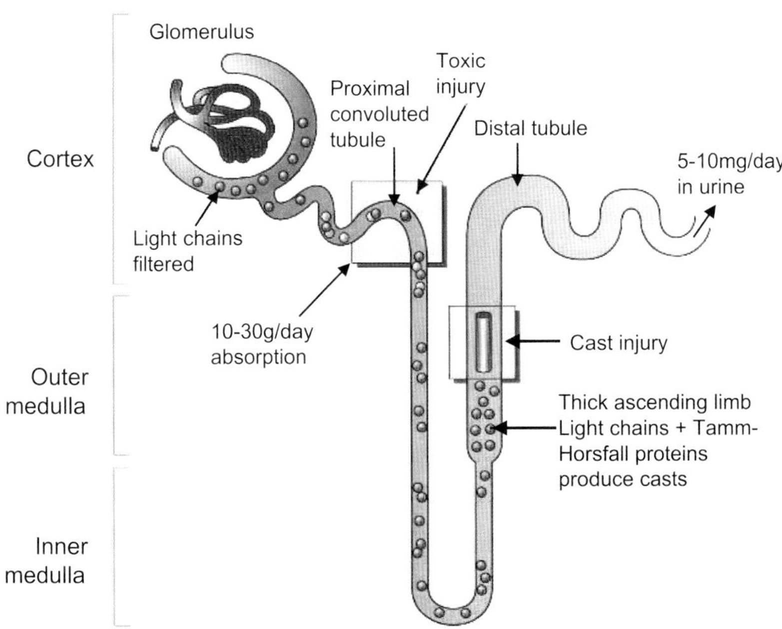

Figure 3.7. Nephron showing filtration, metabolism and excretion of FLCs. (Courtesy of R Johnson and J Feehally).[11]

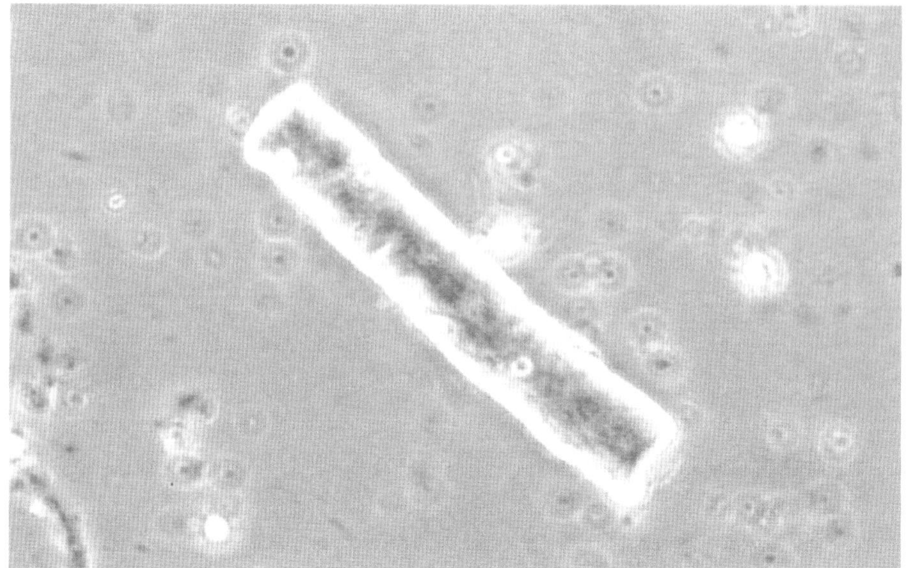

Figure 3.8. Waxy cast from the urine of a patient with multiple myeloma. (Courtesy of R Johnson and J Feehally).[11]

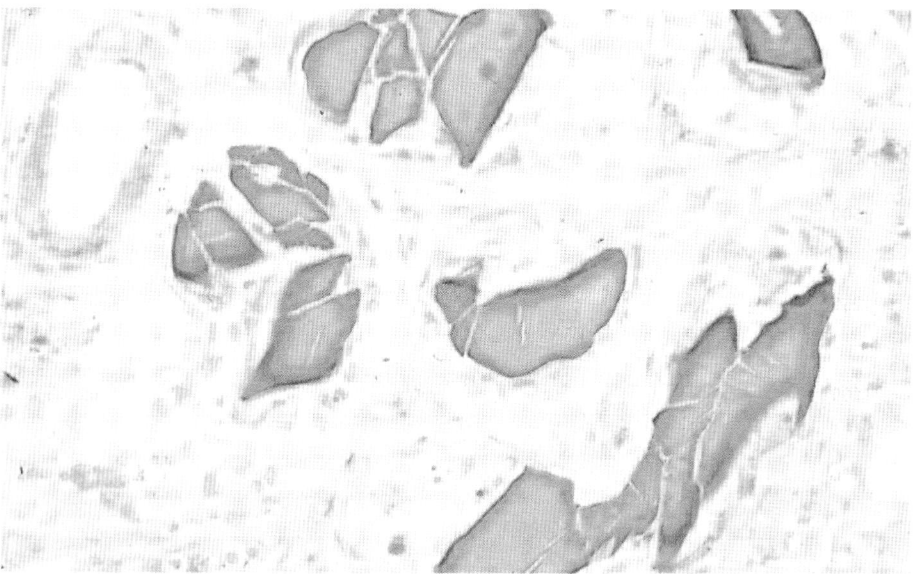

Figure 3.9. Monoclonal FLCs stained by immunoperoxidase anti κ antibodies in the distal tubules of a patient with myeloma kidney. (Courtesy of R Johnson and J Feehally).[11]

typical mucosal defence mechanism to prevent infectious agents entering the body. The 500mg of FLCs produced per day by the normal lymphoid system, therefore, flow through the glomeruli and are completely processed by the proximal tubules.[4]

Modest amounts of FLCs may be found in the urine of normal individuals. If the proximal tubules of the nephrons are damaged or stressed (such as in hard exercise), filtered FLCs may not be completely metabolised. Small amounts may then enter the urine. Although important as markers of general renal function and glomerular function in particular, serum creatinine and cystatin C cannot detect such minor degrees of nephron dysfunction.

As noted above, κ FLC monomers are cleared three times faster than dimeric λ molecules because of their smaller size.[12] Although κ production rates are twice that of λ, its faster removal ensures that the actual serum concentrations are approximately 50% lower *(Chapters 5 and 20)*.

Because of the huge proximal tubule metabolism, the amounts of FLCs in urine, even when production is considerably increased, are more dependent upon renal function than synthesis by the tumour. As a consequence, serum and urine FLC concentrations may not be similar during the evolution of LCMM. This is shown in a hypothetical patient in Figure 3.10. The red line shows the steady increase in sFLCs as the tumour grows over the first 12 months. When synthesis of FLCs exceeds 10-30g/day (greater than 30 times normal) there is an overflow proteinuria and large amounts of FLCs enter the urine. This is normally when patients with LCMM are identified.

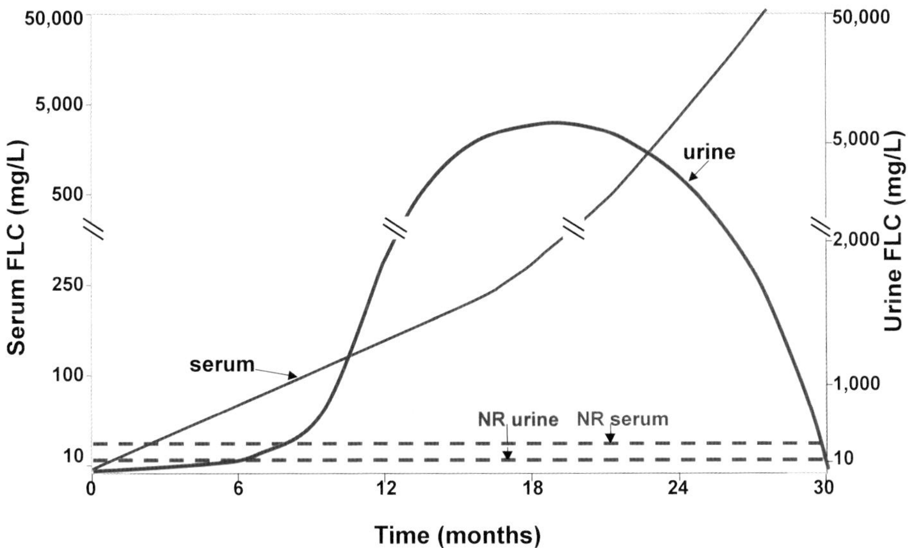

Figure 3.10. Changes in serum and urine free light chain concentrations during the evolution of a hypothetical patient with light chain multiple myeloma.

The FLCs that overwhelm the proximal tubules' absorption mechanisms enter the distal tubules and may cause inflammation or precipitate as casts. These can block the flow of urine causing the death of the respective nephrons (*Figures 3.8 and 3.9*).[11,13-16] Rising concentrations of sFLCs are filtered by the remaining nephrons leading to a vicious cycle of accelerating renal damage with further increases in sFLCs.

This process lengthens the serum half-life of the FLCs so that concentrations rise rapidly, in contrast to urine excretion, which falls as the patients develop terminal renal failure and is zero when the patients become aneuric (*Figure 3.10*). Consequently, the levels of serum and urine FLCs diverge during the later stages of the disease. While increasing serum concentrations indicate disease progression, falling urine concentrations may falsely suggest disease stabilisation or improvement. Thus, Nowrousian et al. showed that urine FLC excretion decreased at high sFLC concentrations if there was significant renal impairment.[17] In a similar manner, urine concentrations may increase as renal function improves with treatment of the tumour.

Understanding the toxic effects of FLCs on renal function and FLC concentrations in serum and urine is important. The inevitable conclusion, from the physiological and pathological mechanisms described above, is that serum is preferable to urine for assessing FLC concentrations in patients with monoclonal FLC diseases.

Summary: Serum free light chains:-

1. Contain constant region epitopes that are hidden in intact immunoglobulins.
2. Are produced in excess by plasma cells.
3. Have a half-life of a few hours because of rapid renal clearance.
4. Bind to Tamm-Horsfall protein in the distal tubules and may obstruct urine flow.
5. Are more frequently abnormal in serum than in urine because of renal metabolism.

References

1. **Solomon A.** Light Chains of Human Immunoglobulins. Meth Enzymol 1985; **116**: 101-121.
2. **Waldmann TA, Strober WS, Mogielnicki RP**. The Renal Handling of Low Molecular Weight Proteins II. Disorders of Serum Protein Catabolism in Patients with Tubular Proteinuria, the Nephrotic Syndrome or Uraemia. J Clin Invest 1972; **51**: 2162-2174.
3. **Miettinen TA, Kekki M.** Effect of impaired hepatic and renal function on Bence Jones protein catabolism in human subjects. Clin Chim Acta, 1967; **18**: 395-407.
4. **Russo L, Bakris GL, Comper WD.** Renal handling of Albumin: A critical Review of Basic Concepts and Perspective. Am J Kidney Dis 2002; **39**: 899-919.
5. **Abraham GN, Waterhouse C.** Evidence for defective immunoglobulin metabolism in severe renal insufficiency. Amer J Med Sci 1974; **268**: 227-233.
6. **Wochner RD, Strober W, Waldmann TA.** The role of the kidney in the catabolism of Bence Jones proteins and immunoglobulin fragments. J Exp Med 1967; **126**: 207-221.
7. **Maack T, Johnson V, Kau ST, Figueredo J, Sigulem D**. Renal filtration, transport and metabolism of low-molecular-weight proteins A review. Kid Int 1979; **16**: 251-270.
8. **Ying W-Z, Sanders PW.** Mapping the Binding Domain of Immunoglobulin Light Chains for Tamm-Horsfall Protein. Am J Path 2001; **158**: 1859-1866.
9. **Sanders PW, Brooker BB, Bishop JB, Cheung HC.** Mechanism of intranephronal proteinaceous cast formation by low molecular weight proteins. J Clin Invest 1990; **85**: 570-576.
10. **Sanders PW, Brooker BB.** Pathobiology of Cast Nephropathy from Human Bence Jones Proteins. J

Clin Invest 1992; **89**: 630-639.

11. Winearls CG. Myeloma kidney. In: Comprehensive Clinical Nephrology; 2nd Edition. Chapt 17. Eds Johnson RJ, Feehally J. Pub: Mosby 2003.

12. Arfors K-E, Rutlil G and Svensjo E. Microvascular transport of macro-molecules in normal and inflammatory conditions. Acta Physiol Scand, Suppl., 1979; **463**: 93-103.

13. Alexanian R, Barlogie B, Dixon D. Renal failure in multiple myeloma. Pathogenesis and prognostic implications. Arch Intern Med 1990; **150**: 1693-1695.

14. Knudsen LM, Hippe E, Hjorth M, Holmberg W, Westin J. Renal function in newly diagnosed multiple myeloma - A demographic study of 1353 patients. Eur J Haematol 1994; **53**: 207-212.

15. Winearls CG. Acute myeloma kidney. Kidney Int 1995; **48**: 1347-1361.

16. Abbott KC, Agodoa LY. Multiple myeloma and light chain-associated nephropathy at end-stage renal disease in the United States: patient characteristics and survival. Clinical Nephrology 2001; **56**: 207-210.

17. Nowrousian MR, Brandhorst D, Sammet C, Kellert M, Daniels R, Schuett P, Poser M, Mueller S, Ebeling P, Welt A, Bradwell AR, Buttkereit U, Opalka B, Flasshove M, Moritz T, Seeber S. Serum Free Light Chain Analysis and Urine Immunofixation Electrophoresis in Patients with Multiple Myeloma. Clin Cancer Res 2005; **11** (24): 8706-8714.

Test questions

1. Is Bence Jones proteinuria, 'overflow', 'glomerular' or 'tubular' in origin?

2. What are the normal half-lives of serum IgG and serum FLCs?

3. Serum albumin concentrations are reduced in patients with nephrotic syndrome with gross proteinuria. Are serum FLC concentrations also reduced in these circumstances?

4. Which protein binds FLCs in the distal tubules?

5. Do urine FLC concentrations always increase alongside rising serum FLC concentrations?

Answers

1. Overflow proteinuria (page 19).

2. IgG is 21 days and FLCs 2-6 hours (page 16).

3. No, nephron damage from any cause increases serum FLC concentrations because glomerular filtration is always impaired (page 16).

4. Uromucoid or Tamm-Horsfall protein (Page 17).

5. No. If there is significant renal impairment, urine FLC excretion falls (Page 20).

Chapter 4

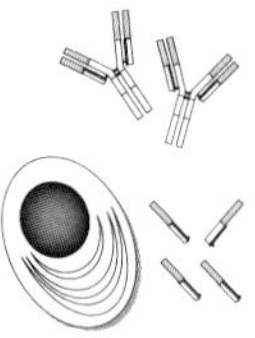

Methods for free light chain measurement

4.1. Laboratory assays for free light chains

There are numerous assays for monoclonal FLCs in urine.[1-4] Some, such as protein precipitation, are simple screening tests but are insensitive and non-specific,[5,6] while others are more sensitive but laborious and may be difficult to interpret.[7-11]

An ideal test for FLCs would have the following characteristics:-

- Sensitive diagnostic assay that identifies all patients producing monoclonal FLCs
- Quantitative measurement of FLCs and κ/λ ratios for monitoring patients
- High specificity with no interference from intact immunoglobulins
- Inexpensive to perform and easy to interpret
- Measures FLCs in serum (*see Chapter 3*)
- Can be performed on a variety of laboratory instruments *(Chapter 27)*

In the light of these requirements some commonly used tests for FLCs are analysed in Table 4.1. Each assay has features that are satisfactory, to some degree or other, but all fail to detect FLCs in serum at concentrations within the normal range (3-25mg/L); or even at concentrations that are several times higher than the normal range. Dipstick assays, based upon dye uptake, are particularly unreliable for measuring cationic proteins such as FLCs and should not be used.

One modern solution to the problems of inadequate assay specificity and sensitivity is to use antibody-based methods. The following chapter describes the development of serum FLC immunoassays and their validation on a variety of laboratory analysers.

	Advantages	**Disadvantages**
Total urine protein	Simple, inexpensive, widely used	Sensitivity inadequate for free light chain detection
Urine dipsticks	Simple, inexpensive, widely used	Sensitivity inadequate for free light chain detection[12,13]
Serum protein electrophoresis	Simple manual/semi-automated method Well established, inexpensive Monoclonal bands visualised Quantitative results with scanning	Insensitive (<500-2,000mg/L). Cannot detect free light chains at low concentrations. Subjective interpretation of results
Urine protein electrophoresis	Simple manual/semi-automated method Well established, inexpensive Monoclonal bands visualised Sensitive in concentrated urine (10mg/L) Quantitative results with scanning	Subjective interpretation of results Urine may require concentration with possible protein loss[14,15] False bands from concentrating urine[16-19] Heavy proteinuria obscures results Cumbersome 24-hour urine collections[20]
Immunofixation electrophoresis on serum and urine	Well established Good sensitivity for serum and very sensitive for concentrated urine (5-30mg/L)	Non-quantitative Serum sensitivity (~150mg/L) inadequate for normal serum FLC levels Manual/semi-automated technique Expensive use of antisera
Capillary zone electrophoresis	Automated technology Quantitative	Less sensitive (~400mg/L) than immunofixation electrophoresis for serum FLC[21-24]
Total serum κ/λ **assays**	Automated immunoassay	Specificity inadequate for detecting many patients with light chain multiple myeloma[25]

Table 4.1. Comparison of different assays for FLCs.

4.2. Development of free light chain immunoassays

A. Production of free light chain antisera

It is essential that FLC antibodies have high specificity and affinity. The following description is an outline of the procedures involved in their development. Sheep were immunised with κ or λ molecules that had been purified from urines containing Bence Jones proteins. The resultant antisera were adsorbed against purified IgG, A and M monoclonal proteins and then affinity purified against mixtures of the respective FLCs that had been immobilised onto Sepharose. Antisera requiring further adsorption, as judged by the tests described below, were recycled through the adsorption and testing procedures until satisfactory.

B. Antisera specificity

Specificity is the most important aspect of the immunoassays and was evaluated using several techniques.

1. Immunoelectrophoresis

The antibodies were purified until they showed no cross-reactions by immunoelectrophoresis with the alternate FLC and intact immunoglobulin molecules *(Figure 4.1)*.

2. Western blot analysis

This sensitive technique was used to assess the reactivity of the antisera against immunoglobulin fragments and FLC polymers. The results showed that both κ and λ FLC antisera reacted strongly with two closely migrating bands at 25-30kDa and weakly with several larger and smaller molecular weight fragments. Similar staining patterns were observed using monoclonal antibodies. The FLC antisera were readily able to detect monomers and dimers of both κ and λ molecules (*Figure 4.2*).

3. Haemagglutination assays

These assays are far more sensitive than immunoelectrophoresis and provide better assessment of specificity. Sheep red blood cells were sensitised with individual FLCs, and purified IgG, IgA and IgM and tested against the FLC antisera. The results showed that κ and λ FLC antibodies reacted with the appropriately labelled cells at >1:16,000 dilution and at <1:2 against cells coated with the alternate FLCs or intact immunoglobulins (*Figure 4.3*).

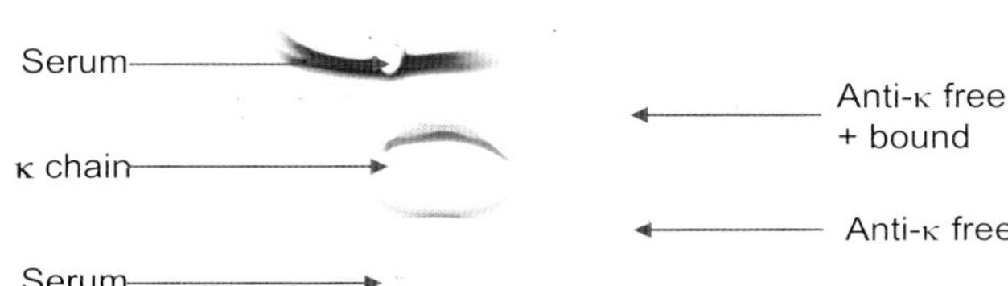

Figure 4.1. Immunoelectrophoresis showing the specificity of κ FLC antisera.

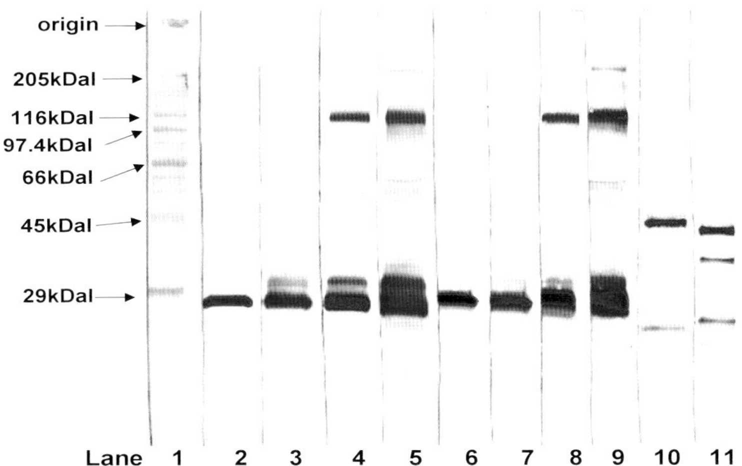

Figure 4.2. Western blots showing the specificity of the polyclonal FLC antisera compared with monoclonal antibodies and the reaction of polyclonal antisera against FLC monomers and dimers separated by non-reducing SDS-PAGE. (Lane 1, molecular weight markers. Lanes 2 & 3, urine containing κ FLCs and 4 & 5, normal serum all probed with mono- and polyclonal anti-κ. Lanes 6 & 7, urine containing λ FLCs and 8 & 9, normal serum probed with mono- and polyclonal anti-λ. Lanes 10 & 11, polyclonal FLC antisera reacting with monomers and dimers of κ and λ).

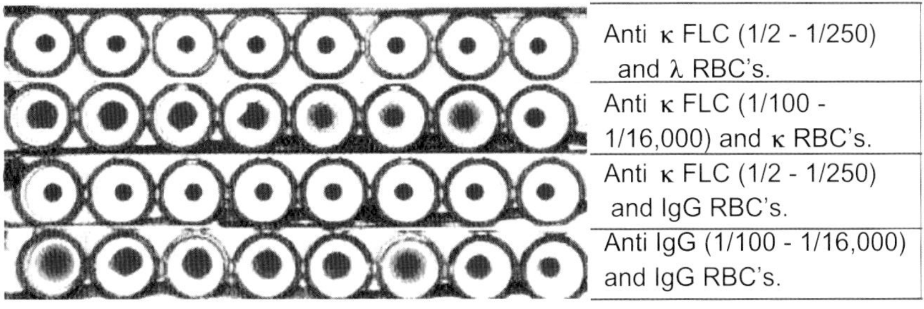

Figure 4.3. Haemagglutination assays showing the specificity of κ FLC antisera against red blood cells (RBC) coated with purified FLCs and IgG.

4. Nephelometry

Latex-conjugated FLC antisera were tested for specificity by nephelometry. Potentially interfering substances were added to serum containing known concentrations of FLCs and the changes in values indicated the effect on the assays (*Figure 4.4*).

Overall, the specificity assessments showed that FLC antisera had minimal reactivity with light chains on intact immunoglobulins and other potentially interfering substances.

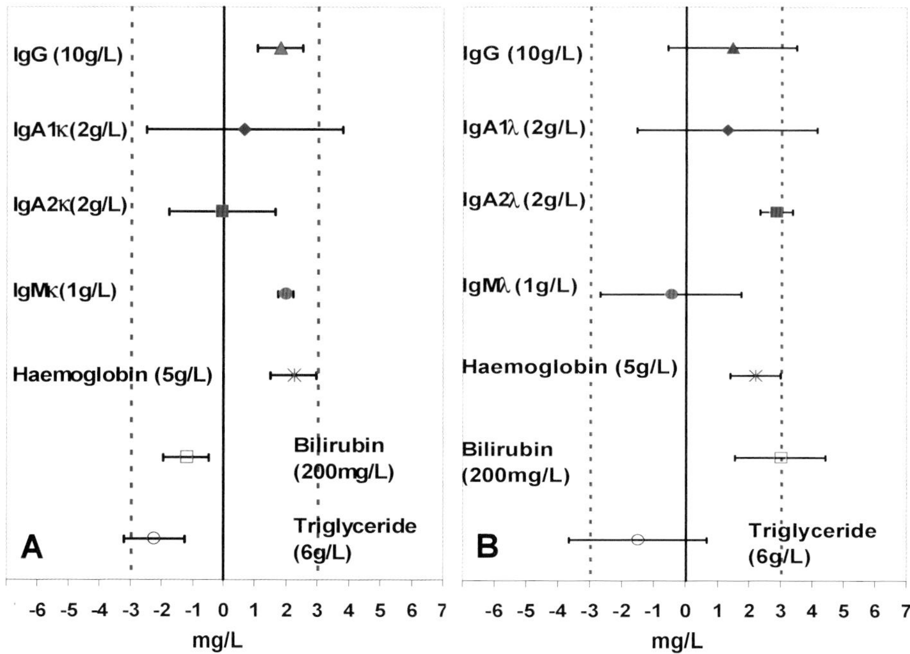

Figure 4.4. Specificity of (A) κ and (B) λ FLC antisera assessed by interference with the results of typical nephelometric assays upon the addition of various substances. Mean and 95% confidence limits for each added substance is shown.

C. Accuracy and standardisation

Accuracy is defined as the closeness of achieved results compared with their absolute values. Unfortunately, international standards do not exist for FLC measurements, so there are no reference points from which to assess the accuracy of results. Furthermore, each monoclonal light chain is unique with its own special set of surface epitopes, so accurate measurements are difficult to obtain. Nevertheless, the light chain constant region domains have little structural variability, so they are good antibody targets.

In order to ensure accurate FLC immunoassays, a suitable basis for standardisation and calibration was required. It was considered that polyclonal FLCs should be used in order to minimise any potential problems that might arise from the use of unique monoclonal proteins.[26] This was achieved in the following manner *(Figure 4.5)*:

1. Production and accurate quantification of pure polyclonal, 'primary' FLC standards.
2. Production of secondary and 'working' reference materials. Comparison with the primary standards.
3. Production of calibration materials for use in the FLC assays that were referenced against the 'working' standards.
4. Analysis of a variety of normal and abnormal samples using a reference nephelometric method.
5. Comparison of results from other instruments with the reference method.

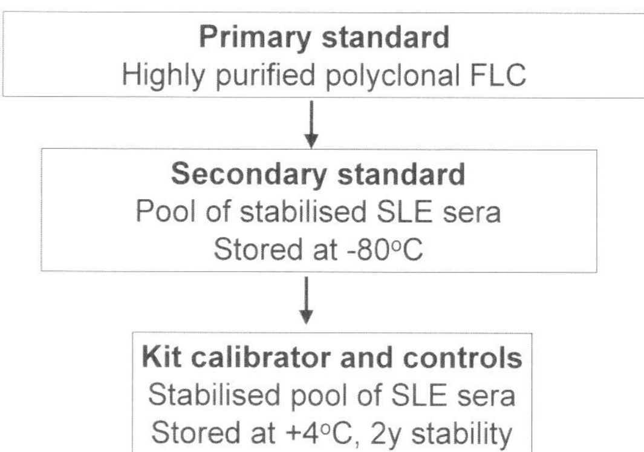

Figure 4.5. Flow chart for the production of standards for serum FLC immunoassays.

The various materials were manufactured and purified in accordance with established procedures.[27] Each primary FLC preparation was found to be greater than 99% pure by silver-stained SDS-PAGE while the alternate FLC was not detected by haemagglutination inhibition and dot blot assays. The amino acid content of each primary standard was then determined in order to produce an accurate estimation of the protein content.

Secondary reference materials were prepared from pools of different monoclonal κ and λ proteins *(Figure 4.5).* These were not considered ideal for use as working calibrators, so additional reference materials were prepared from sera that contained elevated polyclonal FLCs.

The pure FLC preparations were used to assign κ and λ concentrations to the secondary reference preparations. Subsequently, κ and λ values were assigned to the serum pool by nephelometry. Each stage of the value transfer was completed at three dilutions and repeated three times. All protein preparations were stabilised and stored at -80°C until required. The final FLC values for the 'working' reference preparations were 46mg/L for κ and 71.4mg/L for λ. These calibration values were used for all subsequent laboratory and clinical studies.

D. Assay sensitivity (*also see Chapter 6*)

Assay sensitivity (the lowest limit of antigen detection) is somewhat dependent upon the types of sample measured. FLC assays can detect less than 0.5mg/L of κ and λ FLCs in undiluted, clear urines and CSF. Serum sensitivity is typically 5-fold less because of interference from lipids and other light-scattering particles (*Table 4.2)*. Concentrations at 2-3mg/L are below the normal range so the FLC immunoassays allow extreme κ/λ concentration ratios to be established with considerable accuracy. This is important for monitoring patients under treatment because FLC concentrations may be below the normal range. Additional sensitivity for urine and CSF measurements can be obtained by judicious adjustments of the concentrations of the reactants *(Chapter 22).*

	Kappa	Lambda	Diagnostic requirement
SPE	500-2,000mg/L	500-2,000mg/L	monoclonal band
IFE	150-500mg/L	150-500mg/L	monoclonal band
Free light chains	1.5mg/L	3.0mg/L	abnormal κ/λ ratio

Table 4.2. Representative sensitivity levels of frequently used FLC assays.

E. Assay ranges

The measuring ranges of the FLC assays are dependent upon two factors: the slope of the respective calibration curve and the portion selected for the assay *(Figures 4.6 and 4.7)*. The latter should be chosen to allow the maximum number of normal and abnormal clinical samples to be measured at the initial sample dilution. A typical analytical range for κ is 3-150 mg/L and for λ, 5-200 mg/L *(Chapter 27)*. Samples containing higher concentrations require further dilution *(see Antigen excess, below)*.

Patients with bone marrow suppression may have low concentrations of the alternate FLC where the precision of the calibration curves is relatively poor. Consequently, some consideration should be given to the accuracy of κ/λ ratios that include low FLC concentrations *(Chapter 26)*.

F. Antigen excess

Antigen excess causes immunoassays to underestimate very high concentrations of antigen. Some instruments will identify antigen excess situations and recommend sample redilution. In the case of FLC measurements, sample concentrations can range from <1mg/L to >100,000mg/L. This is a greater range than almost all other serum protein tests. Consequently, very high levels may be underestimated on some instruments because of antigen excess. Historically, it was even suggested that this problem invalidated accurate FLC measurements.[28]

This is an important issue. During the development of the FLC assays, results indicated satisfactory detection of antigen excess at up to 200 mg/L for κ and λ using monoclonal FLCs *(Figure 4.8)*. Subsequently, monoclonal FLCs from 304 patients were assessed on the Behring BNII. At a 1:20 serum dilution, six high samples were incorrectly identified as moderately elevated and a further two were identified as normal. When the samples were tested at a dilution of 1:100, all of the eight troublesome samples were correctly identified as highly elevated. Subsequent assays have been modified to use a starting serum dilution of 1:100.[29] FLC assays on other instruments have been designed to prevent incorrectly low results due to antigen excess occuring in any of the samples.

Overall, the results of the antigen excess studies indicate that patients with high concentrations of FLCs will rarely be misclassified.[30] However, samples with FLC structural variations may still be problematical and show antigen excess problems at fairly low concentrations *(see Amyloid disease, Chapter 15)*.

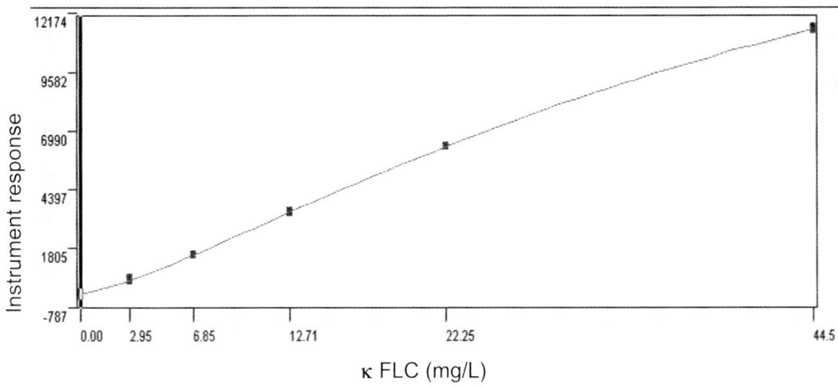

Figure 4.6. Calibration curve for κ FLC using the Roche Modular P.

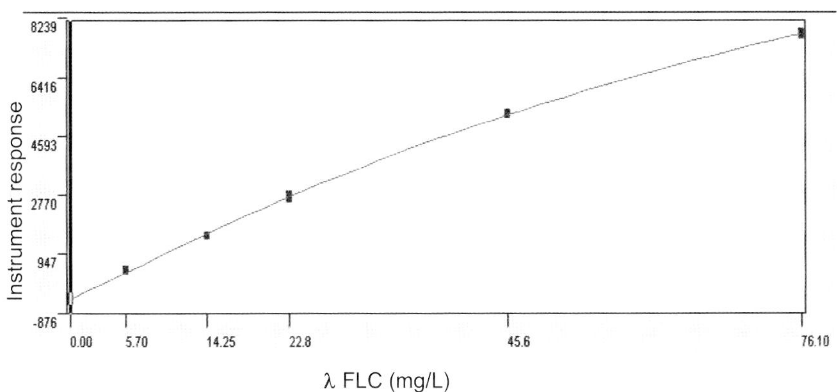

Figure 4.7. Calibration curve for λ FLC using the Roche Modular P.

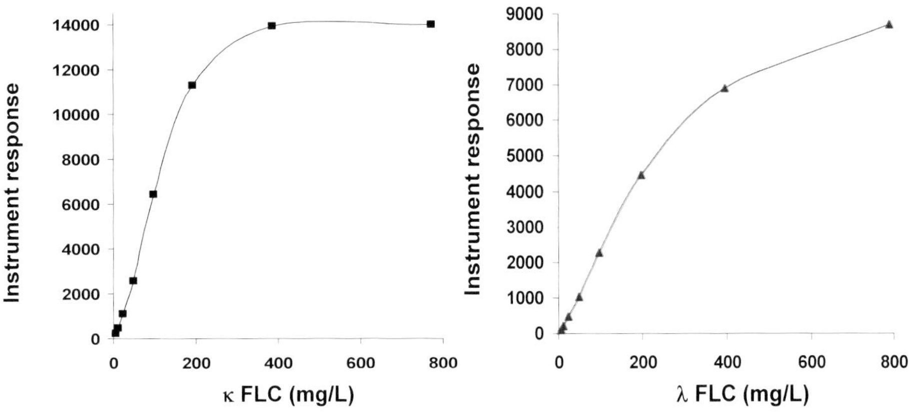

Figure 4.8. Demonstration of antigen excess capacity for FLC assays using monoclonal proteins. Addition of high concentrations of the patients' sera caused the assays results to plateau.

G. Precision

The precision of the sFLC assays is good with percentage coefficients of variation typically less than 10%. However, samples measured at low concentrations, the use of poorly maintained instruments and inexperienced operators may produce results that are less than ideal. Typically, assay precision deteriorates from intra-assay to inter-assay, and the worst is inter-instrument. Results of precision studies assessed at different parts of the measuring ranges are shown in Table 4.4. Further details are available for individual instruments *(Chapter 27).*

H. Linearity

Assays are considered to be linear when the results obtained from measurement of a sample at a series of dilutions are equivalent to the results expected from the original measurement. Non-linearity is due to a number of factors including: poor antibody specificity; inability of the antibody to recognise different forms of the antigen; non-specific assay interference from lipids or fibrin; unsuitable materials for the calibrators or standards etc. Assessment of linearity forms an important part of immunoassay development.

FLC assays are potentially prone to non-linearity. The target antigens are monoclonal proteins which exist as a number of sub-groups, in polymeric forms and contain unique combinations of hypervariable regions. Inevitably, these features cause non-linearity in some samples. Examples of good linearity are shown in Figure 4.9.

I. Free light chain polymerisation

FLC molecules are usually monomers or dimers but higher polymeric forms exist.[31-35] They act as multiantigenic targets in immunoprecipitation assays which may lead to over-estimation of antigen concentrations. This occurs in patients with NSMM who have undetectable concentrations of serum FLCs by IFE but high concentrations by

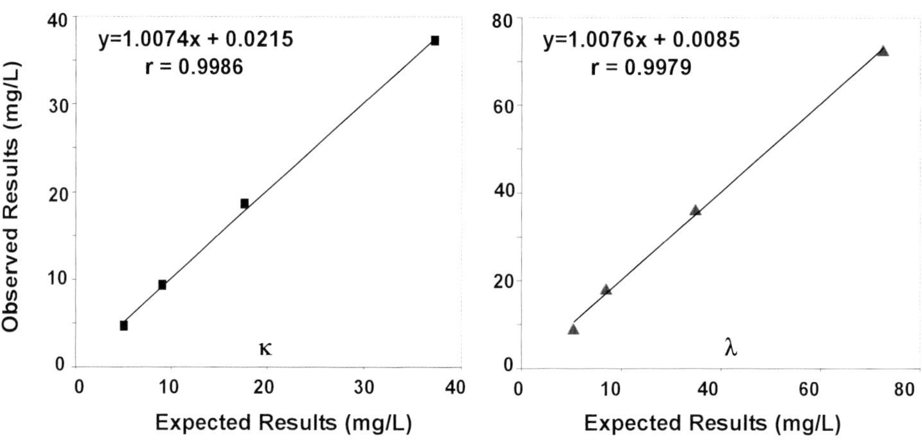

Figure 4.9. Linearity of (A) κ and (B) λ assays on an Hitachi 911.

nephelometry *(Chapter 9)*. Sö lling indicated that with his assays, monomers and dimers were detected equally using antibodies against whole light chains,[34,35] but antibodies directed only against FLC epitopes preferentially detected dimers.[36]

The effect of polymerisation on FLC quantification was recently studied using purified proteins and the new FLC antisera. FLC monomers, dimers and polymers were obtained from patients with MM and FLC concentrations were compared with total protein measurements. It was apparent that dimers were over-estimated by 1.5-fold and higher polymers by 1.5 to 3.5-fold.[37] However, an over-estimation of 10-fold would be necessary to explain the discrepancy between nephelometry and protein electrophoretic measurements in some myeloma sera. Binding to other proteins in serum may be partially responsible.

An additional factor is that SPE tests can underestimate FLC concentrations. Variable polymerisation may cause 'smearing' of monoclonal bands on the gels rendering them less visible, thereby suggesting normality *(Figure 9.2)*. Whatever the explanation, it might be difficult to develop FLC assays that measure all molecular forms equally. Perfect quantification will be elusive.

J. Stability

FLC molecules are very stable in serum and urine *(Figure 4.10)*. Tencer et al.,

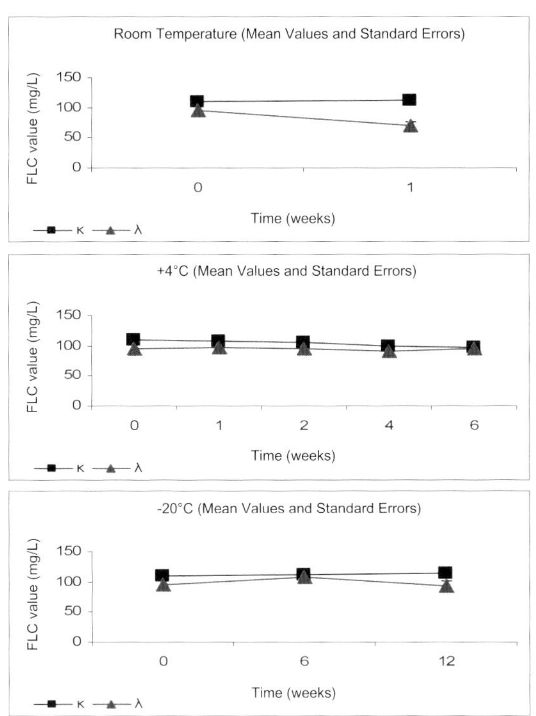

Figure 4.10. Stability of FLCs over different times and at different temperatures.

showed that there was little variation in the concentrations of FLCs in samples stored at -20°C, over a two year period.[38,39] We have found similar concentrations of FLCs in both fresh and old normal sera stored for 20 years at -20°C. Clearly, these results indicate that FLCs do not dissociate from intact immunoglobulins, or fragment, over prolonged periods.

Stability of the FLC antisera is also important. "Open-vial stability" refers to the shelf-life of the antisera after their first use. This may be short because pipetting procedures can introduce contaminants into the vials. These react with the remaining antisera and reduce its activity. Care should be taken not to contaminate antisera vials with sera from previously pipetted samples.

K. Serum and plasma comparisons for free light chain assays

Some laboratories prefer to analyse blood proteins in plasma rather than sera. A study was performed to directly compare the concentrations of FLCs in plasma and serum. 50 paired serum and plasma samples from blood donors and 20 paired samples from patients with MM were studied on a Beckman Immage, a BNII and a Hitachi 911. Plasma samples were collected in acid citrate dextrose or heparin and the sera were prepared by adding fibrin. Figures 4.11 and 4.12 and Table 4.3 show comparison data obtained on different instruments.[40]

4.3. Comparison of assays on different instruments

It is possible to measure serum FLC concentrations on many commonly used laboratory instruments. A list of currently available kits is given in Chapter 27. Comparison of FLC results using an Hitachi 911 and a Beckman Immage are shown in Figure 4.13. Table 4.4 is intended only as an overview.

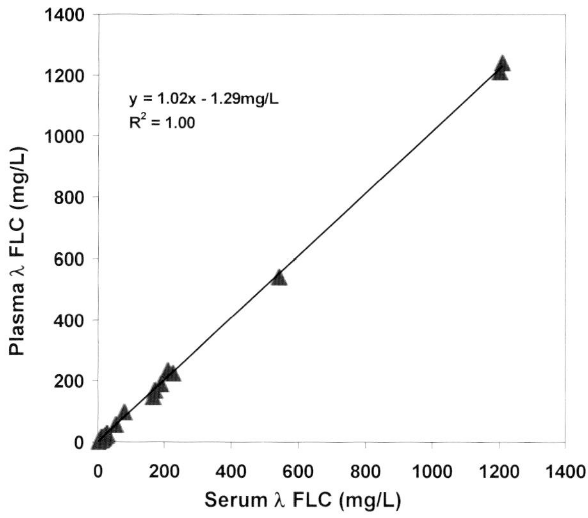

Figure 4.11. Comparison of serum and acid citrate dextrose plasma samples from 50 blood donors and 20 MM patients using a Beckman Immage.

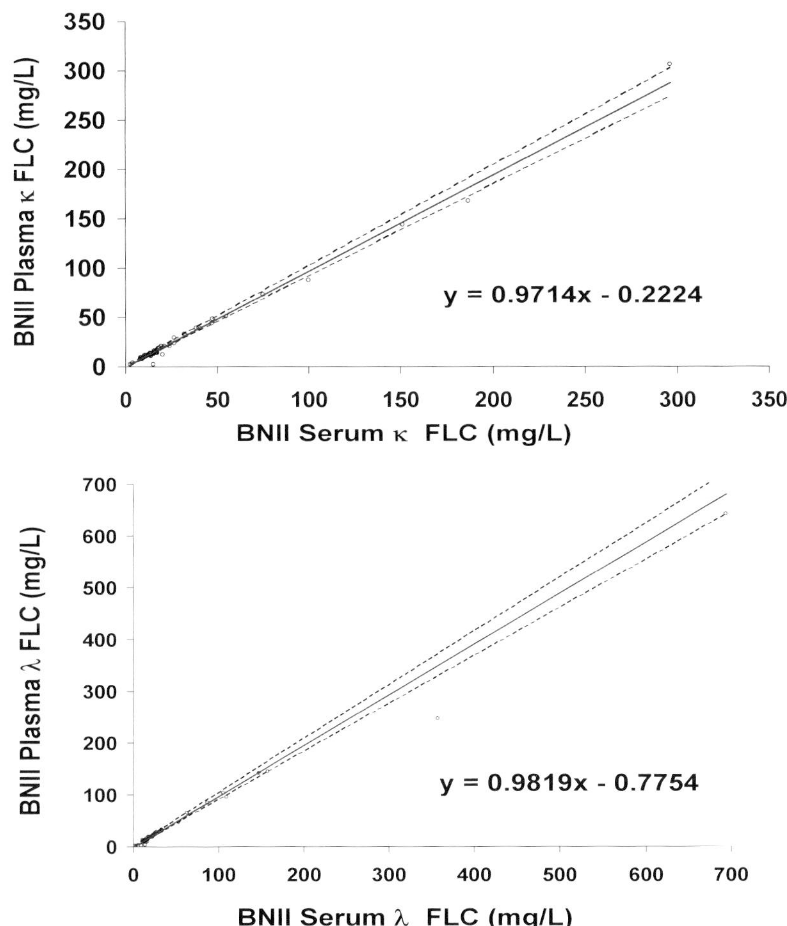

Figure 4.12. Comparison of serum and heparinised plasma samples from 50 blood donors and 20 myeloma patients on a Dade-Behring BNII.

	IMMAGE		BNII		Hitachi 911	
	Kappa FLC	Lambda FLC	Kappa FLC	Lambda FLC	Kappa FLC	Lambda FLC
Slope	1.01	1.02	0.97	0.94	1.02	1.01
Intercept	-0.85	-1.29	0.63	4.37	-0.35	-1.71
Correlation	1.00	1.00	0.99	1.00	1.00	1.00

Table 4.3. Comparison of serum and ACD plasma free light chain concentrations from 50 blood donors and 20 myeloma patients.

4.4. Quality control of free light chain antisera and kits

Maintaining batch-to-batch consistency is essential as the assays may be used for monitoring individual patients over many years. Effective quality control is ensured using a variety of techniques, two of which are briefly described here. External quality assurance schemes are described in Chapter 28.

Specificity is controlled by comparing a set of test results from each new batch of antiserum with results from previous batches. Typically, the panel of samples includes normal sera, sera with elevated polyclonal FLCs and myeloma sera. The results are compared using regression analysis and are considered acceptable when they fall within a defined set of criteria *(Figure 4.14)*.

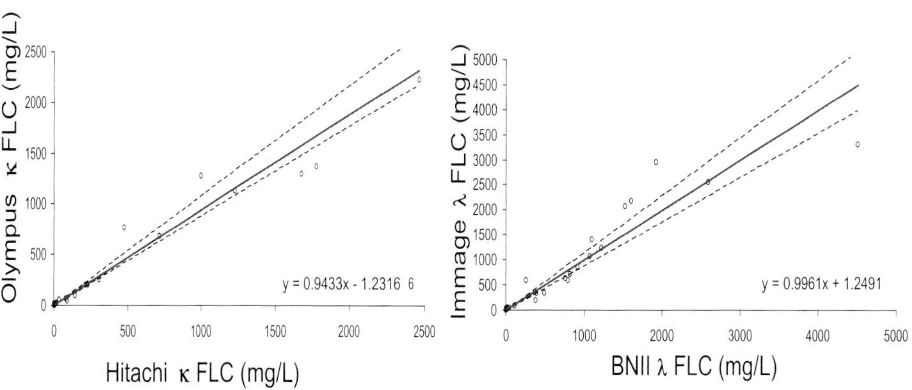

Figure 4.13. Comparison of serum samples on different instruments for kappa (left) and lambda (right).

	Dade Behring BN™II & BN ProSpec	Beckman Coulter IMMAGE®	Roche Modular P	Olympus AU™ Series
Sensitivity (mg/L)	κ 1.2 : λ 1.7(1/20)	κ 3.0 : λ 4.0 (1/5)	κ 1.6 : λ 1.8 (1/2)	κ 1.2 : λ1.2 (1/2)
C.V. (Intra-)	2.5-8.1%	1.9-4.7%	1.4-5.5%	0.7-2.0%
(Inter-)	4.7-8.4%	2.9-9.2%	5.7-9.5%	1.4-3.8%
Antigen excess	Good	Good	Satisfactory	Satisfactory
Analytical time	18 minutes	10 minutes	10 minutes	8.5 minutes
Samples per hour	30	40	200	100
Higher dilutions	Automatic	Off-line if high	Off-line if high	Off-line if high
Utility	Closed systems	Open system	Open system	Open system

Table 4.4. Summary of the characteristics of FLC assays on different platforms. (C.V. = coefficient of variation in precision studies. Numbers in brackets refer to sample dilutions). *See Chapter 27 for more details.*

Once suitable antisera have been selected and attached to latex particles, the other kit components are selected and assembled. Similar materials are used for calibrators and controls and comprise sera containing high concentrations of polyclonal FLCs. The first step is to assign a value to the kit calibrators using the working reference material. This is achieved using 100 separate assays and 10 separate calibration curves. The second step is to assign values to the control reagents using similar procedures.

Analytical comparisons are also made using normal sera. A typical evaluation on 30 normal samples produced the following results: mean κ = 10.8mg/L (range 4.5 - 17.1mg/L), mean λ = 18.0mg/L (range 8.2 - 31.7mg/L), mean κ/λ ratio = 0.58. Inter-instrument agreement is also important with results from two instruments shown in Figure 4.13.

4.5. Scale-up of antiserum production

Scale-up involves producing larger batches of antisera by immunising more sheep and using larger and more automated laboratory equipment. The polyclonal reagents have to be adsorbed to complete specificity and then affinity purified by passage through large chromatography columns. This is controlled using an AKTA biopilot system that can automatically load, wash, elute and collect antibody peaks (*Figure 4.15*). Large volume batches of antisera are advantageous in terms of quality control assessment, assignment of reference values, kit production and cost control.

In the life-cycle of diagnostic tests, the FLC immunoassays are still in their infancy. Improvements will be seen in sensitivity, specificity, reactivity, utility, costs, etc. This will allow the tests to be available to all physicians, laboratories and patients who need serum FLC measurements.

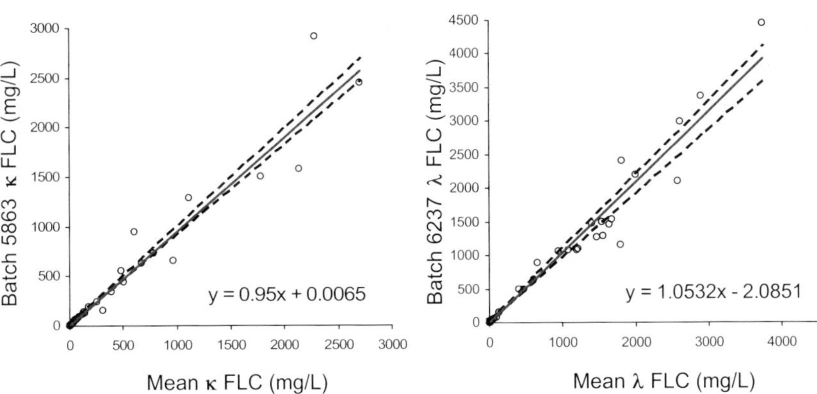

Figure 4.14. Comparison of results obtained from two batches of kits with the mean results from previous analyses. (The mean results were obtained from an average of 12 assays over 6 batches of reagent. The samples included 30 normal sera and 30 myeloma sera of various immunoglobulin types).

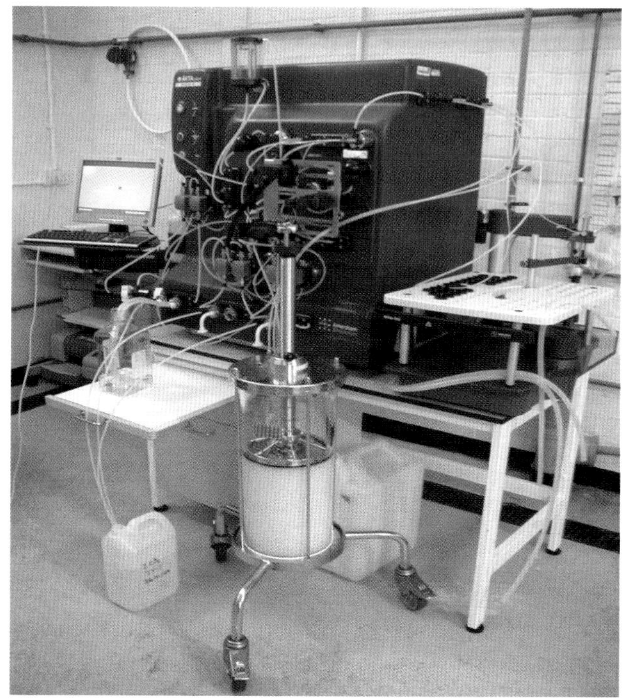

Figure 4.15. AKTA biopilot system for controlling column chromatography.

Summary: Free light chain immunoassays have the following features:-

1. Highly specific for serum and urine FLCs.
2. 1000 times more sensitive than serum electrophoretic tests.
3. Give better precision than electrophoretic tests.
4. Provide quantitative results.
5. Are performed on routine laboratory instruments.

References

1. **Beetham R**. Detection of Bence Jones protein in practice. Ann Clin Biochem 2000; **37**: 563-570.
2. **Keren DF.** Procedures for the Evaluation of Monoclonal Immunoglobulins. Arch Pathol Lab Med 1999; **123**: 126-132.
3. **Le Bricon T, Erlich, Bengoufa D, Dussaucy, Garnier J-P, Bousquet B.** Sodium dodecyl sulfate-agarose gel electrophoresis of urinary proteins: application to multiple myeloma. Clin Chem 1998; **44**: 1191-1197.
4. **Wong WK, Wieringa GE, Stec Z, Russell J, Cooke S, Keevil BG, Lockhart S.** A comparison of three procedures for the detection of Bence-Jones proteinuria. Ann Clin Biochem 1997; **34**: 371-374.
5. **Chambers RE, Bullock DG, Whicher JT**. Urinary Total Protein Estimation - Fact or Fiction?. Nephron 1989; **53**: 33-36.
6. **Lott JA, Stephan VA, Pritchard KA Jr.** Evaluation of the Coomassie Brilliant Blue G-250 method for urinary protein. Clin Chem 1983; **29**: 1946-1950.
7. **Aguzzi F, Gasparro G, Bergami MR, Merlini M.** High-sensitivity electrophoretic method for the detection of Bence Jones protein and for the study of proteinuria in unconcentrated urines. Ann Clin Biochem 1993; **30**: 287-292.

8. Backer ET, Brand A. Detection of Bence-Jones protein in serum by immunoblotting. Ann Clin Biochem 1996; **33**: 132-138.

9. Heys AD, Norden AGW, Fulcher LM, Flynn FV. Bence Jones protein detection: a rapid immunoblotting technique for routine use on unconcentrated urine. Ann Clin Biochem 1986; **23**: 571-576.

10. Martin SM, Kohn J. The sensitivity of gold staining in the detection of Bence Jones proteinuria. Ann Clin Biochem, Suppl 1987; **24**: 120-122.

11. Pascali E, Pezzoli A. The Clinical Spectrum of Pure Bence Jones Proteinuria. Cancer 1988; **62**: 2408-2415.

12. Fine JD, Rees ED. Bence Jones protein detection and implications. N Eng J Med 1974; **290**: 106-107.

13. Penders J,Fiers T, Delanghe JR. Quantitative evaluation of urinalysis test strips. Clin Chem 2002; **48**: 2236-2241.

14. Ala-Houhala I, Marrku T, Parviainen MT, Paternack A. A comparison of three different methods of concentration of urinary proteins. Clin Chim Acta 1984; **142**: 339-342.

15. Lindstedt G, Lungberg P. Loss of tubular proteinuria pattern during urine concentration with a commercial membrane filter cell (Minicon® B-15 System). Clin Chim Acta 1974; **56**: 125-126.

16. Bailey EM, McDermott TJ, Bloch KJ. The Urinary Light-Chain Ladder Pattern. Arch Pathol Lab Med 1993; **117**: 707-710.

17. Harrison HH. The "Ladder Light Chain" or "Pseudo-Oligoclonal" Pattern in Urinary Immunofixation Electrophoresis (IFE) Studies: a Distinctive IFE Pattern and an Explanatory Hypothesis Relating it to Free Polyclonal Light Chains. Clin Chem 1991; **37**: 1559-1564.

18. Hess PP, Mastropaolo W, Thompson GD, Levinson SS. Interference of Polyclonal Free Light Chains with Identification of Bence Jones Proteins. Clin Chem 1993; **39**: 1734-1738.

19. MacNamara EM, Aguzzi F, Petrini C, Higginson J, Gasparro C, Bergami MR, Bianchi G, Whicher JT. Restricted Electrophoretic Heterogeneity of Immunoglobulin Light Chains in Urine: a cause for confusion with Bence Jones Protein. Clin Chem 1991; **37**: 1570-1574.

20. Brigden ML, Neal ED, McNeely MD, Hoag GN. The Optimal Urine Collections for the Detection and Monitoring of Bence Jones Proteinuria. Am J Clin Path 1990; **93**: 689-693.

21. Bossuyt X, Bogaerts A, Schiettekatte G, Blanckaert N. Detection and classification of paraproteins by capillary immunofixation/subtraction. Clin Chem 1998; **44**: 760-764.

22. Bossuyt X, Marien G. False negative results in detection of monoclonal proteins by Capillary Zone Electrophoresis. Clin Chem 2001; **47**: 6: 1477-1479.

23. Bossuyt X, Schiettekatte G, Bogaerts A, Blanckaert N. Serum protein electrophoresis by CZE 2000 clinical capillary electrophoresis system. Clin Chem 1998; **44**: 749-759.

24. Katzmann JA, Clark R, Sanders E, Landers JP, Kyle RA. Prospective study of serum protein capillary electrophoresis immunotyping of monoclonal proteins by immuno-subtraction. Am J Clin Path 1998; **110**: 503-9

25. Boege F. Measuring Bence Jones Proteins with Antibodies Against Bound Immunoglobulin Light Chains: How Reliable are the Results? Eur J Clin Chem Clin Biochem 1993; **31**: 403-405.

26. Carr-Smith HD, Edwards J, Showell P, Drew R, Tang LX, Bradwell AR. Preparation of an immunoglobulin free light-chain reference material. Clin Chem 2000; **46**: 6: No. 699,pA180.

27. Bradwell AR, Carr-Smith HD, Mead GP, Tang LX, Showell PJ, Drayson MT, Drew R. Highly sensitive automated immunoassay for immunoglobulin FLCs in serum and urine. Clin Chem 2001; **47**: 673-680.

28. Graziani MS, Merlini G. Measurement of free light chains in urine. Clin Chem 2001; **47**: 2069.

29. Carr-Smith HD, Showell P, Bradwell AR. Antigen excess assessment of free light chain assays on the Dade-Behring BNII nephelometer. Clin Chem 2002; **48**:6 supplement; A-71 No.A23.

30. Bradwell AR, Drayson MT, Mead GP. Measurement of Free Light Chains in Urine (*letter - reply*). Clin Chem 2001; **47**: 11: 2069-2070

31. Berggard I, Peterson PA. Polymeric Forms of Free Normal κ and λ Chains of Human Immunoglobulin. J Biol Chem 1969; **244**: 4299-4307.

32. Diemert MC, Musset L, Gaillard O, Escolano S, Baumelou A, Rousselet F, Galli J. Electrophoretic study of the physico-chemical characteristics of Bence-Jones proteinuria and its association with kidney damage. J Clin Pathol 1994; **47**: 1090-1097.

33. Abraham RS, Charlesworth MC, Owen BAL, Benson LM, Katzmann JA, Kyle RA. Trimolecular Complexes of λ Light Chain Dimers in Serum of a Patient with Multiple Myeloma. Clin Chem 2002; **48**: 1805-1811.

34. Sölling K. Polymeric Forms of Free Light Chains in Serum from Normal Individuals and from Patients with Renal Diseases. Scand J Clin Invest 1976; **36**: 447-452.

35. Sölling K, Sölling J and Lanng Nielsen J. Polymeric Bence Jones Proteins in Myeloma Patients with Renal Insufficiency. Acta Med Scand 1984; **216**: 495-502.

36. Heino J, Rajamaki A and Irjala K. Turbidimetric measurement of Bence Jones proteins using antibodies against free light chains of immunoglobulins. Scand J Clin Lab Invest 1984; **44**: 173-176.

37. Mead GP, Stubbs PD, Carr-Smith HD, Drew R, Drayson MT, Bradwell AR. Nephelometric measurement of serum free light chains in nonsecretory myeloma. Clin Chem 2002; **48**: No.A70, pA23.

38. Tencer J, Thysell H, Andersson K, Grubb A. Stability of albumin, protein HC, immunoglobulin G, k- and λ- chain-immunoreactivity, Orosomucoid and α1-antitrypsin in urine stored at various conditions. Scand J Clin Lab Invest 1994; **54**: 199-206.

39. Tencer J, Thysell H, Andersson K, Grubb A. Long-term Stability of Albumin, Protein HC, Immunoglobulin G, κ and λ-immunoreactivity, Orosomucoid and α1 -antitrypsin in Urine Stored at -20°C. Scand J Urol Nephrol 1996; **31**: 67-71.

40. Smith LJ, Long J, Carr-Smith HD, Bradwell AR. Measurement of immunoglobulin free light chains by automated homogeneous immunoassay in serum and plasma samples. Clin Chem 2003; **49**: No.D-58, pA106.

Test questions

1. *Why do dye uptake tests for proteinuria fail to detect FLCs accurately?*
2. *How much more sensitive are immunoassays for FLCs than SPE?*
3. *Are serum FLCs unstable?*
4. *What is a typical assay precision for FLC tests?*

Answers

1. *The dyes do not bind readily to cationic proteins such as FLCs (page 22).*
2. *Approximately 1,000 -fold (pages 27-28).*
3. *No. Analysis of frozen samples, even 20 years old, show normal light chain levels (page 31).*
4. *5-10%. (Page 34).*

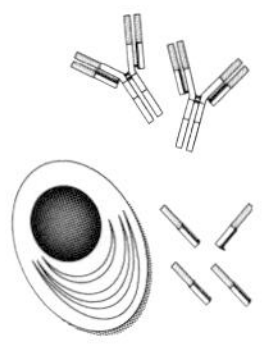

Chapter 5

Free light chain normal ranges and reference intervals

5.1. Serum free light chain normal ranges

Normal range data for sFLCs have been published many times. Results considered to be the most reliable are shown in Table 5.1. Serum results using polyclonal antibodies have varied considerably, indicating a degree of cross-reactivity with bound light chains in some of the assays. Perhaps not surprisingly, assays using monoclonal antibodies have also produced varied results, the discrepancy between two reports for κ FLC being more than 10-fold.[6,10] It is unclear whether the variations were due to specificity, calibration or matrix differences, or a combination of these factors.

The most detailed study of FLC concentrations in normal individuals was published by Katzmann et al.,[12] and showed similar results to those previously reported by Bradwell et al.[11] The same assay procedures were used in both studies but a wider age range of individuals was studied by Katzmann et al.[12] Serum samples were obtained from 127 healthy blood donors (21-62 years) and 155 older, normal individuals (51-90 years). A summary of the median values and reference ranges in the Katzmann study is

		Serum		Urine	
Publication	**Date**	**Kappa**	**Lambda**	**Kappa**	**Lambda**
Waldmann[1]	1972	-	-	-	2.3 (SD±1.1)[ab]
Sölling[2]	1975	13.2(SD±3.8)[a]	10.6(SD±3.1)[a]	3.2(SD±1.2)[ab]	1.1(SD±0.4)[ab]
Hemmingsen[3]	1977	-	-	1.2(0.0-6.8)[bc]	0.8(0.0-2.4)[bc]
Robinson[4]	1982	-	-	3.1(1.9-7.1)[bc]	1.45(0.7-3.4)[bc]
Brouwer[5]	1985	16.2 (CV 9%)[c]	41.4 (CV 10%)[c]	1.8(0.2-7.5)[c]	0.75(0.15-2.1)[c]
Axiak[6]	1987	1.2(0.8-7.5)[d]	-	4.9(3.0-8.0)[d]	-
Wakasugi[7]	1991	7.1(SD±4.3)[c]	5.0(SD±2.7)[c]	-	-
Nelson[8]	1992	10.0(1.6-15.2)[d]	3.0(0.4-4.2)[c]	-	-
Wakasugi[9]	1995	20.6(SD±6)[ce]	16.2 (SD±8.6)[ce]	-	-
Abe[10]	1998	16.6 (SD±6.1)[d]	33.8 (SD±14.8)[d]	2.96(SD±1.84)[d]	1.07 (SD±0.69)[d]
Bradwell[11]	2001	8.4 (4.2-13)[cef]	14.5(9.2-22.7)[cef]	5.5(0.39-15.1)[cefg]	3.17(0.81-10)[cefg]
Katzmann[12]	2002	7.3(3.3-19.4)[cef]	12.7(5.7-26.3)[cef]	-	-

Table 5.1. Publications reporting normal serum and urine FLC concentrations (mg/L unless stated otherwise).[11] ([a]polyclonal antibody against total light chains, [b]urine FLCs in mg/24 hours, [c]polyclonal antibody against FLCs, [d]monoclonal antibody against FLCs, [e]latex reagent, [f]95% range, [g]early morning urine samples).

shown in Tables 5.1 and 5.2.

The results of κ and λ measurements for all individuals are shown in Figure 5.1.[12] There were no significant differences between results obtained using either fresh or frozen sera but there was a trend to higher concentrations in elderly people *(Figure 5.1 and Table 5.3)*. This occurred for both FLCs and also for the renal function marker, cystatin C, that was measured in the same samples. Calculations of cystatin C/FLC ratios and κ/λ ratios on each sample normalised the elevated values *(Figure 5.1, c,e,f)*. Therefore, the higher FLC values seen in older people can be explained by small reductions in glomerular filtration rate.[13-15]

An alternative method of presenting the normal range data is shown in Figure 5.2. This shows the serum κ and λ results for each person plotted on a logarithmic scale. This form of data presentation inherently includes the κ/λ ratios and is useful for visualising results from individual patients. It also allows easy comparison between different disease groups and is used extensively in the clinical comparisons described later.

One curious discrepancy between the results of Katzmann et al.[12] and most earlier results is that serum κ concentrations are lower than serum λ, whereas traditionally it was considered to be the other way around, with κ levels higher than λ *(Table 5.1)*. Since there are nearly twice as many κ as λ–producing lymphoid cells, this observation had seemed reasonable. Certainly, the total serum κ and λ levels reflect the normal ratio of κ to λ FLC synthesis (*Table 5.2*).

A plausible explanation for the inverted serum κ/λ ratio relates to the kinetics of FLC clearance. Since κ molecules are normally monomeric (25kDa), their renal clearance is faster than dimeric λ molecules (50kDa), consequently they accumulate less in serum. Calculation of the κ/λ clearance rate from serum and urine FLC concentrations ([κ urine]/[λ urine] ÷ [κ serum]/[λ serum]) produced a result of 3.0.[11] In a study on the movement of dextran polymers across capillary membranes, it was shown that molecules of 20kDa were cleared 3.2 times faster than 37kDa molecules.[16] Admittedly, polysaccharides are different in charge, shape and flexibility from globular proteins of similar molecular weight, but differential glomerular filtration probably accounts for the inverse κ/λ ratios. This may not have been observed in some of the earlier FLC studies because of poor antisera specificity.

The κ/λ ratio is the most important factor when distinguishing monoclonal from polyclonal increases in sFLCs. The latter result from increased synthesis or decreased renal clearance of normal FLCs *(Chapters 20-21)*. These two processes increase both κ and λ concentrations equally, thereby maintaining a fairly constant κ/λ ratio. In patients

	Free light chains	**Total light chains**
Kappa (95% range)	7.3mg/L (3.3-19.4)	2,520mg/L
Lambda (95% range)	12.7mg/L (5.7-26.3)	1,430mg/L
κ/λ ratio (100% range)	0.6 (0.26-1.65)	1.78 (mean)
κ/λ ratio (95% range)	(0.31-1.2)	N/A

Table 5.2. Median values and ranges for free and total light chain concentrations and κ/λ ratios in the sera of 282 normal individuals.[12]

with renal failure, the half-life of both FLCs is prolonged from a few hours to several days, so concentrations increase 20-fold or more. However, κ/λ ratios remain within fairly narrow limits. In contrast, in monoclonal gammopathies only one of the FLC concentrations increase. Thus, κ/λ ratios distinguish monoclonal from polyclonal diseases.

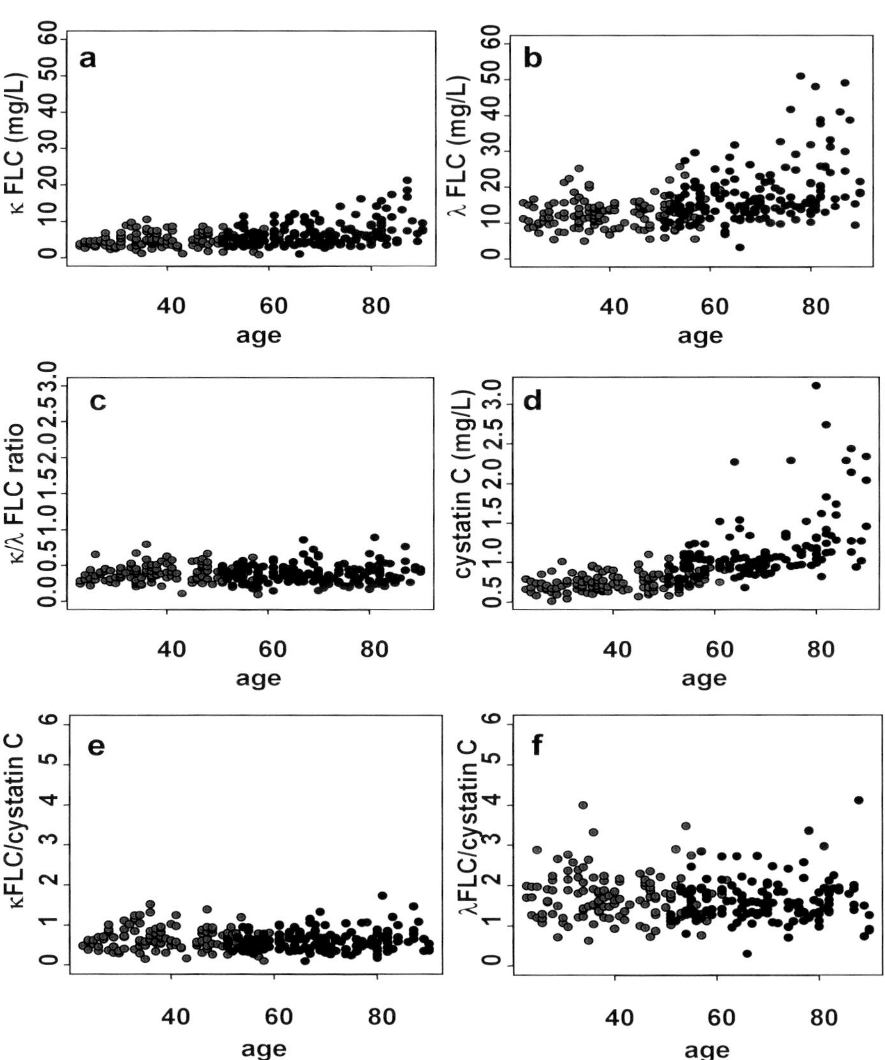

Figure 5.1. (a) κ, (b) λ and (c) κ/λ ratios versus age (years) in 282 normal serum samples together with (d) cystatin C results in the same patients. sFLC/cystatin C ratios (e) and (f) show no change with age, confirming renal deterioration as the cause of increased sFLC levels in elderly individuals. (red = fresh sera, black = frozen sera).[12]

Age, years	κ FLC, mg/L	λ FLC, mg/L	FLC, κ/λ
20-29	6.3	12.4	0.49
30-39	7.2	13.6	0.55
40-49	7.5	12.8	0.58
50-59	6.4	11.3	0.59
60-69	6.9	11.8	0.70
70-79	8.0	11.9	0.65
80-90	9.1	15.1	0.64

Table 5.3. Median values for sFLCs and κ/λ ratios in different age groups.[12]

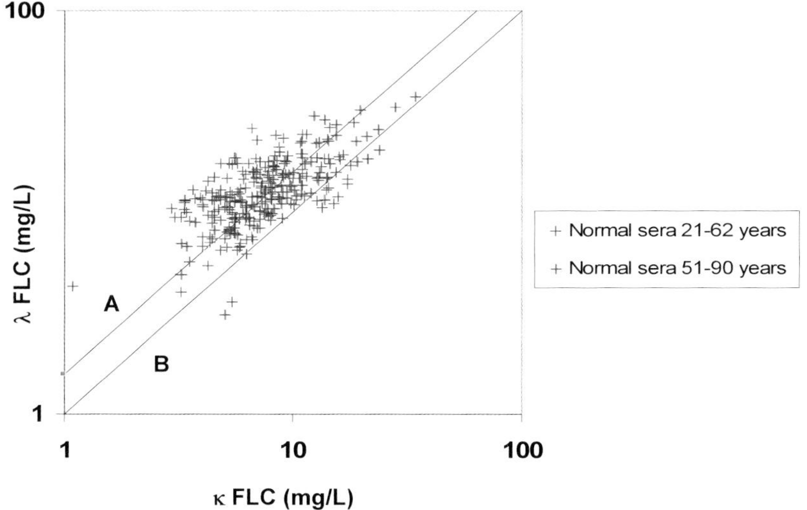

Figure 5.2. κ and λ FLC concentrations in 282 normal sera.[12] A: axis at the normal κ/λ ratio of 0.6. B: axis at a κ/λ ratio.of 1.00.

While decreasing renal function has little influence on κ/λ ratios, there is, nevertheless, a small but observable effect. This arises from the removal of FLCs by other mechanisms *(Chapter 3.4)*. As renal clearance falls the proportion of FLCs cleared by non-renal mechanisms increases. Since this is by pinocytosis of serum, there is no distinction between κ and λ removal rates. Hence, κ/λ ratios increase with deteriorating renal function and are highest in complete renal failure *(Chapter 20)*. The data in Table 5.3 show the rising κ/λ ratios in normal elderly individuals who have reduced glomerular filtration. This is an important issue when evaluating borderline κ/λ ratios and may require the use of accurate markers for glomerular filtration when monitoring patients with changing renal function *(Chapter 20)*.

When screening symptomatic patients in a hospital setting, many ill patients will have renal impairment and/or inflammatory conditions leading to increased polyclonal sFLC concentrations. An example of such borderline results, seen in the context of a screening study, is shown in Figure 5.3.[17]

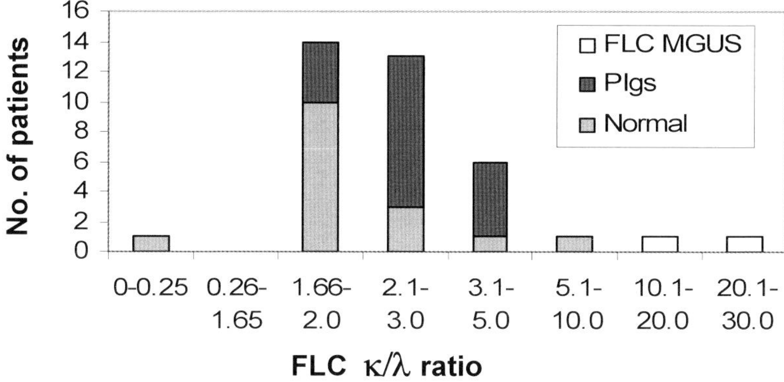

Figure 5.3. Frequency of borderline κ/λ ratios (37 in total) identified in a routine screening study for monoclonal gammopathies in 925 hospitalised patients. PIgs: polyclonal immunoglobulins (Courtesy of J Forsyth).[17]

5.2. Utility of serum free light chain assays for disease diagnosis

Using the reference intervals and diagnostic ranges shown above, the utility of sFLC measurements was assessed for identifying monoclonal FLC gammopathies (*Table 5.4*).[12] Sensitivity, specificity, positive predictive value (PPV), negative predictive value (NPV) and accuracy were estimated for the sFLC κ/λ ratios on the basis of both the central 95% interval and a diagnostic range that included 100% of normal results. Accuracy was calculated as the proportion of individuals classified correctly. PPV and NPV were calculated assuming a 15% prevalence of monoclonal proteins in the samples submitted for monoclonal protein studies. The patients in these studies are described in Chapter 6 for IFE and the respective chapters for MM, AL amyloidosis, LCDD and polyclonal hypergammaglobulinaemia. In the small group of samples selected, sFLC measurements had a higher sensitivity than IFE for detecting small concentrations of monoclonal sFLCs *(Chapter 6)*.

The normal range data reported by Katzmann et al[12]. is the most detailed yet published and has been generally adopted.

5.3. Urine free light chain normal ranges

In general, values in urine have been similar in all studies and have included random, 24-hour and early morning samples. Furthermore, κ concentrations were higher than λ in all the publications. This consistency suggests that the reported uFLC concentrations are reasonably accurate. Presumably, results are similar because normal urine contains insufficient amounts of intact immunoglobulin molecules to interfere with accurate FLC quantification (*Table 5.1*). The higher uFLC levels shown in the study by Bradwell et al.,[11] were explained by the use of early morning urine samples, which are typically 2-3-fold more concentrated than 24-hour urine samples. The mean (±SD) free κ concentration was 5.4 ± 4.95mg/L (n = 66; range, 0.36-20.3mg/L; 95% confidence interval, 0.39-15.1mg/L), and the mean (± SD) free λ concentration was 3.17 ± 3.3mg/L (n = 66; range, 0.81-17.3mg/L; 95% confidence interval, 0.81-10.1mg/L) (*Figures 5.4 and 5.5*). The mean κ/λ ratio was 1:0.54 (95% confidence interval, 1:2.17-1:0.25). The mean normal uFLC excretion was 3.7 mg/g of creatinine for κ and 2.0mg/g of creatinine for λ. There was a positive but nonsignificant correlation of urine creatinine concentrations with κ (r = 0.22) and λ (r = 0.17) measurements.

As expected, the range of uFLC concentrations was wider than for serum and κ/λ ratios were more variable. Presumably, this reflects minor differences in renal handling, urine dilution and variations in mucosal secretion of FLCs. The wider range of normal uFLC concentrations is another argument in favour of serum measurements.

	Reference Interval (0.3-1.2)		**Diagnostic range (0.26-1.65)**	
	Estimate	**95% CL**	**Estimate**	**95% CL**
Sensitivity %	98	91-100	97	89 - 100
Specificity %	95	92 -98	100	98 - 100
PPV %	78	65 - 89	100	91 - 100
NPV %	100	98 - 100	99	97 - 100
Accuracy %	96	93 - 98	99	98 - 100

Table 5.4. Comparison of reference intervals and diagnostic ranges for sFLCs and κ/λ ratios.[12] (Sera from the 282 reference individuals and 25 polyclonal hypergammaglobulinaemia patients as well as 66 sera from AL amyloidosis, LCDD and MM patients were used to calculate utility. (CL: confidence limits).

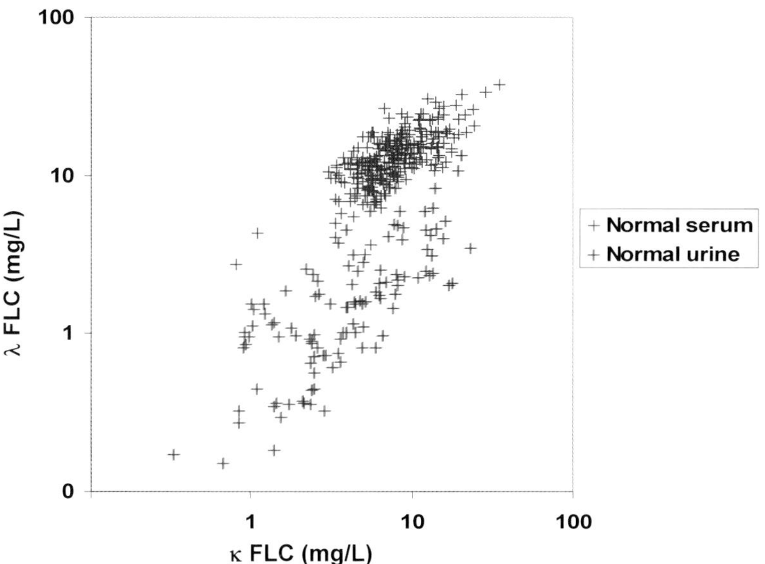

Figure 5.4. Comparison of FLC measurements in serum (*from Figure 5.2)* and early morning urine samples from healthy individuals.[11]

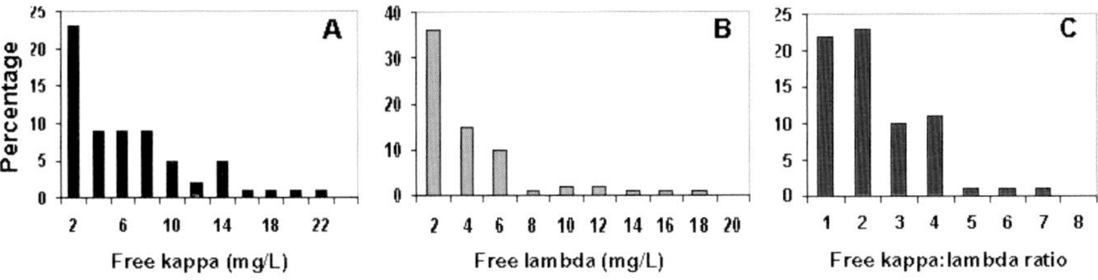

Figure 5.5. Frequency distributions of FLC κ (A), λ (B) and κ/λ ratios (C) in 66 normal urines.[11]

Summary: In sera from normal individuals:-

1. sFLC concentrations and κ/λ ratios are maintained within narrow limits.
2. sFLC concentrations increase slightly with age due to reduced glomerular filtration.
3. Serum κ/λ ratios increase slightly in renal failure *(also see Chapter 20.2).*
4. sFLC concentrations are less variable than in urine.

References

1. **Waldmann TA, Strober WS, Mogielnicki RP**. The Renal Handling of Low Molecular Weight Proteins II. Disorders of Serum Protein Catabolism in Patients with Tubular Proteinuria, the Nephrotic Syndrome or Uraemia. J Clin Invest 1972; **51**: 2162-2174.
2. **Sölling K.** Free light chains of Immunoglobulins in Normal Serum and Urine Determined by Radioimmunoassay. Scand J clin Lab Invest 1975; **35**: 407-412.
3. **Hemmingsen L, Skaarup P**. Urinary Excretion of Ten Plasma Proteins in Patients with Febrile Diseases. Acta Med Scand 1977; **201**: 359-364.
4. **Robinson EL, Gowland E, Ward ID, Scarffe JH.** Radioimmunoassay of free light chains of immunoglobulins in urine. Clin Chem 1982; **28** (11): 2254-2258.
5. **Brouwer J, Otting-van de Ruit M, Busking-van der Lely H.** Estimation of free light chains of immunoglobulins by enzyme immunoassay. Clin Chim Acta 1985; **150**: 257-274.
6. **Axiak SM, Krishnamoorthy L, Guinan J, Raison RL**. Quantitation of free κ light chains in serum and urine using a monoclonal antibody based inhibition enzyme-linked immunoassay. J Imm Methods 1987; **99**: 141-147.
7. **Wakasugi K, Sasaki M, Suzuki M, et al.** Increased concentrations of free light chain lambda in sera from chronic hemodialysis patients. Biomater Artif Cells in Immobil Biotechnol. 1991; **19:** 97.
8. **Nelson M, Brown RD, Gibson J, Joshua DE**. Measurement of free kappa and lambda chains in serum and the significance of their ratio in patients with multiple myeloma. Br J Haemat 1992; **81**: 223-230.
9. **Wakasugi K, Suzuki H, Imai A, Konishi S, Kishioka H.** Immunoglobulin free light chain assay using latex agglutination. Int J Clin Lab Res 1995; **25**: 211-215.
10. **Abe M, Goto T, Kosaka M, Wolfenbarger D, Weiss DT, Solomon A.** Differences in kappa and lambda (κ:λ) ratios of serum and urinary free light chains. Clin Exp Imm 1998; **111**: 457-462.
11. **Bradwell AR, Carr-Smith HD, Mead GP, Tang LX, Showell PJ, Drayson MT, Drew R.** Highly sensitive automated immunoassay for immunoglobulin free light chains in serum and urine. Clin Chem 2001; **47**: 673-680.
12. **Katzmann JA, Clark RJ, Abraham RS, Bryant S, Lymp JF, Bradwell AR, Kyle RA**. Serum Reference Intervals and Diagnostic Ranges for Free κ and Free λ Immunoglobulin Light Chains: Relative Sensitivity for Detection of Monoclonal Light Chains. Clin Chem 2002; **48**: 1437-1444.
13. **Deinum J, Derkx FHM.** Cystatin C for estimation of glomerular filtration rate? The Lancet 2000; **356**: 1624-1625.

14. Cockcroft DW, Gault MH. Prediction of creatinine clearance from serum creatinine. Nephron 1976; **16**: 31-41.

15. Sölling K. Normal values of free light chains in serum in different age groups. Scand J Clin Lab Invest 1977; **37**: 21-25.

16. Arfors K-E, Rutlil G, Svensjo E. Microvascular transport of macro-molecules in normal and inflammatory conditions. Acta Physiol Scand, Suppl., 1979; **463**: 93-103.

17. Forsyth JM, Hill PG, Rai BS, Mayne S, Mead GP. Serum Free Light Chain Measurement Can Replace Urine Electrophoresis in the Detection of B Cell Proliferative Disorders. Blood 2005; **106** (11): 5081: p352b.

Test questions

1. Why is the normal κ/λ ratio inverted in serum compared with urine?

2. How do κ/λ ratios correct for age-related increases in sFLC levels caused by decreases in glomerular filtration rates?

3. Is clonality preferably defined numerically, as κ/λ ratios, or by visualising a monoclonal band on electrophoretic gels?

Answers

1. Because the smaller monomeric κ molecules are cleared faster by the kidneys and enter the urine more readily than dimeric λ molecules (page 40).

2. The non-tumour sFLC acts as a marker of glomerular filtration rate so the ratio eliminates the effect of deteriorating renal function (page 41-42).

3. Arguably numerical κ/λ ratios are better than semi-quantitative, visualised bands particularly if they are faint (Chapter 6).

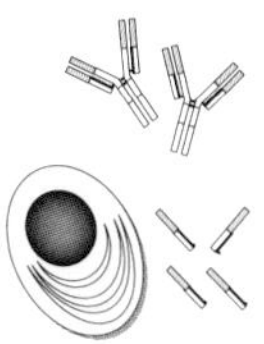

Chapter 6

Comparison of clinical assays for free light chains

There are many factors that need to be taken into account when deciding upon the most appropriate methods for measuring monoclonal FLCs. Requirements for the assays include sensitivity, accuracy, speed, cost, reliability, hands-on time, etc. A number of publications have compared different FLC assays and many of the important features are discussed in other chapters. This chapter is concerned only with a comparison of the sensitivity of routine clinical laboratory assays for FLC detection - arguably the most important issue.[1,2]

6.1. Serum and urine protein electrophoresis (SPE and UPE)

SPE is the standard screening method for MM and is usually based upon scanning

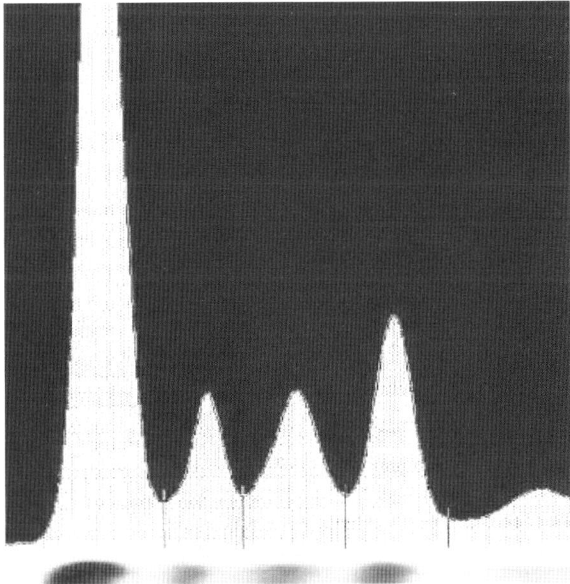

Figure 6.1. Normal SPE. (Courtesy of RA Kyle and JA Katzmann).

agararose electrophoretic gels after the serum proteins have been separated, fixed and stained. A normal SPE is shown in Figure 6.1 and a monoclonal immunoglobulin is shown in Figure 6.2.

The sensitivity of SPE for FLC detection is between 500mg/L and 2,000mg/L depending upon whether or not the monoclonal protein migrates alongside beta proteins.[3] SPE is negative for FLCs in all patients with NSMM, the majority of patients with AL amyloidosis and many patients with LCMM and other plasma cell dysrasias (*Chapters 8, 9 and 15)*.

Examples of sera containing medium to high concentrations of FLCs are shown in Figure 6.3. Most show the typical electrophoretic abnormalities of monoclonal bands and hypogammaglobulinaemia. Sample No 2, however, appears normal yet the λ FLC concentration is elevated 50-fold. This is typical of many serum samples that are sent to the laboratory with a diagnosis of, *"possible multiple myeloma - please investigate"*. Current practice would require testing a urine sample, but this is typically only available for 30-40% of the patients. sFLC assays would avoid the need for testing urine in all of the nine patients shown *(Chapter 24)*. Screening sera by SPE and sFLCs is a simple and sensitive strategy for identifying new patients with monoclonal gammopathies and avoids the need for for urine tests *(Chapter 23)*.

UPE is much more sensitive than SPE since urine can be concentrated many times (*Figure 6.4*). Thus, FLCs in urine can be detected at <10-20mg/L, although most laboratories claim a detection limit in the region of 40-50mg/L. In practice, high concentrations of background proteins and 'ladder banding' of polyclonal FLCs prevent attainment of the ideal sensitivity. Furthermore, some patients with LCMM produce only small amounts of FLCs so that little, if any, passes the reabsorptive surface of the renal proximal tubules. These patients may, therefore, have undetectable levels of uFLCs.

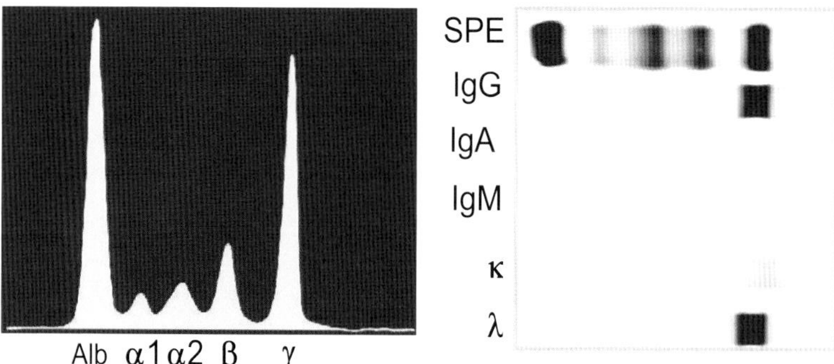

Figure 6.2. SPE and IFE of a serum IgGλ monoclonal protein. Also identified is a small amount of polyclonal IgG with its associated κ and λ staining, and virtually no IgA or IgM. (Courtesy of RA Kyle and JA Katzmann).

6.2. Serum immunofixation electrophoresis (IFE)

Serum IFE is approximately 10-fold more sensitive for FLCs (150-500mg/L) than SPE but still considerably less sensitive than FLC immunoassays. One particular disadvantage of IFE is that it cannot be used to quantify monoclonal immunoglobulins because of the presence of the precipitating antibody. IFE is also rather laborious to perform and visual interpretation may be difficult. A typical result on a sample containing a substantial amount of IgGλ monoclonal protein, is shown in Figure 6.2.

In a study from The Mayo Clinic,[4] it was shown that all of 46 serum samples with low concentrations of monoclonal FLCs were correctly identified by FLC immunoassay

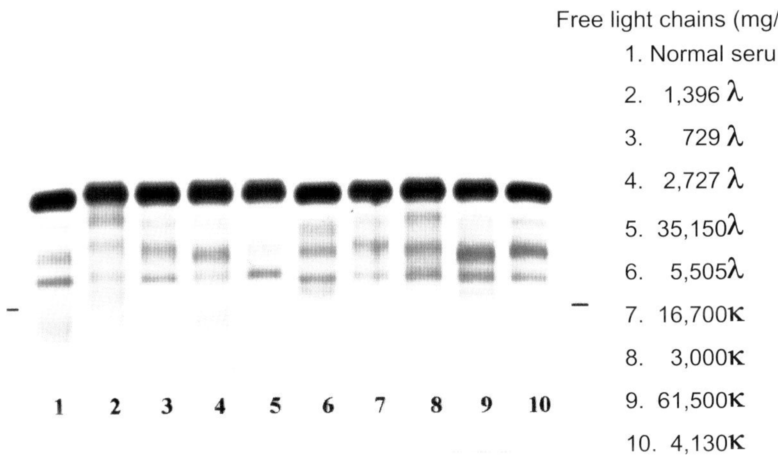

Figure 6.3. SPE in 9 patients with LCMM and one normal sample compared with the concentrations of sFLCs (mg/L). Some samples appear relatively normal by SPE but sFLC concentrations are grossly abnormal in all samples.

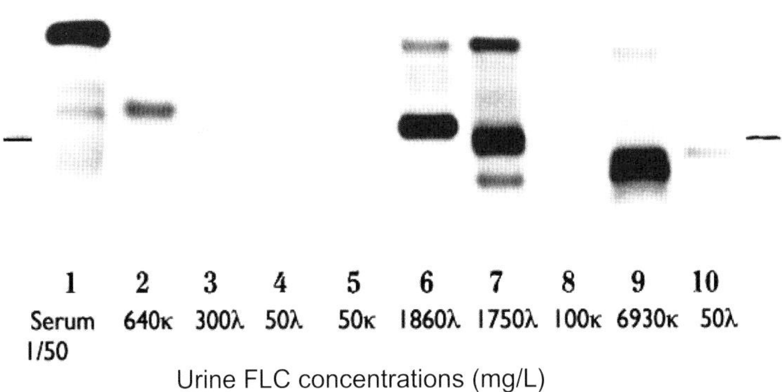

Figure 6.4. UPE in 9 patients with LCMM and one normal serum sample compared with measurements of urine FLCs by immunoassay.

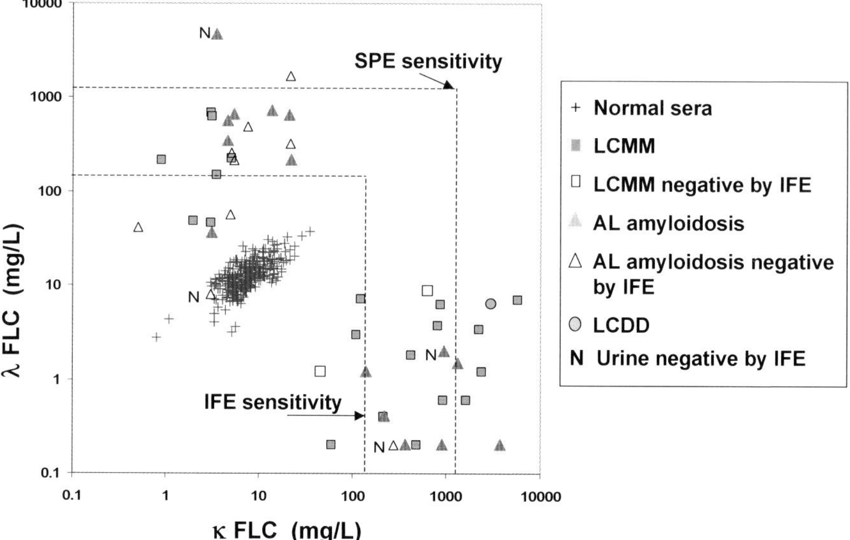

Figure 6.5. FLC concentrations in sera containing monoclonal FLCs that were 'difficult to detect' by IFE.

(*Figure 6.5*). IFE was less sensitive and detected FLCs in some of the sera only after multiple assays and at different sample dilutions. The study included serum samples from patients in whom IFE was only positive for uFLCs. (One sample, shown in Figure 6.5, was negative by serum and urine IFE and sFLC immunoassay).

The high sensitivity of the FLC assays is dependent upon assessing the individual FLC concentrations and the κ/λ ratios. Tumour suppression of the normal plasma cells in the bone marrow reduces the concentrations of the alternate FLC and, thereby, enhances the sensitivity of the κ/λ ratio. The alternate FLC concentrations and hence the κ/λ ratios, are important aspects of the diagnostic accuracy of sFLC immunoassays.

Figure 6.5 shows that there is a poor correlation between sFLC concentrations and the detection of monoclonal proteins by IFE. This may be due to polymerisation of the FLCs, which prevents the formation of visible, narrow monoclonal bands during SPE. This has been observed in patients with NSMM (*Chapter 9*) and probably occurs in most MM sera. However, rare serum samples from patients with AL amyloidosis and LCDD may be negative by sFLC assays but positive by IFE. This indicates that sFLC assays and IFE should be used as complementary diagnostic tests in occasional patients with AL amyloidosis *(Chapter 15).*

6.3. Capillary zone electrophoresis (CZE)

CZE is used in many clinical laboratories for serum protein separation and is able to detect most monoclonal immunoglobulins. However, when compared with IFE, CZE fails to detect monoclonal proteins in 5% of positive samples.[5-7] These so called 'false negative' results encompass low-concentration and 'hidden' monoclonal proteins (e.g. in the transferrin peak).

Marien et al.,[8] compared the sensitivity of sFLC assays and CZE for the detection of low concentration monoclonal immunoglobulins. Frozen sera from 55 patients, previously shown to contain monoclonal proteins by IFE, but negative by CZE, were assessed by immunoassays for FLCs. They included both intact immunoglobulin and FLC monoclonal proteins.

The results showed that all 21 samples from patients with LCMM had abnormal FLC results (*Figure 6.6*). In addition, 13 out of 33 samples from patients with intact monoclonal immunoglobulins had abnormal FLC ratios (not shown). These patients had MGUS and B-cell derived malignant diseases. FLC immunoassays were, therefore, more reliable than CZE for detecting LCMM and identified many abnormal samples in patients from other disease groups. Similar findings were recently reported from Bakshi et al., in a monoclonal protein screening study *(Chapter 23)*.[7]

Figure 6.6 indicates that several samples with FLC concentrations greater than 1,000 mg/L were not detected by CZE. Under ideal conditions the sensitivity of this technique may be better but it is still substantially less than IFE. However, CZE does at least provide a quantitative measure of the monoclonal proteins whereas IFE does not.

6.4. Total κ and λ immunoassays

Unfortunately, immunoassays for total κ and λ are sometimes used to identify patients with LCMM. This is in spite of warnings by The College of American Pathologists and

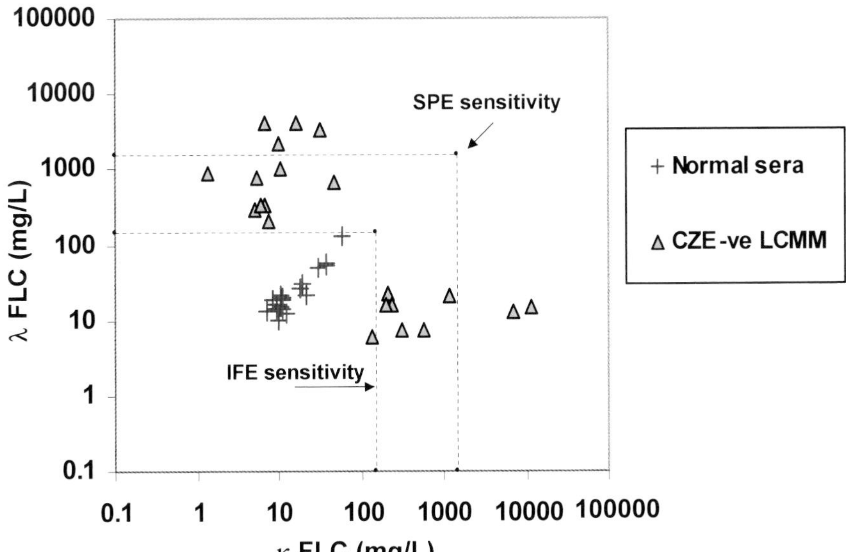

Figure 6.6. Serum κ and λ FLC concentrations in 20 control samples and 21 samples that were normal by CZE but had monoclonal proteins by IFE. (Courtesy of X Bossuyt).

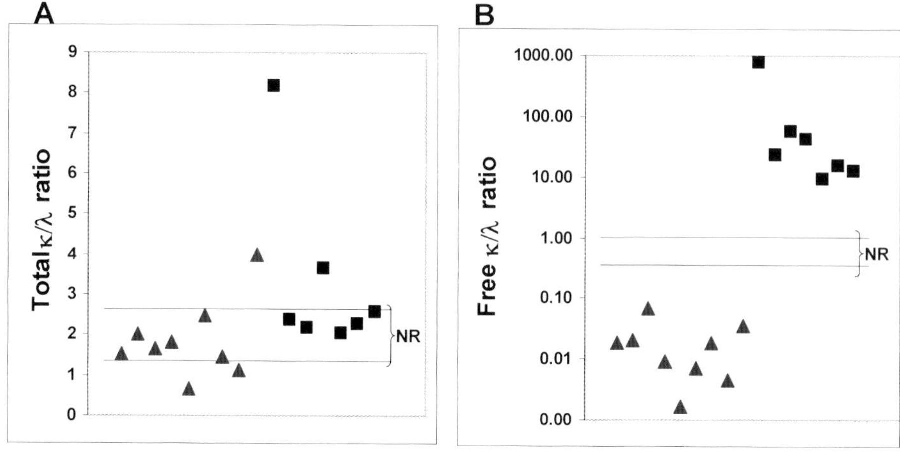

Figure 6.7. Comparison of total serum light chains (A) and sFLC κ/λ ratios (B) for identifying patients with κ and λ LCMM. κ patients: black squares; λ patients: blue triangles. The red triangle is a misclassifed sample. Normal range limits are shown.

others, that the method is not sensitive enough for routine clinical use.[1] Indeed, samples containing many grams of FLCs may be completely missed using this technique.

The sensitivity of sFLC assays and total κ and λ assays were compared in a study by Marien et al.[8] 16 serum samples from patients with LCMM were investigated (samples from the CZE study described above). Total κ and λ concentrations were measured using Beckman-Coulter reagents on the Immage nephelometer. All samples were abnormal by FLC assays. This compared with only 5 of the 16 samples by total κ and λ assays, and one λ patient was misclassified as κ (*Figure 6.7*).

6.5. Urine tests for free light chains

There are many methods for detecting urine FLCs some of which are outlined in Chapter 4. Serum immunoassays are preferable because urine is a poor fluid for assessing FLC concentrations *(Chapter 3).* As shown by Nowrousian et al.,[9] significant amounts of sFLCs are necessary to cause FLC proteinuria in patients with MM. In that study, median monoclonal serum κ and λ concentrations were 113mg/L and 278mg/L respectively, before Bence Jones proteinuria occured. However, this section is only concerned with comparison of urine laboratory methods. Clinical comparisons of assay sensitivity are described in Chapter 24.

Herzog and Hoffman compared the sensitivity of 3 different urine protein tests (*Table 6.1*) with serum and urine FLC immunoassays in 33 patients with MM who had Bence Jones proteinuria by IFE.[10] Six of the patients were light chain only MM while 28 patients had intact monoclonal immunoglobulins in the serum with additional uFLC excretion. 15 of the latter patients also excreted intact monoclonal immunoglobulins into the urine. Results showed that sFLC κ/λ ratios were the most sensitive analysis and

Analytical technique	Normal ranges	Sensitivity
Serum FLC κ/λ ratio	κ/λ >0.26 to < 1.65	33 out of 33
Urine FLC κ/λ ratio	κ/λ >2.04 to <10.37	29 out of 33
Urine total κ/λ ratio + levels	κ/λ >1 to <5.2 & Tκ+λ<10mg/L	29 out of 32
Urine albumin/total protein	albumin/TP <0.3 & TP <300mg/L	14 out of 31
Urine total protein	total protein <100mg/L	26 out of 32

Table 6.1. Sensitivity of different analytical techniques for FLC detection in 33 patients with MM.[10] (Tκ+λ = total κ + λ concentrations; TP = total protein).

better than uFLC κ/λ ratios *(Table 6.1)*. Total protein tests for FLCs were poor. The reference method for this study was urine IFE and positive results were the basis for sample selection. Other studies have shown that in a clinical setting, sFLC tests are considerably more sensitive than uIFE for identifying patients with residual disease (*Chapters 8-12 and 24*).

A comparison of uIFE and uFLC immunoassays for Bence Jones protein detection was made by Viedma et al.[11] While FLC immunoassays correctly identified many of the positive and negative samples, high background polyclonal FLCs (arising from renal damage) obscured correct interpretation of κ/λ ratios. Hence, uIFE was more accurate for monoclonal protein identification.

Le Bricon et al., analysed the sensitivity of different urine assays for Bence Jones proteins in 20 patients with MM.[12] The urines contained monoclonal intact immunoglobulins and/or monoclonal FLCs. Comparisons were made between assays for total protein (Pyrogallol Red), SDS-agarose gel electrophoresis (sensitivity 50mg/L in unconcentrated urine) and FLC immunoassays (sensitivity <1mg/L). The results confirmed the superior sensitivity of the FLC immunoassays. 6 of the 20 patients were abnormal by the total protein test, 11 by SDS-agarose gel electrophoresis and 16 by FLC immunoassays. 6 samples that were only abnormal by FLC immunoassays are shown in Table 6.2. The immunoassays were particularly helpful for identifying monoclonal

Serum M-protein	Urine protein (mg/L)	Urine free light chains		Urine SDS-AGE
		κ & λ(mg/L)	κ/λ ratio	
IgG kappa	50(mg/L)	92:10	9.2	Negative
IgA kappa	40(mg/L)	28:6	4.7	Negative
IgA lambda	50(mg/L)	7:94	0.07	Negative
IgA lambda	960(mg/L)	66:749	0.09	+/- polyclonal
IgD lambda	100(mg/L)	3:21	0.14	Negative
FLC	1,990(mg/L)	60:21	0.29	+/- polyclonal

Table 6.2. Comparison of urine tests in 6 patients who were negative for monoclonal urine proteins by SDS-agarose gel electrophoresis but were abnormal by FLC.[12] There was a good overall correlation except for sample 6 that probably contained albumin.

FLCs when they were present in low concentrations. There was a reasonable correlation between the quantitative results for the different methods.

Herzum et al., also compared FLC immunoassays with other urine tests for FLCs.[13] The FLC assays showed good precision (<10%), linearity and correlation between different instruments (Hitachi and BNII). However, the assays overestimated the amounts of Bence Jones protein present in urine samples. 37 samples were compared using the following methods: benzethonium chloride, Biuret, modified Biuret and FLC immunoassays. Measurements using immunoassays produced the highest results in 26 of the samples. The Biuret methods had the best correlation with the FLC immunoassays. The Biuret method measures peptide bonds, and it is considered to be a good general assay method for proteins. The good correlation with the FLC test results provides supporting evidence for their accuracy.

6.6. Discordant serum and urine free light chain results.

Quantitation of monoclonal FLCs by electrophoretic methods often produces lower results than FLC immunoassays. H Zitterberg (Goteborg University, Sweden: Personal communication) reviewed the laboratory records from 22 newly diagnosed LCMM patients who presented over a 2-year period. By quantitative electrophoresis, none had more than 3g/L of sFLCs and 19 were below 1g/L. This is in contrast to 50% that were over 3g/L in the study by Bradwell et al., using sFLC immunoassays.[14] Part of the explanation is that urine and serum FLCs are frequently polymerised and this leads to high results by immunoassay (*Chapter 9*). In addition, serum FLCs may bind to α_1 antitrypsin[15] while urine FLCs bind to uromucoid *(Chapter 14)*. Also, the protein tests probably underestimated the concentrations of FLCs to a variable extent.

Although not quantitative, IFE is considered to be the 'gold standard' for identifying monoclonal urine FLCs. Nevertheless, the detection of minor monoclonal bands by this method can be misleading. There are many reasons:-

1. The precipitating antibodies against one or other FLC may not be completely specific and may cross-react with intact immunoglobulins or other urine proteins. This can produce a false positive band with the appearance of a monoclonal FLC.
2. A narrow protein precipitate band can occur at the sample application site on the gel and appear like a monoclonal band.
3. Restricted 'ladder banding' in concentrated samples can give the appearance of monoclonality.
4. Heavy proteinuria containing polyclonal FLCs may produce confusing background staining which obscures correct interpretation of monoclonal FLC bands.
5. An inadequate antibody to one of the FLCs (usually λ) gives the impression that only the alternate FLC is being excreted. Although there may be a broad band, it can suggest monoclonality. This is a fairly frequent occurrence.
6. After transplantation, oligoclonal bands are produced for many months. These may produce confusing results in urine samples and appear monoclonal. sFLC ratios, on the other hand, may be normal.

7. IFE is not quantitative so it is difficult to compare one result with another. The major part of the staining intensity is due to the second antibody (80% or more), so it is not possible to assess the amounts of monoclonal protein present.

Even when a monoclonal uFLC band is visually convincing, it should be evaluated alongside other clinical and laboratory data because it may be inconsequential. As discussed elsewhere, clinically significant monoclonal uFLCs are exceptional when sFLCs are normal. In a study of 110 patients with AL amyloidosis, all but one had serum monoclonal proteins and the remaining patient was negative by all tests including urine analysis *(Table 6.3)*.[16] Isolated, minimal uFLC excretion has usually been considered as clinically insignificant, an opinion that is further supported by this data (*Chapter 19.4, Figure 19.6)*.

Urine IFE may correctly identify monoclonal FLCs when serum analysis is normal, under the following unusual circumstances:-

1. When there is damage to isolated nephrons allowing leakage of monoclonal FLCs into urine. Serum levels, in contrast, may not be raised sufficiently to produce abnormal κ/λ ratios.
2. When monoclonal FLCs are truncated and rapidly cleared. The short serum half-life prevents accumulation in serum but significant levels could be present in urine. This is a very rare occurrence.
3. Abnormal amino-acid sequences might change the shape of the 'hidden', surface epitopes on the FLC constant regions. This might prevent detection by antisera specific for FLCs. However, IFE antisera against the whole FLC structures may detect some remaining, undistorted epitopes and produce positive results.[17] This is a very rare occurrence.
4. If the serum and urine samples are collected at different times, results may be discordant. Normally, serum samples are collected at the clinic but the urine is either collected earlier or is subsequently sent in by post. If the samples are separated by a significant time, even a few days, results may be quite different because of the short serum half-life of FLCs *(Chapter 13)*.

In spite of the possibility that uIFE is more sensitive under some circumstances,

Test	Sensitivity
FLC κ/λ ratio	91%
Serum IFE	69%
Urine IFE	83%
FLC κ/λ ratio and urine IFE	91%
FLC κ/λ ratio and serum IFE	99%
Serum IFE and urine IFE	95%
All three tests	99%

Table 6.3. Comparison of serum and urine tests for identifying 110 patients with AL amyloidosis.[16] Urine tests provided no additional diagnostic benefit.

serum assays provide a reliable basis for assessing true FLC production by the tumour. Detailed physiological, technical and clinical reasons for using sFLC assays rather than urine assays are discussed in Chapter 24.

Summary:

A bar chart comparing the sensitivities of the different FLC assays is shown in Figure 6.8. There is considerable variation in the achieved sensitivities reported in different studies, in part due to the variable position of the monoclonal bands in relation to other proteins. This variation in sensitivity is shown as error bars. Since normal sFLC concentrations are considerably below the detection limit of all electrophoretic methods, some patients will always be missed using these techniques. The numbers of patients and the types of diseases missed by serum electrophoretic tests are shown diagrammatically in Figure 6.9. Again, reports vary in their claims for the achieved levels of sensitivity for electrophoretic tests, but the figure clearly indicates the benefits of the increased sensitivity of sFLC measurements.

References

1. **Kyle RA**. Sequence of Testing for Monoclonal Gammopathies - Serum and Urine Assays. Arch Pathol Lab Med. 1999; **123**: 114-118.

2. **Guinan JEC, Kenny DF, Gatenby PA**. Detection and typing of paraproteins: comparison of different methods in a routine diagnostic laboratory. Pathology 1989; **21**: 35-41.

3. **Bradwell AR, Carr-Smith HD, Mead GP, Tang LX, Showell PJ, Drayson MT, Drew R**. Highly sensitive automated immunoassay for immunoglobulin free light chains in serum and urine. Clin Chem 2001; **47**: 673-680.

4. **Katzmann JA, Clark RJ, Abraham RS, Bryant S, Lymp JF, Bradwell AR, Kyle RA**. Serum

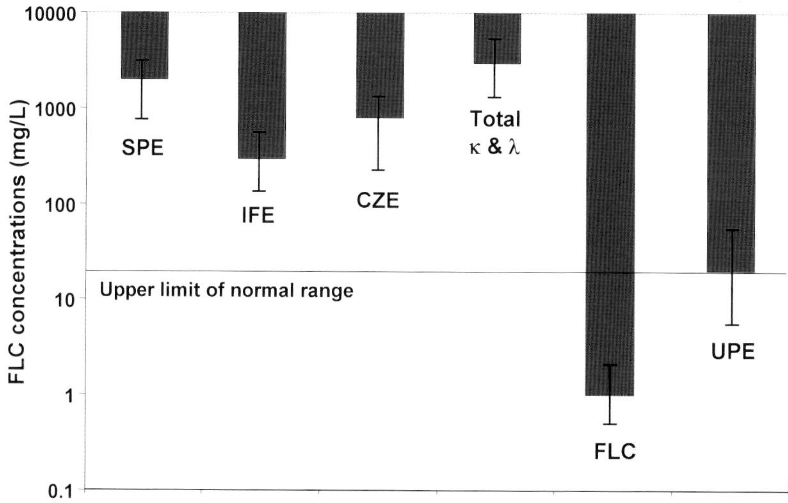

Figure 6.8. Sensitivity of assays for serum FLC quantitation with error bars indicating the different claimed limits.

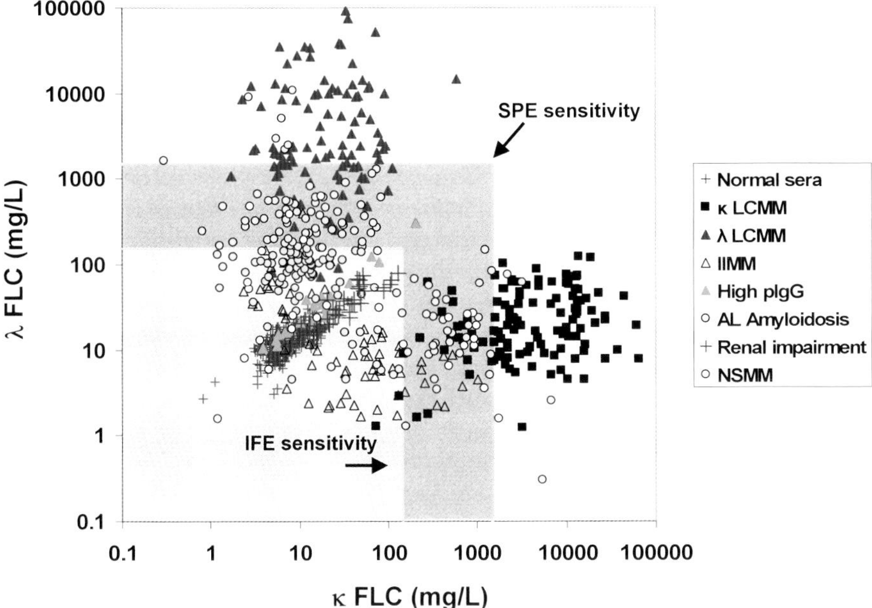

Figure 6.9. κ/λ graph of sFLCs showing samples that would be mis-identified as negative using SPE and IFE. (High pIgG: polyclonal hypergammaglobulinaemia. *For the data on the patient groups see the relevant chapters).*

Reference Intervals and Diagnostic Ranges for Free κ and Free λ Immunoglobulin Light Chains: Relative Sensitivity for Detection of Monoclonal Light Chains. Clin Chem 2002; **48**: 1437-1444.

5. **Katzmann JA, Clark R, Sanders E, Landers JP, Kyle RA.** Prospective Study of Serum Protein Capillary Electrophoresis immunotyping of monoclonal proteins by immuno-subtraction. Am J Clin Path 1998; **110**: 503-509.

6. **Bossuyt X, Mariën G.** False-negative results in detection of Monoclonal Proteins by Capillary Zone Electrophoresis: a Prospective Study. Clin Chem 2001; **47**: 1477-1479.

7. **Bakshi NA, Guilbranson R, Garstka D, Bradwell AR, Keren DF.** Serum Free Light Chain (FLC) Measurement Can Aid Capillary Zone Electrophoresis (CZE) In Detecting Subtle FLC M-Proteins. Am J Clin Path 2005; **124**: 214-218.

8. **Mariën G, Oris E, Bradwell AR, Blanckaert N, Bossuyt X.** Detection of Monoclonal Proteins in sera by Capillary Zone Electrophoresis and free light chain measurements. Clin Chem 2002; **48**: 1600-1601.

9. **Nowrousian MR, Brandhorst D, Sammet C, Kellert M, Daniels R, Schuett P, Poser M, Mueller S, Ebeling P, Welt A, Bradwell AR, Buttkereit U, Opalka B, Flasshove M, Moritz T, Seeber S.** Serum Free Light Chain Analysis and Urine Immunofixation Electrophoresis in Patients with Multiple Myeloma. Clin Cancer Res 2005; **11** (24): 8706-8714.

10. **Herzog W, Hofmann W.** Detection of free kappa and lambda light chains in serum and urine in patients with monoclonal gammopathy. Blood 2003; **102** (11): A5190.

11. **Viedma JA, Garrigos N, Morales S.** Comparison of the Sensitivity of 2 Automated Immunoassays with Immunofixation Electrophoresis for Detecting Bence Jones Proteins. Clin Chem 2005; **51**: 1505-1507.

12. **Le Bricon T, Bengoufa D, Benlakehal M, Bousquet B, Erlich D.** Urinary free light chain analysis by the Freelite immunoassay: a preliminary study in multiple myeloma. Clin Biochem 2002; **35**: 565-567.

13. **Herzum I, Heinz R, Bruder-Burzlaff B, Renz H, Wahl HG.** Reliability of the new Freelite assay

for quantification of free light chains in urine. Clin Chem 2004; **50** (6): Suppl, pA80; C-38.

14. Bradwell AR, Carr-Smith HD, Mead GP, Harvey TC, Drayson MD. Serum test for assessment of patients with Bence Jones myeloma. Lancet 2003; **361**: 489-491.

15. Chapuis-Cellier C, Foray V, Chazaud A, Troncy J. Apparent discrepancies in the quantitation of free light chains in serum of patients presenting with a monoclonal gammopathy. Haematologica 2005; **90** (s1) PO409: p109.

16. Katzmann J, Abraham RS, Dispenzieri A, Lust JA, Kyle RA. Diagnostic performance of Quantitative Kappa and Lambda Free Light Chain Assays in Clinical Practice. Clin Chem 2005; **51** (5): 878-881.

17. Coriu D, Weaver K, Schell M, Eulitz M, Murphy CL, Weiss DT, Solomon A. A molecular basis for nonsecretory myeloma. Blood 2003; **104** (3): 829-831.

Test questions

1. *What is the origin of ladder banding in UPE?*
2. *Which is more sensitive, CZE or SPE?*
3. *Do total serum light chain tests have a useful role in the laboratory?*
4. *Under what circumstances is uIFE unreliable?*
5. *Which is more sensitive - urine FLC immunoassays or uIFE?*

Answers

1. *Oligoclonal FLCs focus separately during electrophoresis (page 48).*
2. *CZE (page 56, Figure 6.8).*
3. *No. FLC immunoassays are better in all respects (page 51).*
4. *There are several reasons listed on pages 54-55.*
5. *Urine IFE (Page 53).*

Section 2

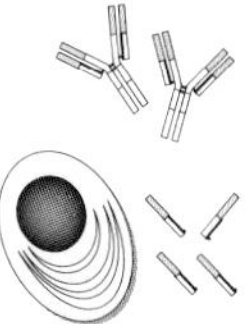

Diseases with monoclonal free light chains

Serum FLC measurements may be useful in any disease that causes abnormal monoclonal or polyclonal light chain concentrations *(Chapter 29)*. The main clinical applications of the assays are in patients with monoclonal gammopathies. Figure 7.0 shows the distribution of clinical diagnoses for monoclonal gammopathies seen at the Mayo Clinic in the USA. Because this data is from a specialist referral centre, general hospitals usually see a different pattern of disease referral with a higher percentage of MM and MGUS and fewer AL amyloidosis patients.

Figure 7.0 shows the approximate annual incidence of the more common monoclonal gammopathies reported in the USA.[1] In the past 5 years there have been many publications covering various aspects of FLCs in MM, AL amyloidosis and other monoclonal gammopathies. The results are reviewed in the following chapters together with suggested FLC investigations that may be of clinical value, but where results have yet to be reported. The clinical utility of sFLC measurements in NSMM and AL amyloidosis is well now established. In LCMM results indicate that serum tests will replace urinalysis for disease diagnosis and monitoring and this may also be true for monitoring patients with IIMM. Many other clinical applications of sFLC assays are

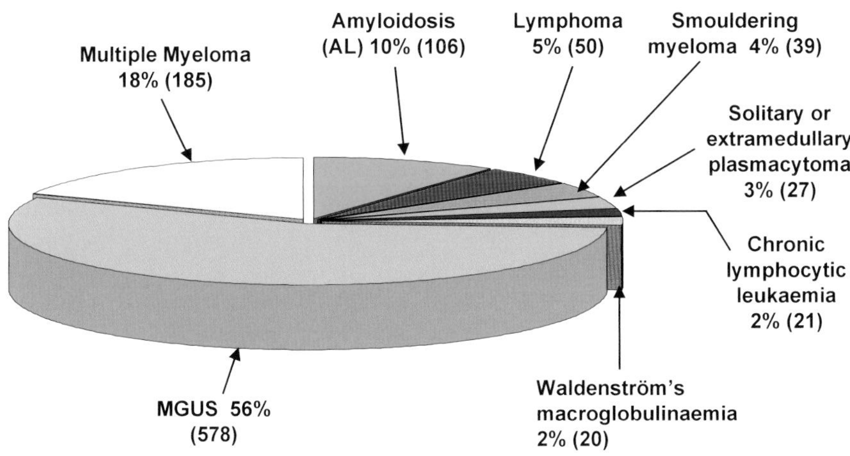

Figure 7.0. Distribution of clinical diagnoses in 1026 patients with a serum monoclonal protein detected at the Mayo Clinic in 1992.[1]

currently under investigation including in patients with solitary plasmacytomas *(Figure 7.01)* and Waldenström's macroglobulinaemia.

References

1. **Blade J and Kyle RA.** Monoclonal gammopathies of undetermined significance. In: Myeloma Biology and Management. Eds: JS Malpas, DE Bergsagel, RA Kyle. Oxford University Press, 1995. New York.

2. **Kyle RA, Rajkumar SV.** Multiple myeloma. N Engl J Med 2004; **351**: 1860-1873.

3. **Malpas JS, Bergsagel DE, Kyle RA, Anderson KC.** Myeloma: Biology and Management. Sanders, Elsevier Inc, USA. 2004.

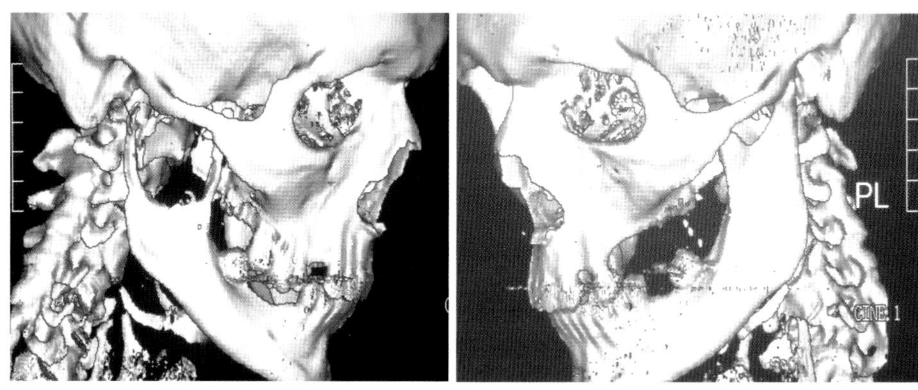

Figure 7.01. Solitary plasmacytoma of the right ramus of the mandible (Courtesy of Ade Olujohungbe , Liverpool, UK).

	Annual Incidence	*Monoclonal proteins	Serum FLC abnormal	Median survival	**Utility of serum FLC
IIMM	10,500	100%	96%	3-4 years	Useful
LCMM	2,000	100%	100%	3-4 years	Important
NSMM	400	0%	>70%	3-4 years	Important
Plasmacytoma	1,000	50%	~80%	>10 years	Useful
AL Amyloidosis	2,500	75-90%	>95%	1-2 years	Important
LCDD	100	90%	90%	3-4 years	Important
Waldenström's	1,000	100%	97%	5 years	Unknown
MGUS	1,000,000	100%	~60%	>12 years	Important
ASMM	250	100%	~90%	5-10 years	Unknown
#B-CLL	10,000	~50%	~20%	~5 years	Unknown

Table 7.0. Incidence of diseases producing monoclonal proteins in the USA.[2,3] * % showing monoclonal proteins by traditional electrophoretic methods. ** Based on current publications. #Other B cell lymphoid malignancies may produce monoclonal immunoglobulins.

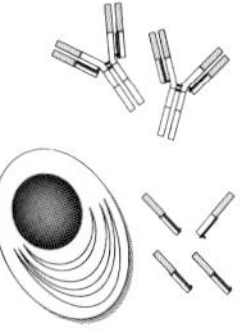

Section 2A. Multiple myeloma

Chapter 7

Multiple myeloma - Introduction

Multiple myeloma (MM) is the 2nd most common form of haematological malignancy after non-Hodgkin lymphoma. In Caucasian populations the incidence is approximately 35 per million per year, it increases with age and there is a slight male preponderance. In the UK there are 2,500-3,000 new cases per year and 15,000 in the USA, with a median survival of 3-4 years. At any one instance, there are 10,000 to 15,000 patients with the disease in the UK and approximately 150,000 world-wide. The incidence of MM in different populations is shown in Table 7.1.

Diagnosis is based on the presence of excess monoclonal plasma cells in the bone marrow, monoclonal immunoglobulins in serum or urine and related organ or tissue impairment such as hypercalcaemia, renal insufficiency, anaemia or bone lesions *(Chapter 25)*. Normal plasma cell content of the bone marrow is about 1% while in MM the content is typically greater than 30% but may be over 90%. Concentrations between 5-10% are equivocal since plasma cell distribution in MM may be patchy or there may be other causes for the plasmacytosis such as chronic infections. Identification of the monoclonal cells is preferably achieved using immunohistochemical staining for κ and λ FLCs *(Figure 3.5)*.

The osteolytic lesions of MM, classically seen in skull X-rays *(Figure 7.1)*, are not a constant feature. Patients may have osteosclerotic bone lesions or no detectable

Location	Men	Women	Location	Men	Women
Argentina	30	21	Japan	18	12
Australia	30	26	Thailand	5	4
Canada	40	27	UK	35	25
Germany	30	25	USA (black)	72	68
India	13	8	USA (white)	40	26

Table 7.1. Annual age-standardised incidence of MM by location per million.[1]

abnormalities. Also, osteolytic lesions may occasionally be seen in other diseases.

The immunoglobulin classes of monoclonal proteins produced by the plasma cell clones reflect their normal frequency in the body. This is shown in Figure 7.2 and is based on more than 2,500 patients entered into the UK MRC multiple myeloma trials from 1980 to 1998.

Reference

1. **Malpas JS, Bergsagel DE, Kyle RA, Anderson KC.** Myeloma: Biology and Management. Saunders, Elsevier Inc, USA. 2004.

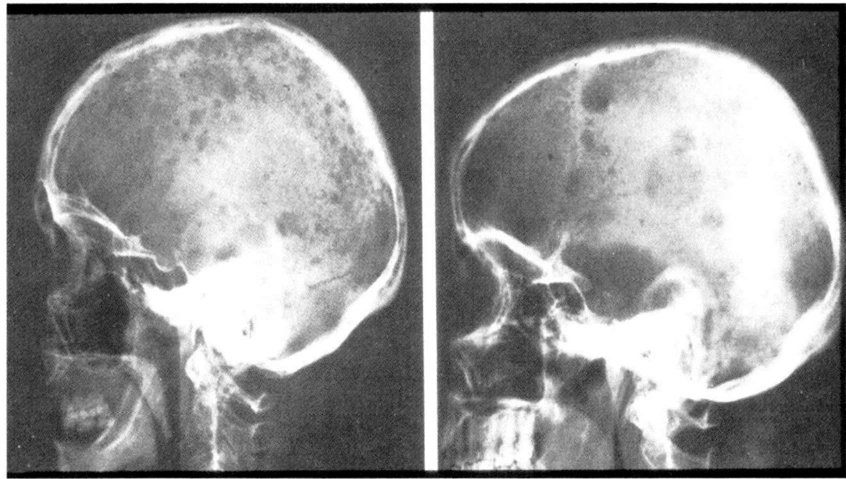

Figure 7.1. Osteolytic lesions in the skulls of 2 patients with multiple myeloma.

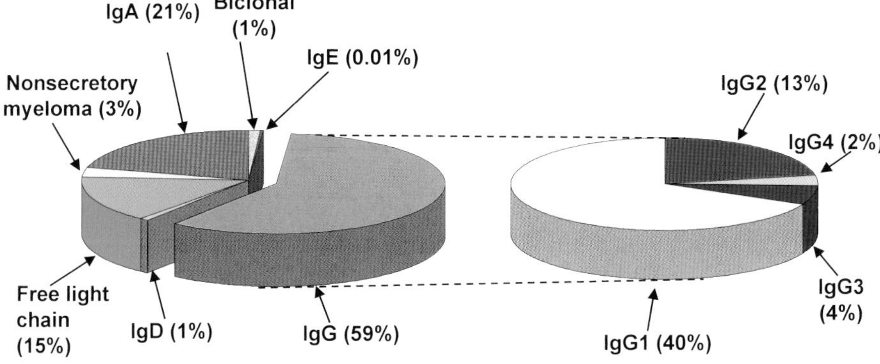

Figure 7.2. Classification of MM based upon monoclonal protein production from the UK MRC Multiple Myeloma trials.

Chapter 8

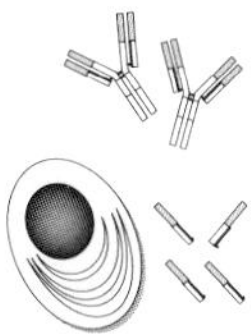

Light chain multiple myeloma

8.1. Diagnosis of light chain multiple myeloma

The typical clinical features of MM, such as bone pain, fractures, renal failure and anaemia alert the physician to the diagnosis. Bence Jones protein in the urine, in the absence of intact monoclonal immunoglobulins in the serum, alongside a positive bone marrow biopsy, confirms the diagnosis. On occasions, clinical symptoms and signs can be obscure so that urine tests for MM are not considered for some time. This leads to delays in diagnosis as indicated by the occasional published case report illustrating the difficulties (*see Clinical Case Histories 1 and 2*).[1,2]

Commonly, the initial screening test for LCMM is SPE. This demonstrates a monoclonal FLC band in approximately 50% of patients and in some of the remainder the serum may show hypogammaglobulinaemia. Serum IFE will demonstrate monoclonal bands in most patients but ultimately a urine test is required to identify and quantitate the monoclonal FLCs. Figure 8.1 shows some typical electrophoretic tests.

Since immunoassays for sFLCs are more sensitive than electrophoresis tests *(Chapter 6)* could they eliminate the need for urinalysis? The answer to this question was published in *The Lancet* in 2003 as a clear, "***Yes***".[3] The study was based on archived sera

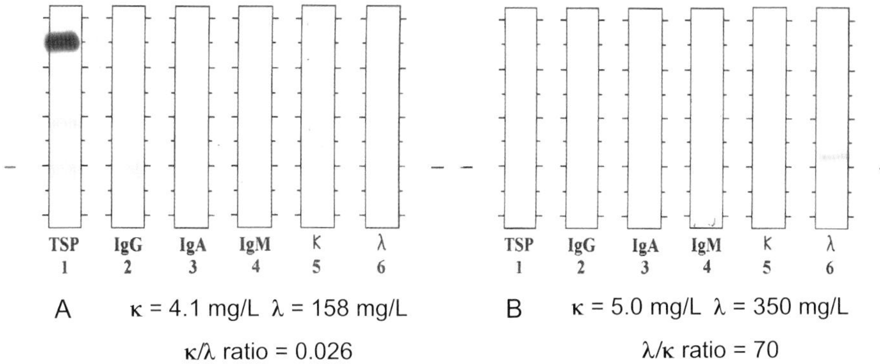

Figure 8.1. Serum and urine IFE on a patient with λ LCMM compared with FLC immunoassay results. SPE and IFE of (A) serum with no abnormality visible and (B) urine showing a λ FLC band.

from 224 patients with LCMM entered into the UK MRC Myeloma trials between 1983 and 1999. The clinical diagnosis of MM had been established using bone marrow plasma cell content, the presence of monoclonal FLCs in the serum or urine (without intact monoclonal immunoglobulins) and the presence of lytic bone lesions.

The results showed that at the time of diagnosis, all patients had abnormal concentrations of the appropriate sFLC (*Figure 8.2*) and abnormal κ/λ ratios. The concentrations were clearly different from FLCs measured in the serum of 282 normal adults (*Chapter 5*). The non-tumour FLCs, produced by normal plasma cells, were also abnormal in many of the patients. Many were either elevated as a result of renal impairment or suppressed because of bone marrow failure. Comparison of results was made with 31 patients who had renal impairment from causes other than monoclonal gammopathies. Characteristically, they had elevations of both FLC types with normal κ/λ ratios (*Chapter 20*).

Similar results were found in a study of 66 patients with MM by Nowrousian et al.[4] Nearly all patients who had uFLCs by IFE had abnormal sFLC κ/λ ratios. Furthermore, more than 60% of patients under treatment, with negative urine tests for Bence Jones protein, had abnormal sFLCs, indicating the additional sensitivity of the serum test. They concluded that assessment of sFLCs was much more sensitive than urine IFE for identifying Bence Jones protein in patients with MM.

In *The Lancet* study mentioned above, all the patients had elevated concentrations of

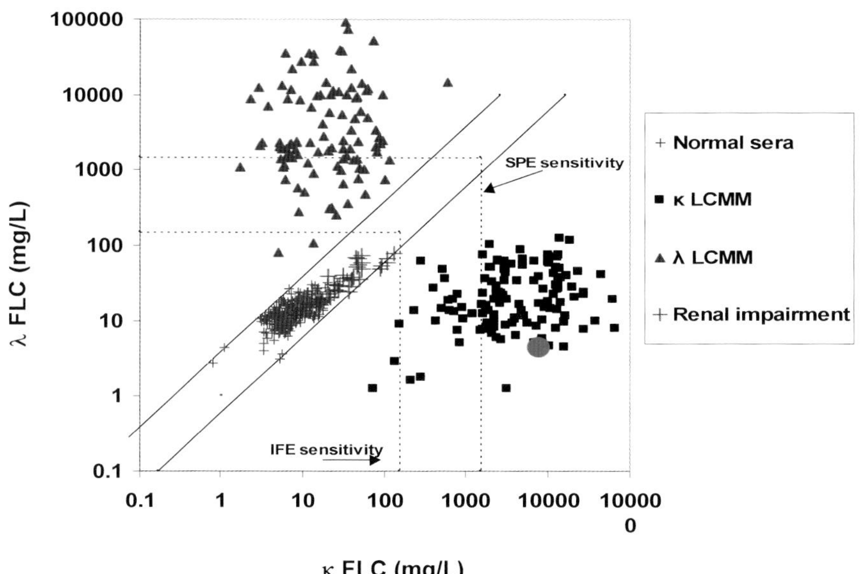

Figure 8.2. Serum FLC concentrations in normal individuals, patients with LCMM and patients with renal impairment *(Chapter 20)*. The diagonal lines separate monoclonal from polyclonal diseases. ●Clinical case No 1.

both serum and urine monoclonal FLCs, so it might be expected that the two would be highly correlated. In fact, there was only a modest association (*Figure 8.3*). This may seem rather surprising, at first glance, but can be explained by the effect of the renal tubular metabolism of FLCs. The amount of FLCs observed in urine is highly dependent upon renal function. If the kidneys are functioning normally, 20-30g can be removed from the glomerular filtrate per day *(Chapter 3)*. Serum and urine FLC concentrations are frequently discordant, with serum being more representative of tumour mass than urine concentrations. The amounts of sFLCs required to produce abnormal urine tests is discussed in Chapter 24.

8.2. Monitoring light chain multiple myeloma

Assays that are useful in disease diagnosis are likely to be useful for disease monitoring and this is particularly true for FLC assays. Not only are immunoassays inherently quantitative but also their precision is considerably better than results from scanning monoclonal bands on electrophoretic gels. Furthermore, serum FLC concentrations better indicate tumour synthesis compared with urine measurements that are largely determined by renal function.

It was shown in Figure 8.3 that there was a poor correlation between serum and urine FLC concentrations at the time of disease diagnosis. In contrast, changes in serum and urine FLC concentrations observed during the course of the disease show a good correlation. This is illustrated in Figure 8.4 in 2 patients from the Mayo Clinic.[5] In both patients the concentrations of FLCs in serum and urine fell following chemotherapy (although in the first patient this was not in parallel, possibly due to inadequate 24-hour urine collections). In the expanded study, a good correlation was found between changes in serum and urine FLC concentrations *(Figure 8.5)*.[5] The authors concluded that sFLC

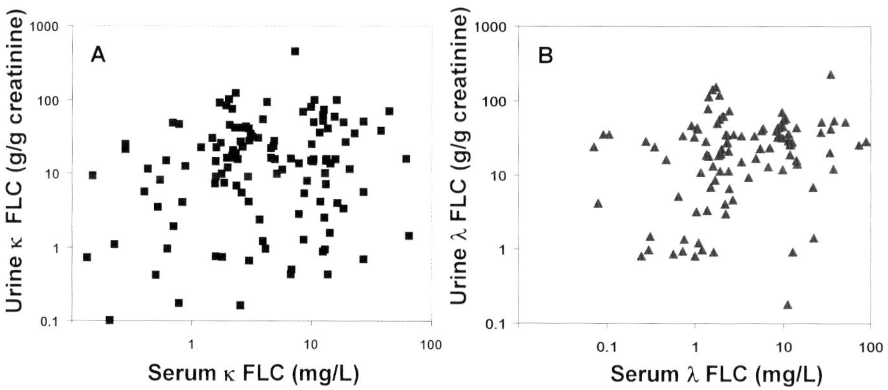

Figure 8.3. Relationship between serum and urine FLCs in 224 patients with LCMM at the time of diagnosis. (A) κ: r=0.29; p=0.0012. (B) λ: r=0.13; p=0.183. Urine FLCs were measured by immunoassay and corrected for urine dilution using creatinine concentrations.

measurements provided a satisfactory alternative to 24-hour urine collections for monitoring patients with LCMM.

In *The Lancet* study,[3] changes in sFLC concentrations were assessed as indicators of responses to treatment. The results showed that 99% of patients (81/82) had reductions in sFLCs compared with 95% (78/82) for the corresponding uFLCs. This indicated a marginally better sensitivity for serum tests when initial responses to chemotherapy were

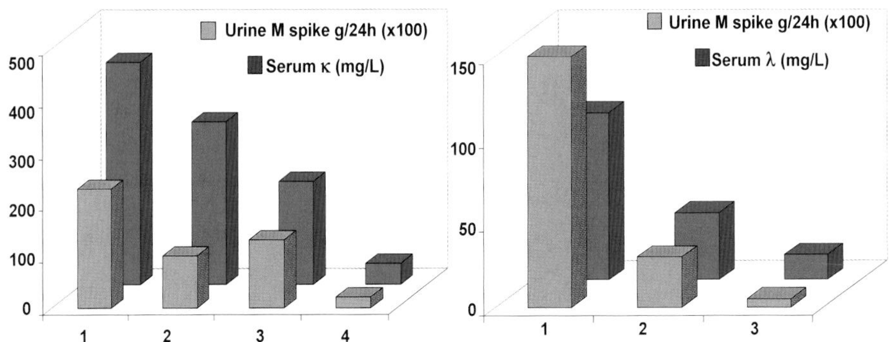

Figure 8.4. Comparison of 24-hour urinary monoclonal protein concentrations and serum FLCs in 2 patients with LCMM, measured at different times after chemotherapy. (Courtesy of RA Kyle and JA Katzmann).[5]

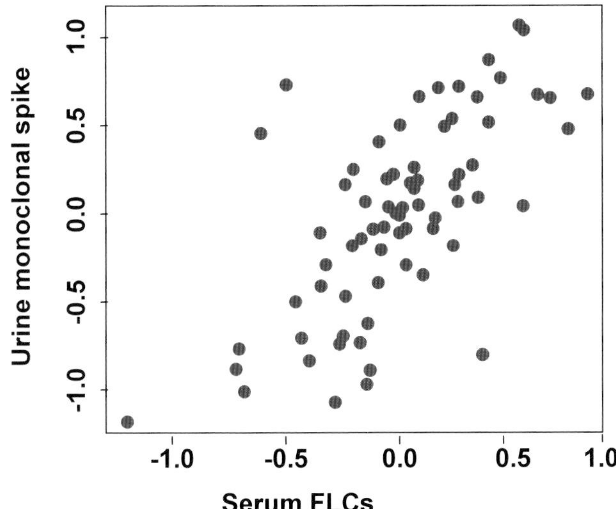

Figure 8.5. Correlation between changes in serum and urine FLCs during the evolution of their disease in 71 patients with LCMM. Initial measurement values were changed to zero and further adjusted logarithmically for comparison purposes (P=0.0001). (Courtesy of RA Kyle and JA Katzmann).[5]

evaluated. However, there were considerable differences when assessing rates of remission. 32% (26/82) of the patients were considered to be in complete remission as assessed by normal uFLC concentrations but this compared with only 11% (9/82) from sFLC levels. In the same clinical trials, 10% of patients with IIMM (117/1189) had complete serological remission. Since the serum responses to chemotherapy were similar in the two groups, the results indicated that uFLC measurements were relatively insensitive for assessing residual disease. This has been substantiated in other studies *(Chapter 12)*.

The discrepancy between serum and urine results is mainly due to metabolism of FLCs in the kidneys (*Chapter 3*). Other factors are the greater sensitivity of the immunoassays and errors in collecting and measuring urine samples *(Chapter 24)*. While changes in serum and urine FLC concentrations generally occur in parallel, sFLCs remain abnormal in many patients when urine is normal. Clinical responses and assessment of residual disease are better judged from sFLC measurements.

Comparisons of serum and urine assays for monitoring LCMM are illustrated for two patients in Figures 8.6 and 8.7 In both patients the uFLC measurements became normal while serum tests remained abnormal.

The results indicate that sFLC measurements have an important role in identifying and managing these patients. FLC tests are being included in the international diagnosis and response guidelines for MM (*Chapter 25*).

A detailed comparison of the use of serum and urine FLC tests is given in Chapter 24.

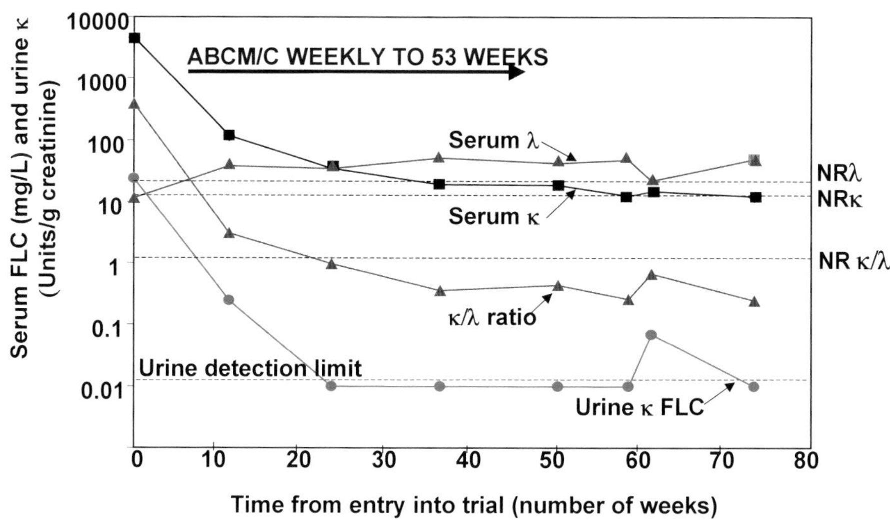

Figure 8.6. Serum and urine FLC levels in a patient with κ LCMM during treatment.

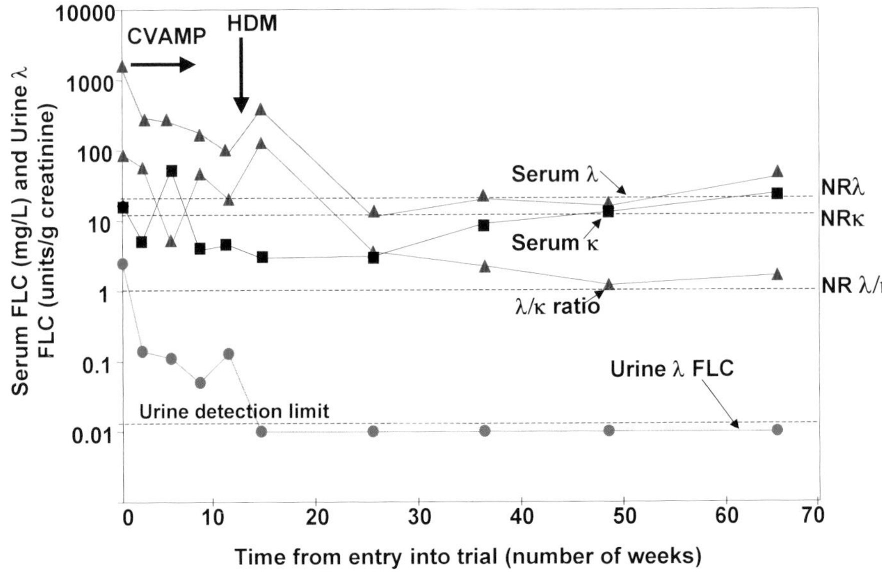

Figure 8.7 Serum and urine FLC levels in a patient with λ LCMM during treatment.

Clinical case history No 1. Unusual clinical features in a patient with light chain multiple myeloma.

A 63-year-old woman attended hospital with severe pain in her right shoulder. An X-ray showed minor erosive changes in the shoulder joint while blood tests were normal apart from a marginally elevated serum calcium at 2.69 mmol/L (NR: 2.08-2.67). An orthopaedic surgeon recommended a hemiarthroplasty. At operation, the head of the humerus was eroded and the glenoid was almost entirely replaced by 'extremely soft bone' suggestive of malignancy or a metabolic cause. The operation was aborted and the tissue was sent for histological examination.

Re-examination of the patient failed to identify any additional clinical features. Investigations showed a normal chest X-ray while the serum calcium had increased further to 3.41mmol/L and she was hypophosphataemic at 0.55mmol/L (NR: 0.67-1.54). Other results included a raised alkaline phosphatase at 234 IU/L (NR: 30-115) and an increased parathyroid hormone related peptide at 9.5 pmol/L (NR: 0.7-1.8) while parathyroid hormone levels were low at 9ng/L (NR: 10-60). A metastatic tumour deposit was considered the most likely cause of her shoulder disease. The search for a primary tumour, however, was unsuccessful: CT scans of the abdomen and thorax were normal, as were the serum cancer markers, CA-199, CA-125 and CEA.

The possibility of MM was considered. Bone histology from the surgically resected specimen showed only osteo-arthritis and osteopenia and there was no excess of plasma cells. A skeletal survey showed only osteoporotic bone with no discrete lytic lesions and no features of MM. Serum and urine electrophoretic tests showed no

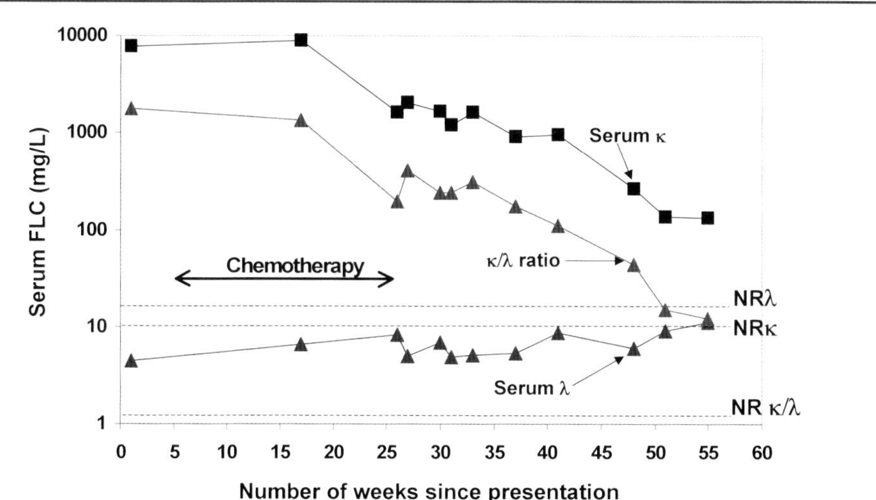

Figure 8.8. Case history No 1. Serum FLC concentrations in a patient with κ LCMM and unusual clinical features.

monoclonal gammopathy but assessment of immunoglobulins by nephelometry revealed hypogammaglobulinaemia: IgG 3.20g/L (NR: 5.3- 16.5), IgA 0.15g/L (NR: 0.8- 4.0) and IgM 0.26g/L (NR: 0.5- 2.0).

In view of the diagnostic difficulties, the recently available sFLC measurements were requested, with the following results:- κ 7,840mg/L (NR: 3.3 - 19.4); λ 4.4mg/L (NR: 5.7 - 26.3); κ/λ ratio 1,782 (NR: 0.26-1.65) (*Figure 8.8*). Urine FLC concentrations by immunoassay were as follows: κ 371mg/L; λ 4.7mg/L; κ/λ ratio 79.

Subsequent bone-marrow aspiration of the iliac crest indicated a high concentration of abnormal plasma cells. This established the diagnosis as κ-secreting LCMM with production of excess parathyroid hormone related peptide leading to hypercalcaemia.

Several months after her initial clinical presentation, the patient was finally treated with chemotherapy. This resulted in a satisfactory reduction of the serum κ FLC concentrations and normalisation of serum calcium. Since then her shoulder however, has remained unstable, although pain free.

Comment. The diagnosis of LCMM can be difficult. In this patient the clinical features were atypical and did not provide a clear lead to the diagnosis, so tests for MM were not considered for some time. When electrophoretic analysis of serum and urine were eventually performed the results showed no monoclonal proteins. Reassessment of the original urine sample, at a later date, showed a low concentration of monoclonal κ by IFE that had been overlooked on the earlier analysis. The final diagnosis was LCMM with limited plasma cell infiltration of the bone marrow.

The response of the tumour to chemotherapy was good. The serum κ FLC concentrations fell for 45 weeks with a half-life of approximately four weeks. The patient is likely to have a good clinical course in the medium term.

Clinical case history No 2. Free light chain breakthrough during relapse of multiple myeloma.[6]

A 56-year-old man was followed for refractory MM grade IIIB (Durie and Salmon classification). The IgGλ monoclonal protein was 69 g/L, at diagnosis, on the scanned SPE gel. Following a bone marrow allograft, SPE and IFE showed a reduction and stabilisation of the IgGλ band at 3.0 g/L.

Three months after the allograft the patient was clinically deteriorating with no change in the IgGλ monoclonal protein band *(Figure 8.9)*. SPE showed a peak in the gamma-region while IFE showed a monoclonal IgGλ but no monoclonal FLC band.

sFLC analysis showed: κ:1.3mg/L: λ:242mg/L: κ/λ ratio: 0.005, clear evidence of the tumour that was not apparent from the monoclonal IgGλ level. The diagnosis was relapse of the MM with FLC breakthrough. The patient died one month later.

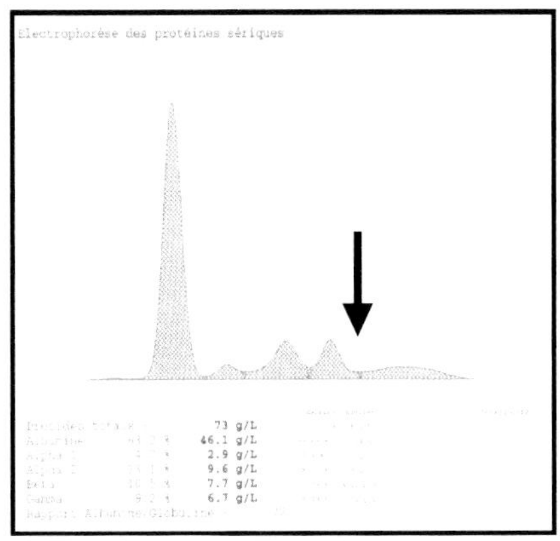

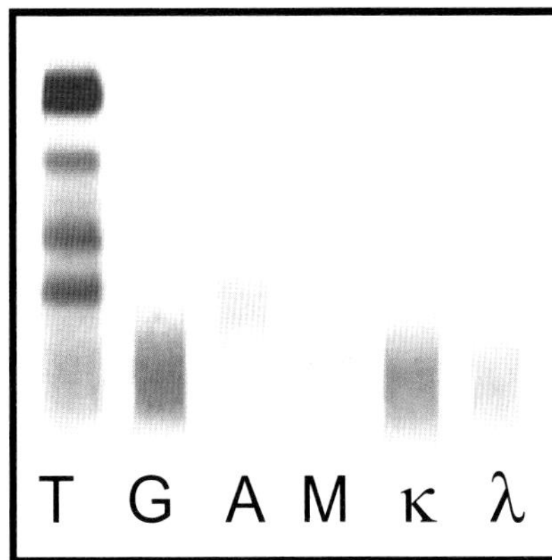

Figure 8.9. Case history No 2. SPE scan and sIFE of the patient during clinical relapse.

Summary: In patients with LCMM, sFLC concentrations are:-

1. Always elevated when urine FLCs are elevated.
2. More sensitive than IFE.
3. A better indicator of minimal residual disease than urine measurements.
4. Able to indicate disease changes more accurately than urine measurements.
5. More easily measured than in urine.
6. Able to provide numerical results compared with IFE.
7. Able to provide additional information about renal and bone marrow function from the alternate FLC concentrations and κ/λ ratios.
8. Useful in the differential diagnosis of patients with bone pain and fractures, unexplained renal disease and other features of MM when urine samples are not available.

References

1. **Brigden ML, Webber D.** Clinical Pathology Rounds: The case of the anaplastic carcinoma that was not - potential problems in the interpretation of monoclonal proteins. Lab Med 2000; **31** (12): 661-665.

2. **Van Zaanen HCT, Diderich PNM, Pegels JG, Ruizeveld De Winter JA.** Nierinsufficientie door neerslag van lichte ketens bij multipel myeloom. Ned Tijdschr Geneeskd 2000; **144**: 2133-2137.

3. **Bradwell AR, Mead GP, Carr-Smith HD, Drayson MT.** Serum test for assessment of patients with Bence Jones myeloma. Lancet 2003; **361**: 489-491

4. **Nowrousian MR, Brandhorst D, Daniels R, Sammet C, Schuett P, Ebeling P, Buttkereit U, Opalka B, Flasshove M, Moritz T, Seeber S.** Free light-chain measurement in serum compared with immunofixation of urine in patients with multiple myeloma. Blood 2003; **102** (11), A5197.

5. **Abraham RS, Clark RJ, Bryant SC, Lymp JF, Larson T, Kyle RA, Katzmann JA.** Correlation of serum immunoglobulin free light chain quantitation with urine Bence Jones protein in Light Chain Myeloma. Clin Chem 2002; **48**: 655-657.

6. **Guis L, Diemert MC, Ghillani P, Choquet S, Leblond V, Vernant JP, Musset L.** The quantitation of serum free light chains: Three case reports. Clin Chem 2004; **50**: Suppl, pA183; F-38.

Test questions

1. How many patients with LCMM will be missed if urine tests for Bence Jones protein are abandoned for serum tests FLC tests?

2. Is the correlation between serum and urine concentrations of monoclonal FLCs good, medium or poor?

3. What is the median concentration of serum monoclonal λ FLCs required to overflow into the urine and produce positive urine FLC tests?

Answers

1. None (page 64).

2. Poor (Figure 8.3).

3. Approximately 300mg/L (Chapter 24, Figure 24.2).

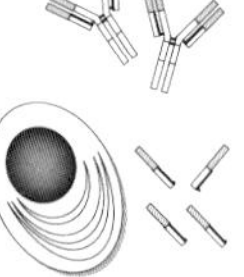

Chapter 9

Nonsecretory multiple myeloma

9.1. Introduction

Nonsecretory multiple myeloma (NSMM) accounts for 1-5% of all MM patients. The disease is characterised by the absence of monoclonal immunoglobulins in serum and urine using electrophoretic tests.[1-3] Nevertheless, monoclonal proteins can usually be demonstrated in the bone marrow plasma cells by immunohistochemical staining. Using high sensitivity tests such as isoelectric focusing, monoclonal proteins have been detected in the sera of some patients.[4] Other patients have tumour cells that produce but do not secrete monoclonal immunoglobulins into the blood. Finally, 10-15% of NSMM patients are true 'non-producers'.[5] In these patients the tumour plasma cells contain no detectable immunoglobulins. As tests for monoclonal proteins have become more sensitive, fewer patients are now classified as NSMM. Yet, even in expert hands, 2-3% of patients with MM have undetectable serum or urine monoclonal immunoglobulins by IFE.[2,6-8]

From a logical standpoint, such patients cannot be producing significant amounts of intact monoclonal immunoglobulins. IgG molecules accumulate in serum with a half-life of 3-4 weeks so production from even small clones of plasma cells is visible as monoclonal bands on SPE gels. In contrast, FLCs have a serum half-life of only 2-6 hours, 100-200 fold less. Clonal production of monoclonal FLCs, therefore, needs to be correspondingly that much greater to produce serum levels similar to those found in IgG producing MM. Hence, more sensitive techniques are required to detect FLC producing clones when they are small or when production is inefficient.

Investigations on urine samples may also be unhelpful because patients with NSMM usually have normal renal function. The modest increases in monoclonal FLC production, typically seen, may not be sufficient to overwhelm the reabsorption capacity of the kidneys and enter the urine *(Chapter 3)*.

9.2. Diagnosis of nonsecretory multiple myeloma

The above arguments suggest that sensitive assays for sFLCs might detect monoclonal proteins in a proportion of patients with NSMM. The results from a large study are shown in Table 9.1.[1]

Archived sera were obtained from patients studied in the UKMRC multiple myeloma trials between 1983 and 1999. Out of 2,323 patients, 64 (2.8%) were diagnosed with NSMM and of these, 28 were selected for study because they had complete clinical records and the appropriate stored serum samples. In all the patients, serum concentrations of κ and λ were compared with results from SPE and IFE tests. The results showed that 19 of the 28 sera had elevated κ or λ FLC concentrations and abnormal κ/λ ratios. A further four samples showed abnormally low levels of one or both FLC. FLC concentrations in the remaining 5 samples were substantially normal (*Figure 9.1, Table 9.1*).

Careful repeat testing of the sera by IFE, using optimal sensitivity (*Table 9.1*), showed

Classification based on serum free light chains		Free κ (mg/L)	Free λ (mg/L)	κ/λ ratio	Bone marrow plasma cells %	Other Results
Normal sera		**3.6-16**	**8-33**	**0.36-1**		
12 elevated free κ and increased κ/λratio	1	1754	1.6	1096	85	IFE κ +/-
	2	1201	3.6	333	82	BJP κ +/-
	3	935	11	85	70	
	4	487	6.6	74	20	
	5	931	13.2	71	>90	IFE κ +/-
	6	730	11.1	65	35	
	7	978	19.4	50	65	
	8	920	26.3	35	14*	
	9	789	25.6	31	>50	BJP κ +/-
	10	480	23.8	20	30	
	11	151	11.5	13	66	Hist κ+ve
	12	79.8	30.8	2.6	50	
7 elevated free λ with reduced κ/λ ratio	13	11.2	196	0.057	20	IFE λ+
	14	2.7	50.9	0.053	74	
	15	2.6	61	0.043	6*	
	16	17.8	624	0.029	8	IFEλ+BJP+/-
	17	3.8	144	0.026	70	
	18	7.7	389	0.019	60	
	19	2.8	481	0.005	29	IFE λ+
4 suppression of either κ, λ or both free light chains	20	4.5	6	0.75	21	
	21	1.2	1.6	0.75	55	
	22	2.4	8.1	0.296	34	
	23	3.6	13.1	0.274	70	
5 κ or λ normal or borderline and normal κ/λ ratios	24	16.2	23.4	0.692	67	
	25	20.7	33	0.627	73	
	26	77	142	0.543	18	IFE λ+
	27	8.3	17.4	0.477	9*	
	28	8.6	25.2	0.341	80	

Table 9.1. Serum FLC concentrations in 28 patients with NSMM.[1] IFE +/- = weak diffuse bands; IFE + = weak narrow band; BJP +/- = low concentrations of urine FLCs; Hist = immunohistochemical confirmation of MM; * = trephine biopsy +ve for MM.

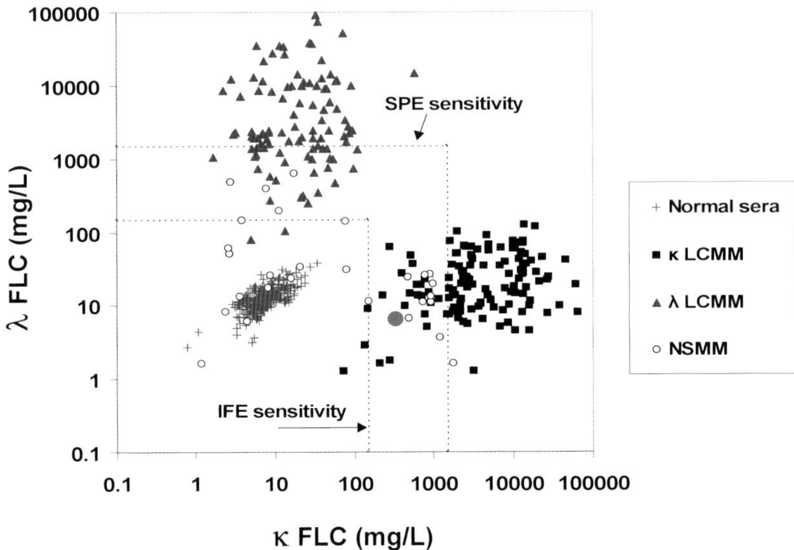

Figure 9.1. Serum FLC concentrations in patients with NSMM compared with normal individuals and patients with LCMM. ●Clinical case No 3.

monoclonal FLCs in 6 of the 28 sera but the monoclonal bands were mostly weak and diffuse. Rather surprisingly, in 9 of the 28 patients no monoclonal bands were seen using IFE even though the immunoassays indicated FLC concentrations of >200mg/L, and some were considerably higher. In many of these samples, the elevated FLC concentrations should have been easily detectable by IFE.

IFE gels applied with sera from 5 of the samples containing high concentrations of κ FLCs are shown in Figure 9.2. These are compared with 3 κ samples from patients with typical LCMM. The FLCs in the NSMM samples failed to focus into the same narrow monoclonal bands seen in the LCMM sera.

Two sera from patients with substantial concentrations of FLCs (980mg/L and 1,700mg/L), were subjected to size-separation gel chromatography and found to contain highly polymerised FLCs (40-200kDa) (*Figure 9.3*). The results suggested that variable polymerisation caused smearing of the monoclonal bands on the SPE gels (*see polymerisation in Chapter 4*) and this could account for their absence or diffuse appearance. Such large polymers would have minimal renal clearance compared with monomeric FLCs. Good renal function would be maintained (typical of these patients) and little FLC would enter the urine. These observations concur with other reports that describe polymerised or structurally abnormal FLCs in some patients with MM.[8,10]

Of additional interest, it was found that diffuse bands were more common in κ producing patients (*Table 9.1*). Hence, λ patients with low FLC production are more likely to produce discrete monoclonal bands and be classified as 'secretory' LCMM. At one time, this dearth of λ patients led to the suggestion that such patients may not exist.

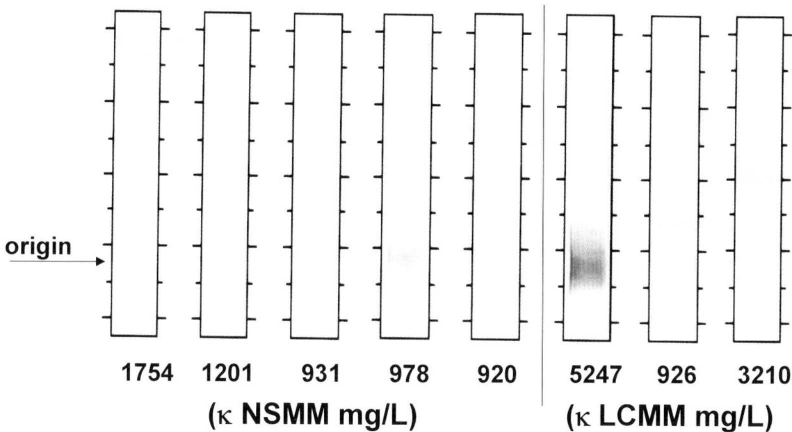

Figure 9.2. Serum IFE from 5 patients with κ NSMM and 3 patients with κ LCMM. Samples were applied at similar FLC concentrations.

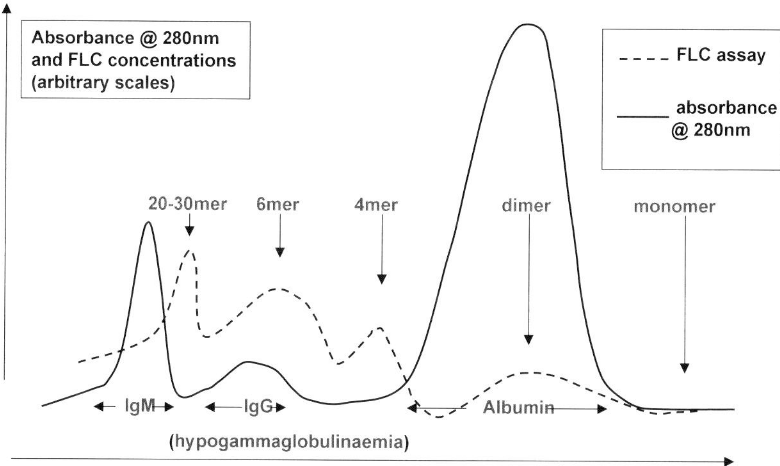

Figure 9.3. Size-separation gel chromatography showing the FLC size variation in a serum sample from a patient with NSMM. The sample contained 1,754 mg/L of κ FLCs by immunoassay but was negative by SPE and IFE.

Moreover, the observed higher frequency of κ polymerisation may explain the 4:1 ratio of κ to λ NSMM patients reported in the literature.[2]

There have been no other large studies on sFLC measurements in NSMM but there have been reports confirming the above observations in smaller groups of patients. Katzmann et al.,[7] recently reported sFLCs in 5 patients with NSMM at diagnosis and all were abnormal. Six others had received high dose therapy and were in clinical remission, a finding supported by the FLC results. Similarly, Cavallo et al. reported 4 of 5 NSMM patients with abnormal FLC concentrations.[8]

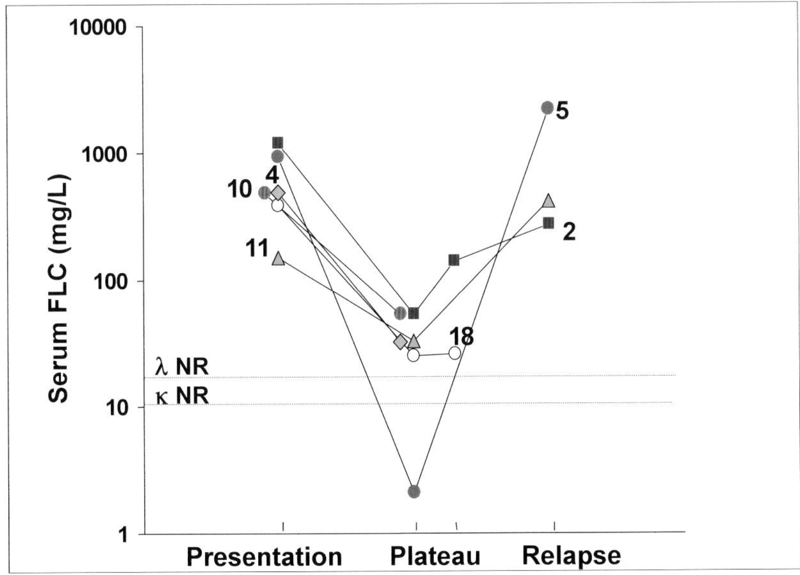

Figure 9.4. Changes in serum FLCs and clinical status in 6 patients with NSMM. (Numbers refer to patients in Table 9.1)[1].

9.3. Monitoring nonsecretory multiple myeloma

Serum FLC concentrations are also important for monitoring disease progress. In an initial study, samples from 6 patients showed elevated sFLC levels at clinical presentation, reduced levels during plateau phase, and increased levels at relapse (*Figure 9.4*). One of the patients showed a discordance between clinical features and sFLC concentrations (No.2). While the patient was in remission from a clinical viewpoint, rising concentrations of FLCs indicated imminent disease relapse.

Many patients with NSMM have been studied prospectively since the assays first became available. Two examples are described below.

Clinical case history No 3. Nonsecretory multiple myeloma with "difficult to assess" symptoms during clinical relapse.

A 38-year-old woman, presented with a fractured rib following mild trauma. Over the following months, the pain subsided but non-specific symptoms including breathlessness, vague chest pains and tiredness persisted. During this time, full blood counts, erythrocyte sedimentation rate (ESR) and biochemistry were all normal as were chest X-rays and lung function tests. In the absence of a diagnosis, the general practitioner considered a psychiatric assessment.

Seven months after the initial presentation, she remained symptomatic and was re-investigated, whereupon bone scans and X-rays showed extensive osseous lesions. Immunoglobulin measurements showed immune paresis, but no serum monoclonal protein was detected. She was noted to have hypercalcaemia (2.85 mmol/L - NR: 2.08-2.67) but had normal renal function. In view of the absence of monoclonal immunoglobulins, MM was still considered unlikely. However, a skull X-ray and CT scan showed osteolytic lesions (*Figure 9.5*) so a skull biopsy was performed which was reported as 'plasmacytoma/NSMM'. She was given chemotherapy comprising ABCM for the following 8 months that resulted in symptomatic relief.

Seven months later and over 2 years after the initial presentation, she re-attended hospital because of chest pains and breathlessness. Again, clinical examination was normal, as were routine biochemistry and haematology tests. Immunology tests showed reduced immunoglobulins but no monoclonal spike. A bone marrow biopsy showed 5% plasma cells that were morphologically normal. Chest X-ray, a ventilation perfusion scan and lung function tests revealed no evidence of pulmonary disease. Blood tests were requested for FLCs, the results of which were: κ 330mg/L, λ 6.5mg/L and κ/λ ratio 51, suggesting recurrence of NSMM *(Figure 9.1 and Figure 9.6 at week 67)*. Doubt was expressed regarding the validity of the results so FLC measurements were repeated 2 and 3 weeks later and showed κ increases to 470mg/L and then 525mg/L with a rising κ/λ ratio, confirming recurrence of the disease.

FLC concentrations were assessed retrospectively from archived samples and then the patient was monitored prospectively. Figure 9.6 shows that κ FLC concentrationhad increased rapidly during the tumour recurrence, with an apparent doubling time of 30 days as indicated by the κ/λ ratio. Serum κ concentration subsequently reduced during VAD chemotherapy prior to high dose melphalan and PBSCT rescue. During the period of relapse the alternate FLC increased in concentration suggesting deteriorating renal clearance of FLCs from impaired glomerular filtration. Serum κ and λ concentrations and the κ/λ ratio returned towards normal, post-transplant, as the patient went into clinical remission. For 2 years following the transplant the patient remained completely well.

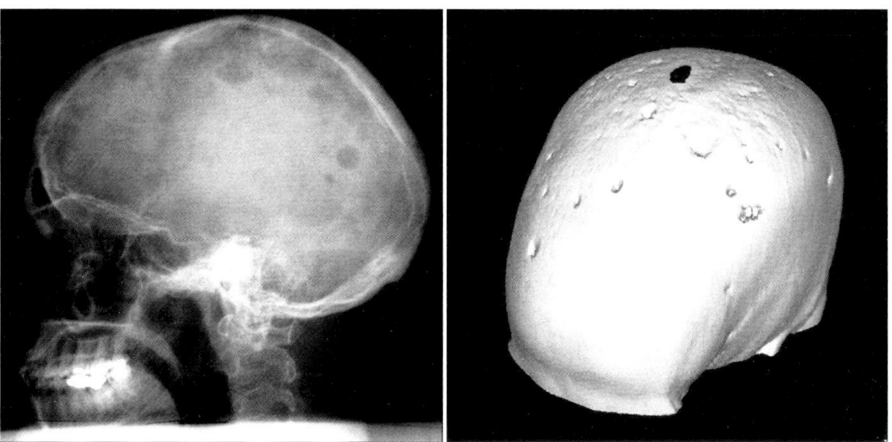

Figure 9.5. X-ray and CT scans of the skull in nonsecretory multiple myeloma.

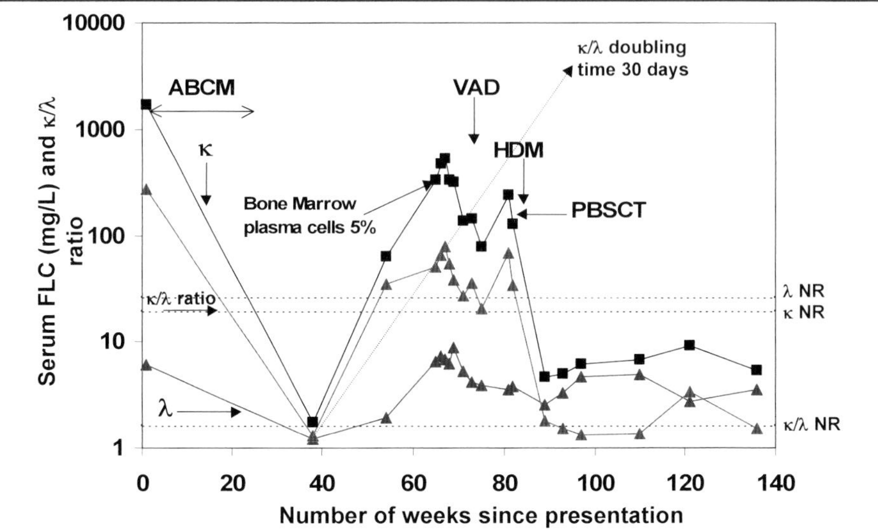

Figure 9.6. Serum FLC concentrations in Patient No 3 during the course of the disease. The changing κ/λ ratio is related to the tumour growth.

Discussion: NSMM is rare, so it is not normally considered when a patient first presents with symptoms but rather when other diseases have been excluded.[6,9] Even then, normal serum and urine tests for monoclonal proteins tend to deceive the diagnostician. When MM is finally thought of, the patient is subjected to a painful bone marrow biopsy, which is not undertaken lightly. Clearly, since sFLC measurements are important they should be requested when the diagnosis of MM is first considered.

While monitoring these patients, repeated serum tests should generally replace other forms of investigation. At present, skeletal surveys using X-rays, MRI or positron emission tomography may be used, together with repeated bone marrow biopsies. None of these tests is likely to provide results that are as representative of the changing total tumour burden as sFLC tests. sFLC concentrations assess FLC production from all of the bone marrow and extramedullary sites. They are likely to be a better reflection of overall tumour activity than bone marrow aspirations or skeletal surveys.

Of additional interest in these patients is the κ/λ ratio. This is a more accurate measure of changing monoclonal FLC production than individual FLC concentrations since the alternate FLC compensates for alterations in glomerular filtration rate. This was apparent during the relapse phase in this patient. After week 40, the alternate FLC gradually increased which suggested impaired renal function from renal deposition of tumour-produced FLCs.

It is also of note that normalisation of the κ/λ ratio had not occurred even 2 years after treatment. This suggests either that the clone of tumour cells persists or that bone marrow function has not completely returned to normal. It is likely that this patient has residual disease *(Chapter 12)*.

Clinical case history No 4. A patient with NSMM/plasmacytoma excluded from clinical trials.

A 37-year-old man with pelvic pain was found to have a solitary plasmacytoma located in the right iliac crest. Bone marrow biopsy of the opposite iliac crest was normal and no monoclonal protein was identified in serum or urine. Treatment comprised surgical resection followed by irradiation (5,000Gy). Subsequently, he remained asymptomatic, but 5 years later a routine skeletal survey showed a thoracic spine lesion at T-2 that was irradiated. Over the following 7 years further painful lesions developed. These were identified using different scanning techniques (particularly PET) and were treated with irradiation or melphalan and prednisolone.

Throughout this period, and in spite of repeated testing, no monoclonal protein was identified by SPE and UPE. Finally, 12 years after the initial presentation FLC immunoassays became available and showed; κ 7.5mg/L, λ 632mg/L and a κ/λ ratio 0.01. These results identified a λ producing tumour with no associated suppression of the κ FLC *(Figure 9.7)*. One month later, λ concentrations had increased to 700mg/L, prompting treatment with thalidomide (50mg/day) and dexamethasone (40mg weekly). Over the subsequent 7 months, serum λ gradually fell to 33mg/L and the κ/λ ratio began to normalise. Based on the FLC results, dexamethasone was reduced to 12 mg per week and he remained well and in complete remission.

Figure 9.7 shows the changes in sFLC concentrations over a 12 month period. The effectiveness of the drugs and the doses required can all be monitored during this period of therapy. This has produced clear benefits for the patient and avoided costly scans and painful bone marrow biopsies. Furthermore, the patient can be entered into clinical trials of new treatments when absence of a disease marker had previously led to his exclusion. The patient has been monitored successfully using sFLC assays for several years since the original tests were performed.

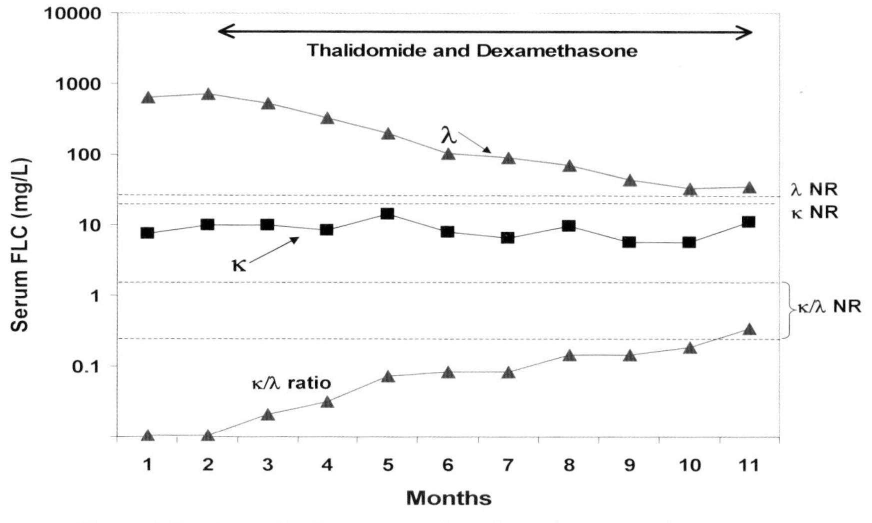

Figure 9.7. Serum FLC concentrations in Patient No 4 during treatment.

Summary: In patients with NSMM, serum FLC measurements:-

1. Are important for diagnosis.
2. Identify relapses and responses to treatment earlier.
3. Allow monitoring without the need for repeated bone marrow biopsies or radiological scans.
4. Allow patients to be included in clinical trials from which they were previously excluded.

References

1. **Drayson MT, Tang LX, Drew R, Mead GP, Carr-Smith HD, Bradwell AR.** Serum free light-chain measurements for identifying and monitoring patients with nonsecretory multiple myeloma. Blood 2001; **97**: 2900-2902.

2. **Blade J, Kyle RA.** Nonsecretory Myeloma, Immunoglobulin D Myeloma and Plasma Cell Leukemia. Hem/Onc Clin N Amer 1999; **13**: 1259-1272.

3. **Dreicer R, Alexanian R.** Nonsecretory Multiple Myeloma. Am J Hematol 1982; **13**: 313-318.

4. **Sheeham T, Sinclair D, Tansey P, O'Donnell JR.** Demonstration of serum monoclonal immunoglobulin in a case of non-secretory myeloma by immunoisoelectric focusing. J Clin Pathol 1985; **38**: 806-809.

5. **Raubenheimer EJ, Dauth J, Senekal JC.** Non-secretory IgA k Myeloma with distended endoplasmic reticulum: a case report. Histology 1991; **19**: 380-382.

6. **Reilly BM, Clarke P, Nikolinakos P.** Easy to See but Hard to Find. N Engl J Med 2003; **348**: 59-64.

7. **Katzmann J, Abraham RS, Dispenzieri A, Lust JA, Kyle RA.** Diagnostic Performance of Quantitative Kappa and Lambda Free Light Chain Assays in Clinical Practice. Clin Chem 2005; **51** (5): 878-881.

8. **Cavallo F, Rasmussen E, Zangari M, Tricot G, Fender B, Fox M, Burns M, Bart Barlogie B.** Serum Free-Lite Chain (sFLC) Assay in Multiple Myeloma (MM): Clinical Correlates and Prognostic Implications in Newly Diagnosed MM Patients Treated with Total Therapy 2 or 3 (TT2/3). Blood 2005; **106**: 11: 3490. P974a.

9. **Abdalla IA, Tabbara A.** Nonsecretory Multiple Myeloma. South Med J 2002; **95**: 761-764.

10. **Coriu D, Weaver K, Schell M, Eulitz M, Murphy CL, Weiss DT, Solomon A.** A molecular basis for nonsecretory myeloma. Blood 2003; **104** (3): 829-831.

Test Questions

1. *Which is more sensitive, serum or urine IFE, for detecting NSMM?*
2. *Why do most so called 'NSMM' patients have excess monoclonal FLCs rather than excess monoclonal intact immunoglobulins?*
3. *Are sFLC tests more accurate than bone marrow assessments of tumour responses?*

Answers

1. *By definition, neither test is positive in NSMM (page 72).*
2. *Because intact immunoglobulins accumulate in serum 100-200 times more than FLCs, for the same tumour production. They can then can be readily detected by insensitive techniques such as SPE (page 72).*
3. *sFLC tests are sometimes the most accurate method of assessing tumour responses to therapy. sFLC concentrations are a consequence of production from all the tumour deposits, rather than from a small part of the tumour that is sampled in a bone biopsy (page 76).*

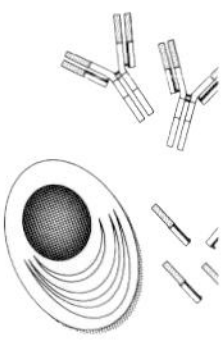

Chapter 10

Intact immunoglobulin multiple myeloma (IIMM)

10.1. Introduction

Approximately 80% of patients with MM produce intact immunoglobulin monoclonal proteins (*Figure 7.2*) of which 46% have excess monoclonal FLCs in the urine by IFE.[1] SPE tests for FLCs are less frequently positive because of their low serum concentrations (although sFLCs may be highly elevated in patients with renal failure).

The first attempt to use sFLC tests in IIMM was by Sölling in 1976. Using column chromatography, FLCs were separated from bound light chains prior to their measurement by antibodies against whole light chains. He showed that monoclonal sFLCs were present in 86% of IIMM patients.[2] It might be expected that highly sensitive serum FLC assays would be abnormal in even more patients.

10.2 Serum free light chains and intact monoclonal immunoglobulins

Mead et al. assessed sFLC concentrations, at the time of presentation, in 314 patients with IgG, 142 with IgA and 36 with IgD MM using archived samples from the UK MRC multiple myeloma trials.[3] Overall, 88% had elevated FLCs with the following breakdown: IgG 84%, IgA 92% and IgD 94%, and in all of 5 IgE patients. Some of the remaining patients had normal or reduced concentrations of FLCs but the κ/λ ratios were abnormal, indicating monoclonality in association with bone marrow suppression. In total, 96% of all MM patients had abnormal FLC concentrations or abnormal κ/λ ratios (*Figures 10.1 to 10.4*). This percentage is higher than previously reported,[1] reflecting the increased sensitivity of the FLC immunoassays and, in particular, the use of the suppressed alternate FLC to identify abnormal κ/λ ratios. It is also of note that there was complete concordance between the monoclonal FLC type identified by κ/λ ratios and IFE *(Figure 10.1)*. This provides an important specificity validation of the FLC immunoassays.

Serum FLC concentrations were higher in IgA than IgG patients but highest in IgD patients (similar to LCMM patients *see Figure 10.2*). The high levels of uFLC excretion and excess of λ compared with κ is typical of IgD patients.[4,5] 5 patients with IgE myeloma are shown in Figure 10.2. Although the number of patients was small, the FLC

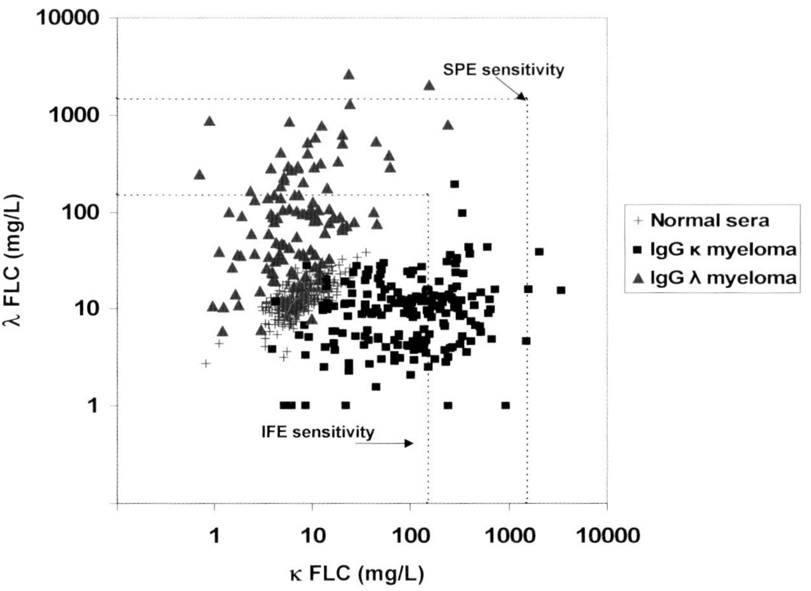

Figure 10.1. Concentrations of FLCs in 314 patients with IgG MM compared with 282 normal sera.

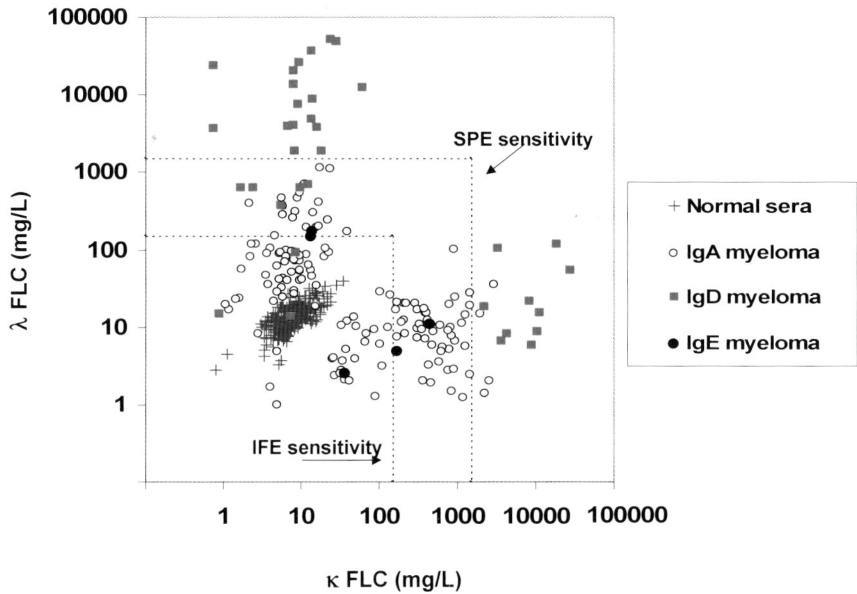

Figure 10.2. Concentrations of sFLCs in 142 IgA, 36 IgD and 5 IgE MM patients compared with 282 normal sera.

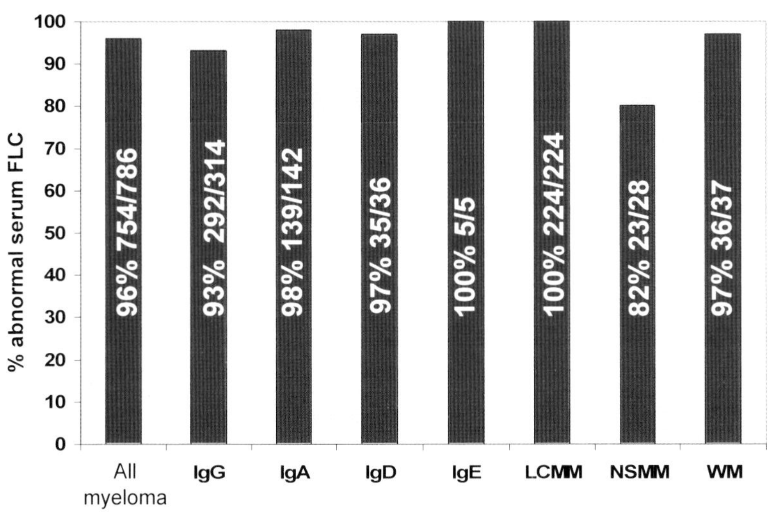

Figure 10.3. Frequency of abnormal sFLC concentrations in patients with different types of MM and Waldenström's macroglobulinaemia (WM).

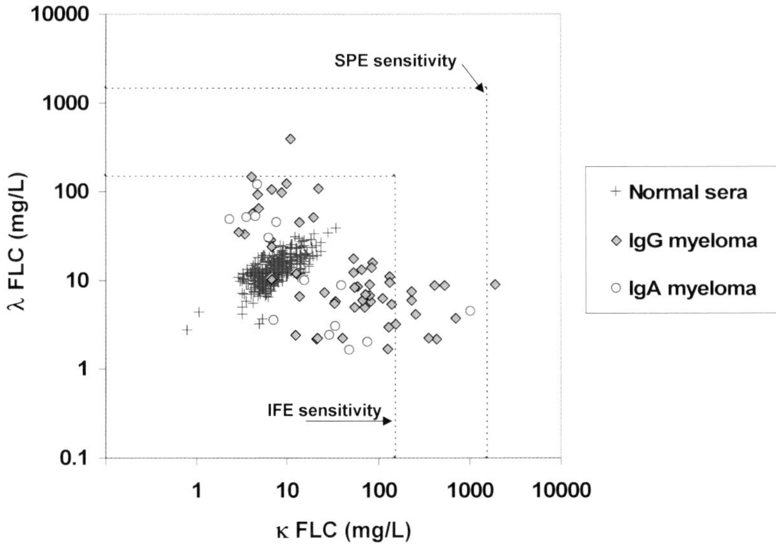

Figure 10.4. sFLCs in 55 IgG and 14 IgA MM patients who had no urine FLC excretion compared with 282 normal sera.

results are presumably representative of the disease.

A subgroup of 69 patients with IIMM (55 IgG and 14 IgA), who had no uFLC excretion (less than 40mg/L), is shown in Figure 10.4. Serum analysis showed that 95% of the patients had abnormal FLC concentrations. It is of note that none of the patients had increased concentrations of the alternate FLC, indicating there was no significant renal impairment. This is in contrast to patients with LCMM.

At clinical presentation there was no correlation between serum creatinine and sFLC levels (as for LCMM - *Figure 8.3)*. There was also no correlation ($R<0.02$) between the FLC levels and intact IgG or IgA monoclonal immunoglobulin concentrations at the time of clinical presentation *(Figure 10.5)*. This is an important issue because it means that ***serum FLC concentrations are an independent marker of the disease process*** in IIMM and provide additional information when monitoring patients.

In this study there was no correlation between FLC concentrations at presentation and survival. However, other studies have shown that the presence of abnormal sFLC κ/λ ratios relates to disease staging *(Chapter 25)*.[6-8] Cavallo et al., showed that sFLC concentrations and abnormal κ/λ ratios were both highly correlated with cytogentic abnormalities and MM staging.[8] Since these are 2 important prognostic factors for both event-free survival and overall survival, sFLCs should have independent predictive power with long-term follow-up.

As sFLC concentrations were normal in some of the patients with IIMM, it is clear that SPE tests are essential for diagnosis. In contrast, sFLC assays are more sensitive for the identification of LCMM and NSMM. Therefore, when MM is suspected the optimum laboratory practice should be to test sera by both SPE and sFLC assays.

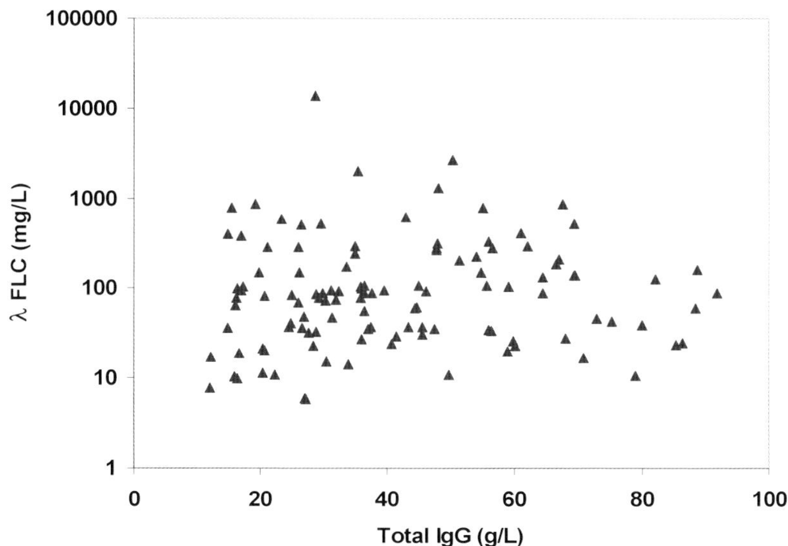

Figure 10.5. Shows the poor correlation between sFLCs and intact monoclonal immunoglobulins in 116 patients with IgGλ MM at the time of diagnosis.

10.3. Monitoring IIMM using serum free light chain concentrations

Normally, patients with IIMM are monitored using serum tests and urine FLCs (when present). Measurement techniques for intact immunoglobulins comprise nephelometry or scanning of monoclonal bands on SPE gels. Nephelometry has the advantages of simplicity and good precision but it has poor accuracy at low concentrations when the normal immunoglobulins are included in the measurements. SPE scanning provides better accuracy if the monoclonal bands are well defined but it is difficult to measure low concentration monoclonal bands that overlie other proteins (typically monoclonal IgA).

Another monitoring problem using intact immunoglobulins is their relatively long half-life. This is 20-25 days for IgG (IgG3 - 8 days), 6 days for IgA, 3 days for IgD and 2 days for IgE. This is in contrast to 2-6 hours for sFLCs. Thus, patients monitored using IgG will show apparently slower responses to therapy than the sFLC levels suggest. The benefits of this short half-life can be harnessed in patients with IIMM.[8-17]

Figure 10.6 shows a patient with MM producing monoclonal IgGκ and monoclonal κ serum FLCs (but no urine FLCs). During the initial therapy, κ concentrations rapidly fell while IgGκ, quantified from SPE gels, gradually returned to normal. The apparent half-life of IgGκ was between 100 and 200 days. (This depended, in part, upon which densitometric scanning device was used: white-light scanners may under-read at high protein concentrations.) The observed response comprised the tumour kill half-life plus the half-life of serum IgG. A similar pattern of sFLC and IgG responses was seen during a subsequent relapse and treatment period.

A slow reduction of monoclonal IgG concentrations is usually observed during

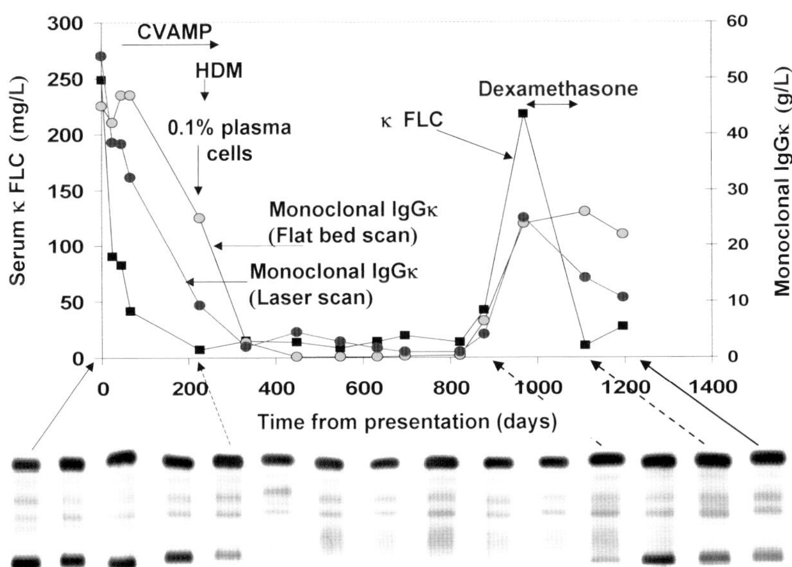

Figure 10.6. Monitoring of a MM patient using IgGκ and κ sFLCs. SPE gels are shown for each sample.

treatment. A further example is given in Figure 10.7 in which the IgGκ half-life was 50 days. In this patient the sFLCs were clearly within the normal range at the first measurement point following treatment, and presumably earlier. Yet chemotherapy was continued for many weeks longer. In such patients it may be preferable to stop chemotherapy when FLC levels have normalised in order to minimise drug side effects.

The fast response of sFLCs to chemotherapy was recently studied by Hassoun et al.[15,16] They found that normalisation of the FLC κ/λ ratio after the first or second cycle was highly predictive of outcome. ***"Since the aim of therapy is to achieve a complete response, assessement of sFLCs after 1 or 2 cycles may be an important milestone in the decision-making for these patients".*** Similar observations were made by Cavallo et al.,[8] and Moesbauer et al.[17] FLC kinetics are further discussed in Chapter 13.

Under other circumstances, sFLC measurements may indicate that a longer duration of chemotherapy is appropriate. Thus, sFLC concentrations may indicate residual disease when intact monoclonal immunoglobulin concentrations have normalised *(Chapter 12).* Also, sFLCs are more sensitive than uFLCs for residual disease. This is typically seen in LCMM. Urine FLCs may normalise while serum concentrations remain abnormal *(Chapter 8).*

10.4. Bone marrow biopsies and serum free light chain concentrations

The value of sFLCs rather than IgG levels for assessing responses in IIMM is

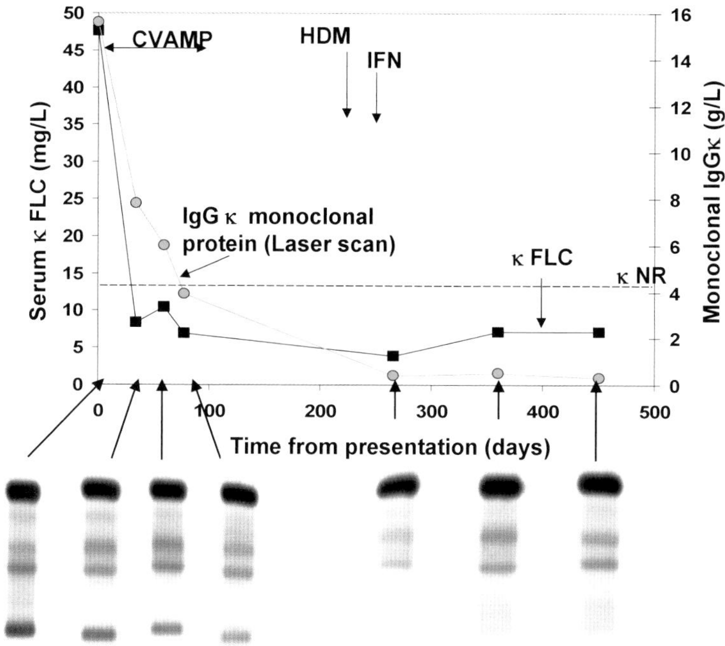

Figure 10.7. Monitoring of MM using IgGκ and κ sFLCs. SPE gels are shown for each sample. IFN = interferon. κNR: upper limit of κ FLC normal range.

apparent from bone marrow samples. During treatment, monoclonal plasma cell counts correlate better with changes in sFLCs (and serum β_2 microglobulin) than intact monoclonal IgG *(Figure 10.8)*.[3] In a study of 51 patients by Mead et al.,[10] *(Table 10.1)*, sFLC concentrations were better than both uFLCs and serum IgG for assessing disease status. Thus, serum IFE showed elevated intact immunoglobulin levels in many patients who had normal bone marrow biopsies, reflecting their slow clearance. 4 patients had abnormal bone marrow biopsies but normal sFLC levels (non-FLC producers). Interestingly, 5 patients had abnormal sFLCs but normal marrows suggesting that the biopsy had been taken from the wrong part of the bone marrow. In a disease with patchy distribution, a serum test that measures protein production from all tumour cells is likely to be highly sensitive for residual disease in some patients.

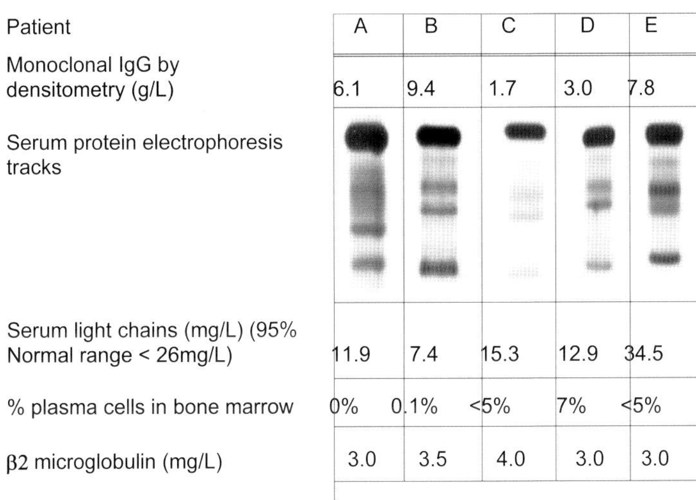

Figure 10.8. Accuracy of different blood tests for assessing bone marrow plasma cell volume in MM. Because of slow catabolism, IgG concentrations lag behind reductions in bone marrow plasma cell content during treatment.

		Bone marrow	
		Normal	**Abnormal**
Serum free light chains	Normal	19	4
	Abnormal	5	47
Urine free light chains	Normal	21	21
	Abnormal	3	30
Serum IFE	Normal	10	5
	Abnormal	14	46

Table 10.1. Comparison of bone marrow plasma cell counts in MM using different tests for monoclonal proteins.[10]

10.5. Recycling of IgG by FcBr receptors

The explanation for the long half-life of IgG relates to its mode of catabolism. Immunoglobulins are removed from serum over 3-4 days by pinocytosis, along with many other serum proteins. The half-life of IgG is, however, prolonged to 20-25 days by FcBr receptors that recycle it back into the blood many times. This extended half-life guarantees that it is an insensitive marker for judging early tumour responses to therapy. In contrast, the half-life of FLCs is only a few hours so that serum concentrations closely match tumour killing rates.

Figure 10.9 compares the sensitivity of the serum responses of monoclonal IgGκ, total IgG and free κ in a patient undergoing chemotherapy. Concentrations of monoclonal κ had reduced by 25-fold at 30 days compared with IgGκ concentrations that only reduced by 3-fold over the same period. The FLC results in this patient *(and others in Figures 10.6 - 10.7)* illustrate the beneficial combination of the short serum half-life together with the large clinical range. In a study of 17 patients, the tumour-produced sFLCs fell 210-fold (range 2.1-1678) whereas the intact immunoglobulin reduction was only 14-fold (1.5-88 fold).[3] The greater range of sFLC concentrations indicates it is more sensitive to small changes in tumour volume than intact immunoglobulin levels. This may be particularly useful when the concentrations of intact monoclonal immunoglobulins are low, making their measurement unreliable.

It is of interest that in some patients the reduction in serum IgG after chemotherapy is faster than its 21-day half-life would suggest. The explanation is unclear, but it is possible that production of FcBr receptors is impaired by chemotherapy. This would

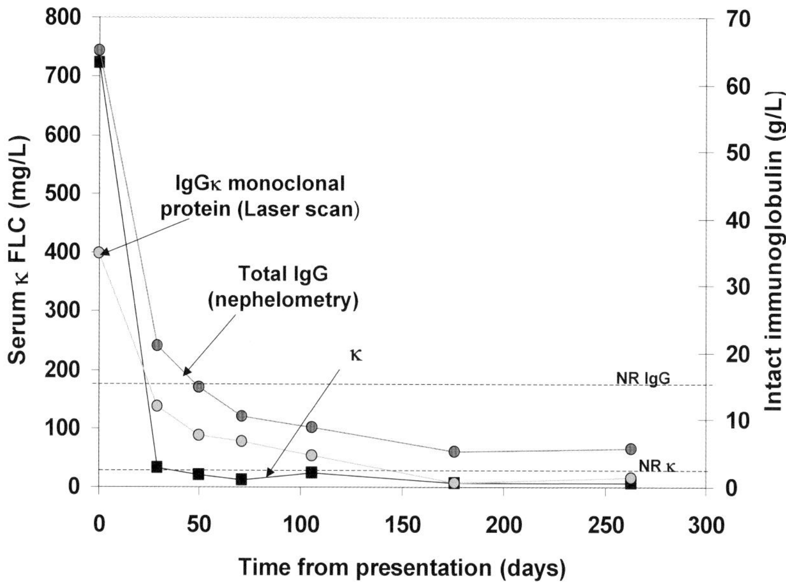

Figure 10.9. sFLCs and IgGκ levels in a patient after chemotherapy. κ concentrations had fallen 8-fold further than the monoclonal IgGκ by day 30.

prevent re-cycling of IgG molecules, thereby reducing their serum half-life.

10.6. Serum free light chain levels during disease relapse

During tumour relapse, concentrations of intact monoclonal immunoglobulins and FLCs generally increase in parallel because of the renewed synthesis of all molecules (*Figure 10.6*). However, sFLCs provide an earlier indication of relapse in 10-15% of patients *(Figure 10.10)*,[11-14] for the following reasons:-

1. When the tumour intrinsically produces large amounts of FLCs and small amounts of intact immunoglobulins the clinical sensitivity of the FLC assay is superior. Since there is little correlation between the production of the two molecules *(Figure 10.5)*, FLC resynthesis will be detectable before that of the intact immunoglobulin monoclonal proteins in some patients.
2. When the monoclonal immunoglobulin production by the tumour has changed to FLCs only.[14] FLC 'breakthrough' is said to occur in 2-5% of patients with modern intensive treatment *(Figure 10.10 and Clinical case history No 2; page 70)*.
3. When relapse occurs within a few months of treatment. In this situation, intact immunoglobulin concentrations are still falling and this hides the early increases from the tumour relapse *(Figure 10.6 after day 1,100 and Figure 13.3)*.

While sFLCs normally increase with other monoclonal proteins during disease relapse, this is not necessarily the case. Any pattern seems possible although patients usually conform to their earlier monoclonal protein expression profile. In some patients, the disease is stable as determined by the levels of intact immunoglobulins but sFLC levels indicate relapse. Others may go into remission but with residual abnormal FLCs. Figure 10.11 shows a patient who was normal by SPE and UPE but who had high λ

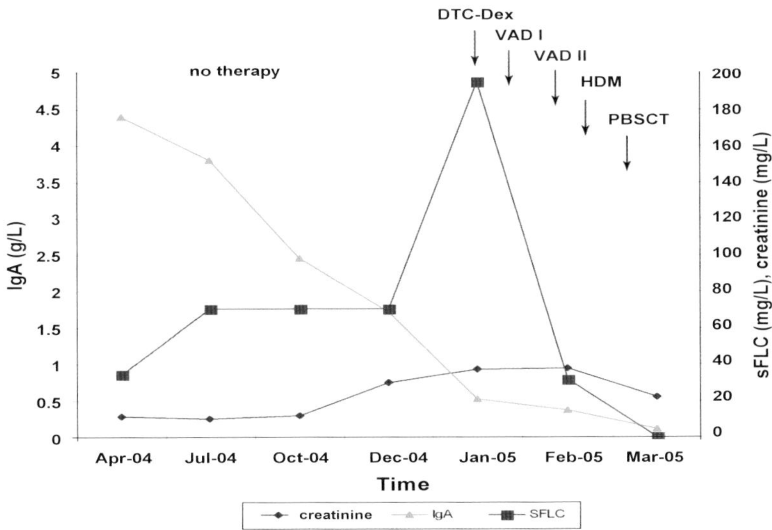

Figure 10.10. Serum λ FLCs and IgAλ in a patient during relapse. Free light chain 'breakthough' was apparent as the IgA clone disappeared (Courtesy of M Engelhardt).[14]

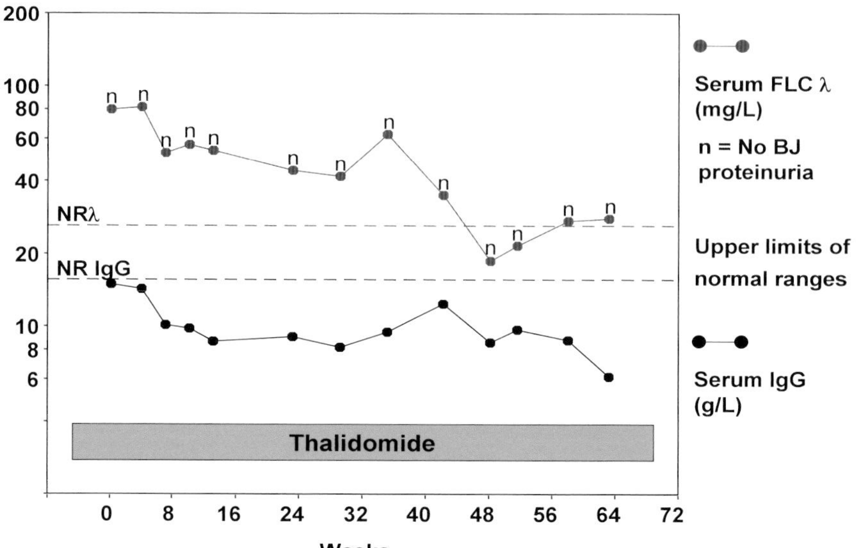

Figure 10.11. A patient treated with thalidomide to normalise λ sFLCs after the IgG monoclonal protein had disappeared. n: no Bence Jones proteinuria by IFE (Courtesy of MR Nowrousian).[6]

sFLC concentrations. A successful response of the FLC to thalidomide was observed over a six-month period. Figure 10.12 shows a patient who was given additional chemotherapy to normalise the sFLCs after intact monoclonal immunoglobulins had become normal by conventional electrophoretic tests.

10.7. Disease stage and serum free light chains

The amounts of FLCs produced by MM cells vary enormously between different patients (although they are closely related to the tumour mass for any individual patient). Therefore, there is only a modest relationship between disease stage and sFLC concentrations. However, on a statistical basis, patients with advanced disease are more likely to have Bence Jones proteinuria or abnormal sFLC concentrations *(Figure 10.13).*[6,8,15,16]

In contrast, β_2 microglobulin is a reliable marker for disease mass when comparing different patients because it is consistently produced by the nucleated MM cells. β_2 microglobulin does share one characteristic with FLCs in that it is rapidly cleared by the kidney. Hence, both are increased in renal impairment. However, the clinical range of β_2 microglobulin is small so that fluctuations are more difficult to interpret, particularly at low concentrations (*Figure 10.14*). Nevertheless, β_2 microglobulin will retain its important role of providing prognostic information and allowing comparison of disease staging in different studies *(Table 25.1).*

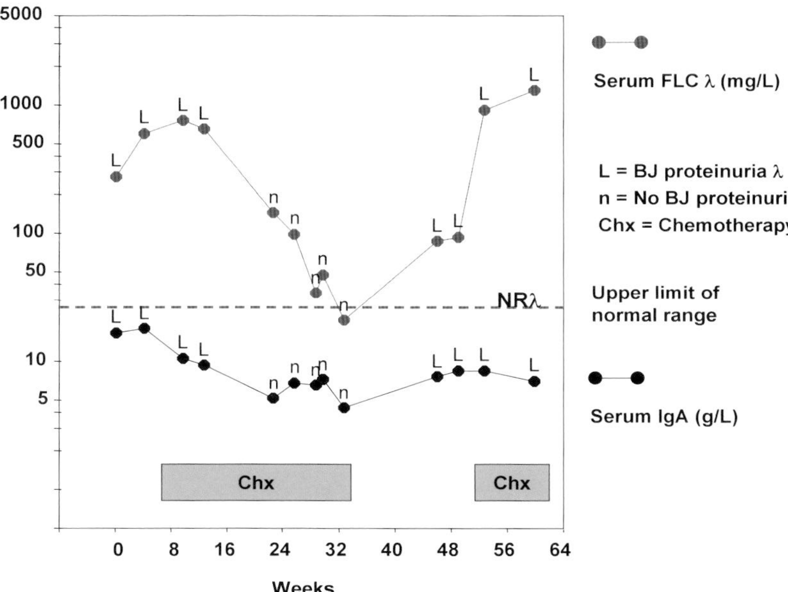

Figure 10.12. A patient treated with additional courses of chemotherapy to normalise sFLCs after other monoclonal proteins had disappeared (Courtesy of MR Nowrousian).[6]

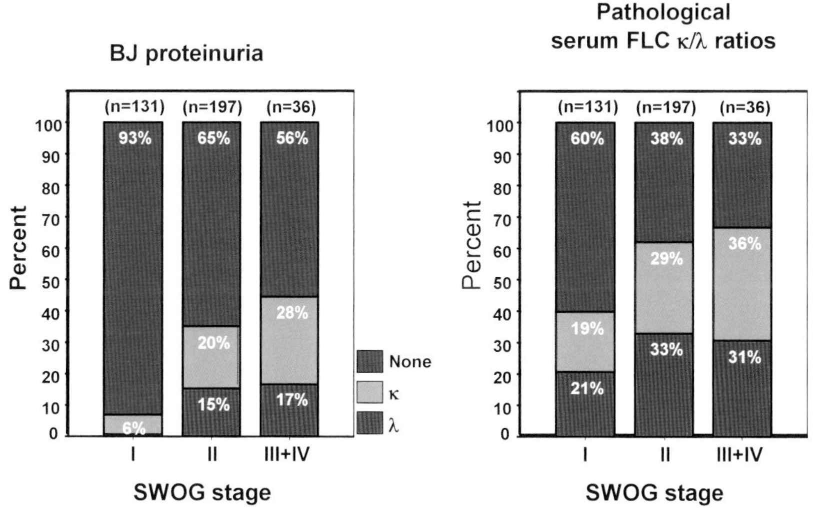

Figure 10.13. Relationship between SWOG disease stage (South West Oncology Group) and the presence of proteinuria or abnormal κ/λ ratios in 289 patients studied in a MM clinic (Courtesy of MR Nowrousian).[6]

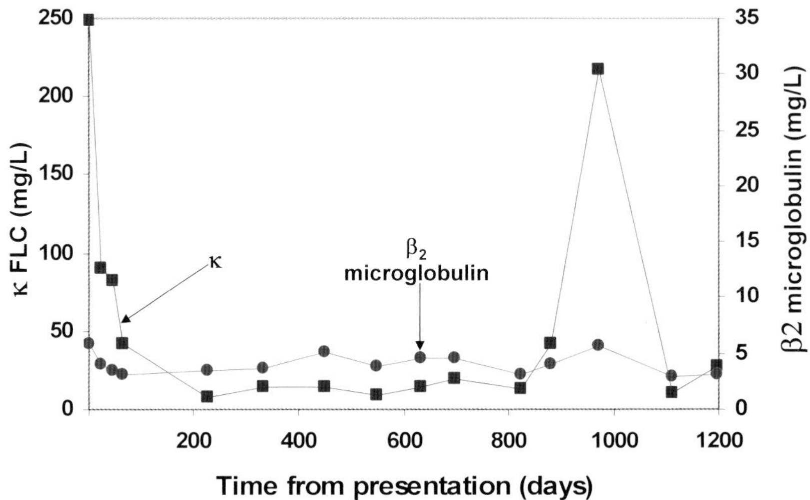

Figure 10.14. Serum κ FLCs and β2 microglobulin during disease monitoring.

Summary: In patients with IIMM, monoclonal serum FLCs:-

1. Are abnormal in 95% of patients at disease presentation.
2. Show no correlation with intact monoclonal immunoglobulin concentrations.
3. Correlate better with bone marrow biopsy data than intact immunoglobulins.
4. Have a short serum half-life that allows detection of early responses or lack of responses to treatment.
5. May show disease relapse when other markers are unchanged.
6. Are nephrotoxic in some patients.
7. Allow distinction between good and poor long-term responses at an early stage and prior to PBSCT.

References

1. **McIntyre OR**. Laboratory investigation of myeloma. In: Malpas JS, Bergsagel DE, Kyle RA (eds); Myeloma Biology and Management, New York, USA, Oxford Medical Publications, 1995, 191-221.

2. **Sölling K, Lanng Nielsen J, Sölling J and Ellegaard J**. Free Light Chains of Immunoglobulins in Serum from Patients with Leukaemias and Multiple Myeloma. Scand J Hematol 1982; **28**: 309-318.

3. **Mead GP, Carr-Smith HD, Drayson MT, Morgan GT, Child JA, Bradwell AR.** Serum free light chains for monitoring multiple myeloma. Br J Haem 2004; **126**: 348-354.

4. **Blade J, Kyle RA.** Nonsecretory Myeloma, Immunoglobulin D Myeloma and Plasma Cell Leukemia. Hem/Onc Clin N Amer 1999; **13**: 1259-1272.

5. **Kanoh T, Niwa Y.** Nonsecretory IgD (kappa) Multiple Myeloma. Am J Clin Path 1987; **88**: 516-519.

6. **Nowrousian MR.** *Personal communication.*

7. **Engelhardt M, Rapple D, Weis A, Bisse E, Thorst G.** Serum Free Light Chain Measurement in Multiple Myeloma Patients Correlate with Known Monoclonal Paraprotein, Disease Stage and Therapy Response. Blood 2004; **104**: 11: 4907.

8. **Cavallo F, Rasmussen E, Zangari M, Tricot G, Fender B, Fox M, Burns M, Barlogie B.** Serum Free-Lite Chain (sFLC) Assay in Multiple Myeloma (MM): Clinical Correlates and Prognostic Implications in Newly Diagnosed MM Patients Treated with Total Therapy 2 or 3 (TT2/3). Blood 2005; **106**: 11: 3490. P974a.

9. **McLaughlin P, Alexanian R.** Myeloma Protein Kinetics Following Chemotherapy. Blood 1982; **60**: 851-855.

10. **Mead GP, Reid S, Augustson B, Drayson MT, Bradwell AR, Child JA**. Correlation of Serum Free Light Chains and Bone Marrow Plasma Cell Infiltration in Multiple Myeloma. Blood 2004: **104**: 11: Abstract 4865.

11. **Tate JR, Grimmett K, Mead GP, Cobcroft R, Gill D**. Free light chain ratios in the serum of myeloma patients in complete remission following autologous peripheral blood stem cell transplantation. Clin Chem 2002; **48** (6): Suppl: E-50: A166.

12. **Tate JR, Mollee P, Gill D.** Serum free light chains for monitoring multiple myeloma. Br J Haem 2005; **128**: 405-406 *letter*

13. **Mead GP, Carr-Smith HD, Drayson MT, Morgan GT, Child JA, Bradwell AR.** Serum free light chains for monitoring multiple myeloma. Br J Haem 2005; **128**: 406-407. *Reply to letter*

14. **Kühnemund A, Liebisch P, Bauchmuller K, Haas P, Kleber M, Bisse E, Schmitt-Graff A, Engelhardt M.** Secondary light chain multiple myeloma with decreasing IgA paraprotein levels correlating with renal insufficiency and progressive disease: Clinical course of two patients and review of the literature. Onkologie 2005; **28** (suppl 3): 165.

15. **Hassoun H, Reich L, Klimek VM, Dhodapkar M, Cohen A, Kewalramani T, Riedel ER, Hedvat CV, Teruya-Feldstein J, Filippa DA, Fleisher M, Nimer SD, Comenzo RL.** The Serum Free Light Chain Ratio after One or Two Cycles of Treatment Is Highly Predictive of the Magnitude of Final Response in Patients Undergoing Initial Treatment for Multiple Myeloma. Blood 2005; **106** (11): 3481: p972a.

16. **Hassoun H, Reich L, Klimek VM, Dhodapkar M, Cohen A, Kewalramani T, Zimman R, Drake L, Riedel ER, Hedvat CV, Teruya-Feldstein J, Filippa DA, Fleisher M, Nimer SD, Comenzo RL.** Doxorubicin and dexamethosone followed by thalidomide and dexamethasone is an effective well tolerated initial therapy for multiple myeloma. Br J Haem 2005; **132**: 155-161.

17. **Moesbauer U, Schieder H, Renges H, Ayuk F, Zander A, Kröger N.** Serum Free Light Chain [FLC] Assay in Multiple Myeloma Patients Who Achieved Negative Immunofixation after Allogeneic Stem Cell Transplantation. Blood 2005; **106** (11): 2023: p572a.

Test Questions

1. *Can sFLC measurements be used as an early marker of relapse in IIMM?*
2. *How often are sFLCs abnormal in IgA multiple myeloma?*
3. *Why might the short half-life of sFLCs be clinically useful?*

Answers

1. In some patients sFLC levels are abnormal before other monoclonal immunoglobulins (page 89).

2. In 98% of patients at clinical presentation (Figure 10.3).

3. It allows an early assessment of treatment response or failure (pages 85-90).

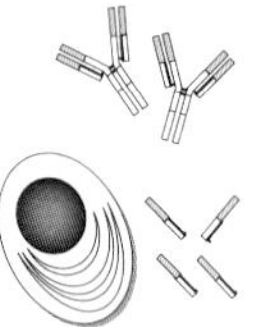

Chapter 11

Asymptomatic (smouldering) multiple myeloma

Patients with asymptomatic or smouldering MM satisfy two of the criteria for MM (monoclonal protein concentrations greater than 30g/L and/or 10% or more monoclonal plasma cells in the bone marrow) but do not have related organ or tissue impairment. These patients were classified in the Durie and Salmon staging system as Grade 1. The time to disease progression is typically 12-32 months so they do not require immediate treatment but they need to be monitored on a regular basis.[1]

Since the presence of urine FLCs in these patients is an adverse prognostic indicator, sFLCs may also be useful.[2,3] Extrapolation from the data of Rajkumar et al., in individuals with MGUS FLCs would further suggest their utility in asymptomatic MM.[4]

In a pilot study by RA Kyle and JA Katzmann at The Mayo Clinic (personal communication), it was shown that of 25 patients with asymptomatic MM, 64% had increased serum κ or λ FLCs while 96% had abnormal κ/λ ratios (*Figures 11.1 and 11.2*). This was later extended to 72 patients. Abnormal sFLC levels were found in 88% of patients but there was no comment on outcome.[5]

Augustson et al.[6] studied 43 patients with asymptomatic MM who had been registered on the UK, MRC multiple myeloma trials between 1980 and 2002. They found that abnormal FLC κ/λ ratios were present in 36 (84%) of the patients while 7 (16%) were normal. In the 26 patients with abnormal ratios who progressed, the median time period was 713 days. This compared with 1,323 days in the 6 patients who progressed that had normal κ/λ ratios. Although there was no significant difference in survival between the

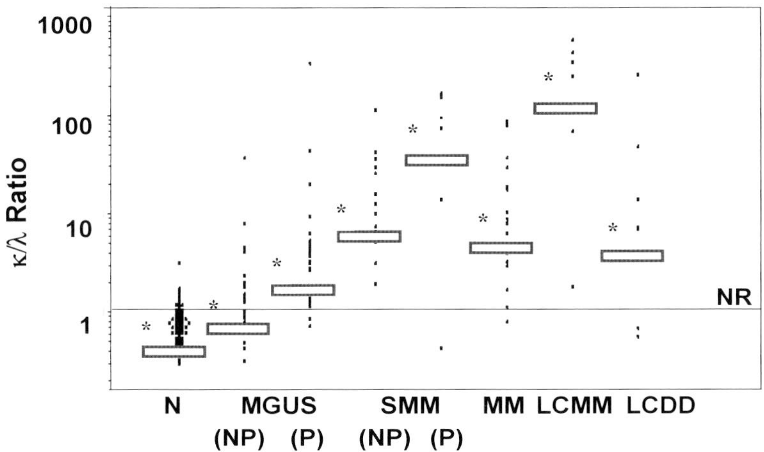

Figure 11.1. sFLC κ/λ ratios in patients with κ producing monoclonal gammopathies. N = Normal sera; P = progression; NP = no progression; * = median. (Courtesy of RA Kyle and JA Katzmann).

two groups ($p<0.13$) the patient numbers were probably inadequate for reliable statistical analysis *(Figure 11.3)*. However, it may be that disease progression is faster in those patients with abnormal sFLCs κ/λ ratios.

While no firm conclusions can be drawn, it is apparent that in the spectrum of disease development from MGUS, through asymptomatic to symptomatic MM, excess monoclonal FLC production becomes progressively more probable.

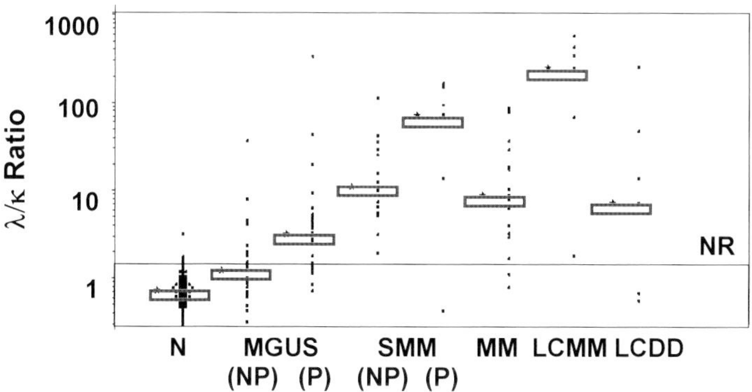

Figure 11.2. sFLC λ/κ ratios in patients with λ producing monoclonal gammopathies. N = Normal sera; P = progression; NP = no progression. (Courtesy of RA Kyle and JA Katzmann).

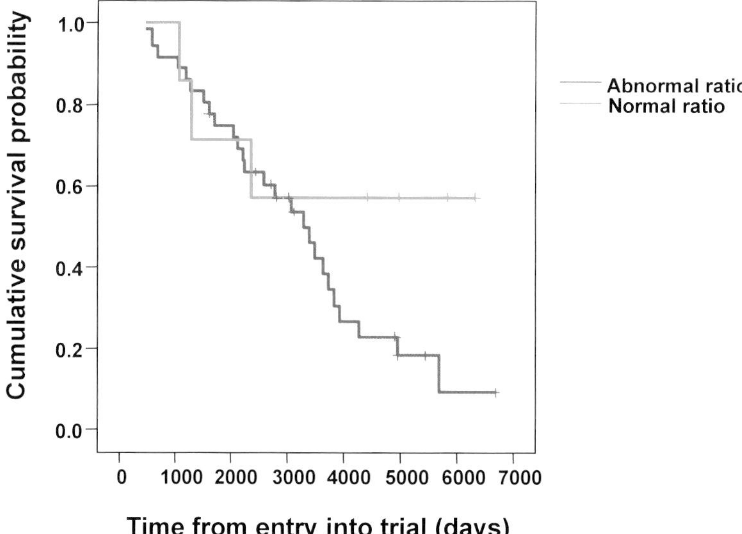

Figure 11.3. Kaplan-Meier plot of survival in 43 patients with asymptomatic MM with and without abnormal κ/λ ratios.[6]

References

1. **Lokhorst H.** Myeloma: Clinical features and diagnostic criteria. In: Myeloma, Eds. J Mehta & S Singhal; Pub: M Dunitz Ltd., London 2002; Chapt 10: 157-158.

2. **Dimopoulos MA, Moulopoulos A, Smith T, Delasalle KB, Alexanian R.** Risk of Disease Progression in Asymptomatic Multiple Myeloma. Amer J Med 1993; **94**: 57-61.

3. **Cesana C, Klersy C, Barbarano L, Nosari AM, Crugnola M, Pungolino E, Gargantini L, Granata S, Valentini M, Morra E.** Prognostic factors for Malignant Transformation in Monoclonal Gammopathy of Undetermined Significance and Smouldering Multiple Myeloma. J Clin Oncol 2002; **20**: 1625-1634.

4. **Rajkumar SV, Kyle RA, Therneau TM, Melton III LJ, Bradwell AR, Clark RJ, Larson DR, Plevak MF, Dispenzieri A, Katzmann JA**. Presence of monoclonal free light chains in serum predicts risk of progression in monoclonal gammopathy of undetermined significance (MGUS). Br J Haem 2004: **127**: 308-310.

5. **Katzmann J, Abraham RS, Dispenzieri A, Lust JA, Kyle RA.** Diagnostic performance of Quantitative Kappa and Lambda Free Light Chain Assays in Clinical Practice. Clin Chem 2005; **51** (5); p878-881.

6. **Augustson BM, Reid SD, Mead GP, Drayson MT, Child JA, Bradwell AR.** Serum Free Light Chain Levels In Asymptomatic Myeloma. Blood 2004; **104** (11): No 4880.

Test Question

1. How frequently are sFLCs abnormal in asymptomatic MM?

Answer

1. In approximately 90% of patients (page 94).

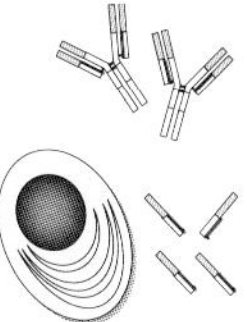

Chapter 12

Serum free light chains for assessing residual disease

12.1. Introduction

Absence of monoclonal proteins after high-dose therapy is prognostic for good survival. Some patients currently considered to be in complete remission by electrophoretic tests might be reclassified as having residual disease by the more sensitive sFLC tests. Two studies have addressed this important question.

12.2. Clinical studies

Sirohi et al. studied sera for sFLCs from 107 MM patients who were in complete remission as assessed by electrophoretic tests (Blade criteria)[1,2] The patients were subsequently monitored and relapse was determined in a conventional manner. Results were as follows: median κ: 14.2mg/L (range 3.08-161); median λ: 16.7mg/L (range 1.9-756); median κ/λ ratio: 0.82 (range 0.06-14.67) (*Figure 12.1*). The ratio was outside the

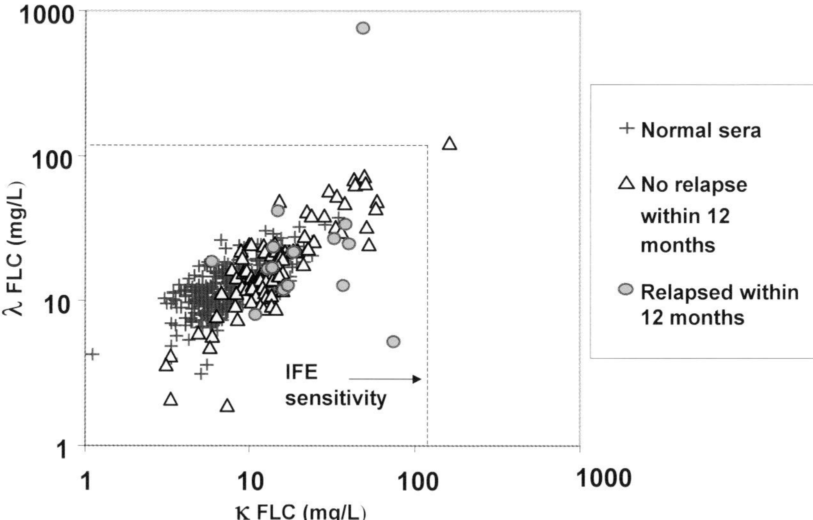

Figure 12.1. Serum FLC concentrations in normal individuals and 107 patients with MM in complete remission, both clinically and by serum and urine IFE.[2]

95% range in 20 patients, of whom 6 had ratios outside the 100% reference range. Patients with ratios outside the 95% range had a 1.3-fold increased risk of progression ($p<0.05$) and patients with results outside the 100% range had a 2.7-fold increased risk ($p<0.01$) (Fisher's exact test). Patients with both FLCs elevated (but normal κ/λ ratios) were considered to have impaired renal function *(Chapter 20)* or disordered immune reconstitution and showed no increased risk of relapse.

Thus, even though intact monoclonal immunoglobulins were undetectable by IFE in all patients, sFLCs were frequently abnormal and predicted worse outcome. The authors concluded that abnormal sFLC κ/λ ratios may be a sensitive marker of residual disease but because of the small numbers of patients, larger studies were warranted.

Reid et al., measured sFLCs in 36 patients with LCMM who were clinically in complete remission or had stable disease *(Figure 12.2 and Table 12.1)*.[3] 17 of the patients had no detectable FLCs in either serum or urine by IFE (Sebia system). However, 11 of these patients had abnormal κ/λ ratios with increased FLC concentrations. In contrast, all 19 patients with abnormal IFE results had abnormal sFLC concentrations. In a further study of 61 patients with IIMM in complete remission by conventional criteria, 17 had abnormal sFLC κ/λ ratios (*Figure 12.3*).[3]

Survival data was available for 23 of the LCMM patients *(from Figure 12.2)*. In this small number of patients results suggested that abnormal FLC ratios might be an adverse prognostic factor (990 vs. 1188 days: $p<0.15$). Similarly, survival data from 21 patients with IIMM *(from Figure 12.3)* indicated that abnormal FLC ratios were an adverse survival factor (891 vs. 1430 days: $p<0.03$). In the combined data of 44 patients, abnormal FLC ratios were highly significant for poor outcome ($P<0.007$) (*Figure 12.4*).

In both studies, sFLC assays were clearly more sensitive than IFE for identifying monoclonal FLCs.[2,3] This should allow more patients with residual disease to be

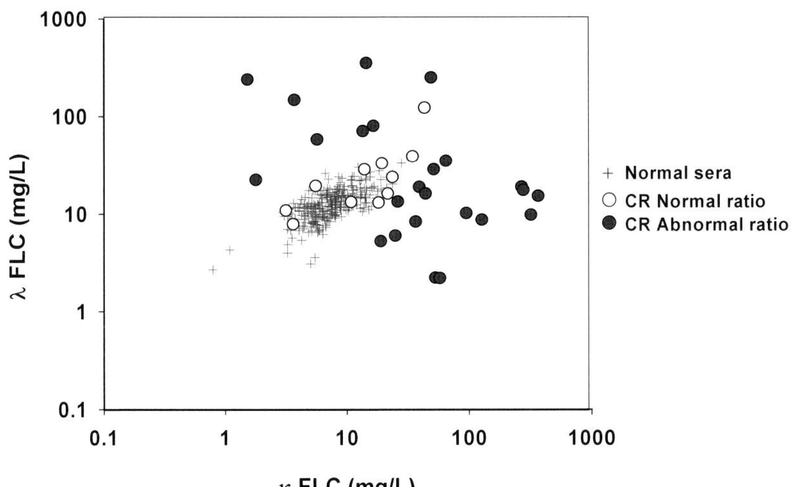

Figure 12.2. Serum FLC concentrations in 36 patients with LCMM in complete remission or with stable disease.[3]

identified. Furthermore, abnormal κ/λ ratios in these patients were predictive of reduced overall survival.

This work was extended by Augustson et al.[4] Patients who received intensive therapy in the UK MRC VIIth Myelomatosis trial were studied following treatment. Patients who were IFE negative had improved progression-free survival and overall survival than those positive by IFE at 6, 9 and 12 months. However, the number of patients available

Patient number	Serum free kappa (mg/L)	Serum free lambda (mg/L)	κ/λ ratio	IFE negativity?
1	13.5	71	0.19	Yes
2	48.9	250	0.2	Yes
3	16.5	80.2	0.21	Yes
4	43.2	123	0.35	Yes
5	13.9	28.7	0.48	Yes
6	19.4	33.1	0.59	Yes
7	10.8	13.3	0.81	Yes
8	34.5	39.1	0.88	Yes
9	23.7	23.9	0.99	Yes
10	51.3	28.7	1.79	Yes
11	26.2	13.4	1.96	Yes
12	44	16.2	2.72	Yes
13	94.6	10.2	9.27	Yes
14	267	19	14.05	Yes
15	275	17.6	15.63	Yes
16	364	15.3	23.79	Yes
17	318	9.81	32.42	Yes
18	6.66	535	0.01	No
19	15.8	581	0.03	No
20	20.9	508	0.03	No
21	8.45	221	0.04	No
22	3.8	105	0.04	No
23	24.9	585	0.04	No
24	27.8	382	0.07	No
25	20	104	0.19	No
26	21	12.9	1.66	No
27	71	14.7	4.8	No
28	529	31.5	16.79	No
29	24	1.24	19.44	No
30	352	15.4	22.86	No
31	920	20.7	44.44	No
32	584	8.03	72.73	No
33	970	12.8	75.78	No
34	3520	36.3	96.97	No
35	1800	13.8	130.43	No
36	3200	12.5	256	No

Table 12.1. Serum FLC concentrations in 36 patients with LCMM and stable disease, following treatment. 17 patients had normal IFE and 19 were abnormal. Abnormal κ/λ ratios are in orange and normal in green.

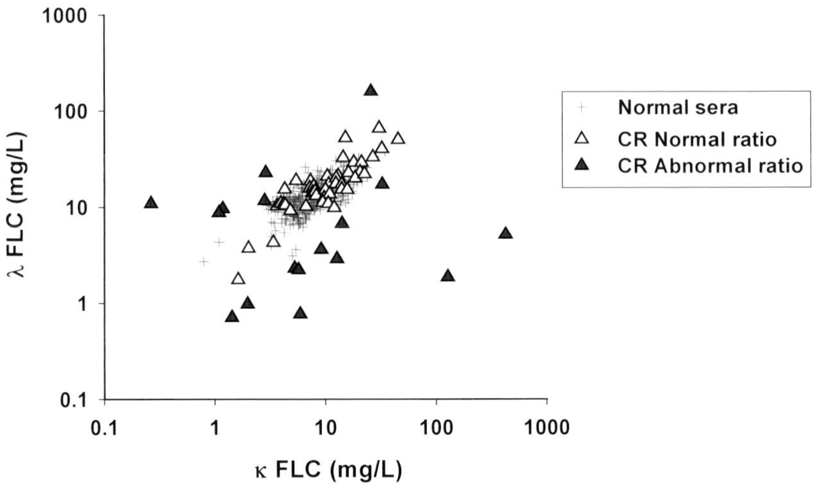

Figure 12.3. sFLC concentrations in 61 patients with IIMM whilst in complete remission, both clinically and by serum and urine IFE.[3] CR: complete response.

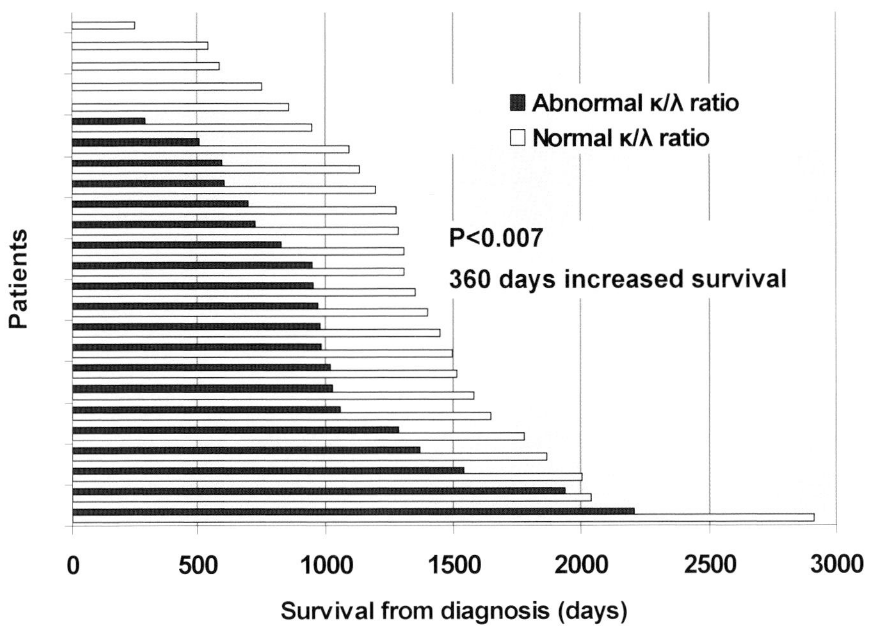

Figure 12.4. Survival of 44 patients with MM who had complete response by conventional criteria, in relation to residual sFLC concentrations.[3]

for analysis was insufficient to reach statistical significance for survival differences.

Moesbauer U et al.[5] evaluated the sensitivity of sFLCs in 26 MM patients in complete remission for early detection of relapse. 12 patients remained negative for all tests throughout the period with concordance between sFLC and IFE. Of 9 patients who sero-converted from IFE negative to positive during follow-up, all had corresponding increases in sFLCs. In 4 of these patients there was a >25 % increase of sFLCs 3 months earlier (median 97 days) than IFE abnormality (due to the high sensitivity of FLC assays). A further 5 patients converted to IFE negativity during follow-up. However, the corresponding sFLC concentrations became normal at a median of 38 days earlier (due to the shorter serum half-life). They concluded that sFLCs detected relapse and remission earlier than IFE and might be a useful guide for additional strategies to prevent clinical relapse (*Figure 12.5*).

Prospective trials assessing the role of sFLC measurements for outcome parameters are ongoing.[6,7] Indeed, some patients with residual disease, as determined only by abnormalities of sFLCs, have been given additional high dose therapy and PBSCT. While evidence for the benefit of this extra treatment is not yet available, it is a logical approach.

12.3. Variations in serum free light chain levels after high dose therapy

When bone marrow myeloma cells have been eradicated with intensive therapy, normal haematopoesis may not return for many months. This may show as minor fluctuations of sFLC concentrations around the normal range. Caution should, therefore, be taken when interpreting the data. Figure 12.6 shows a patient who was monitored for 18 months following treatment. While κ concentrations rapidly normalised, λ concentrations did not recover for over a year, as manifested by the abnormal κ/λ ratios. When assessing residual disease or complete remission the relevance of minor

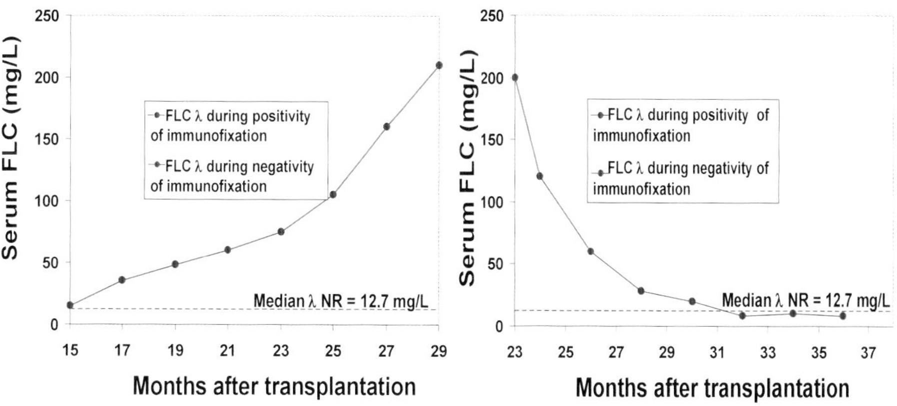

Figure 12.5. Serum FLCs and IFE during the evolution of patients with MM in remission. (A) during relapse and (B) commencement of remission. Earlier changes in sFLCs are apparent in both patients. (Courtesy of N Kroger).[5]

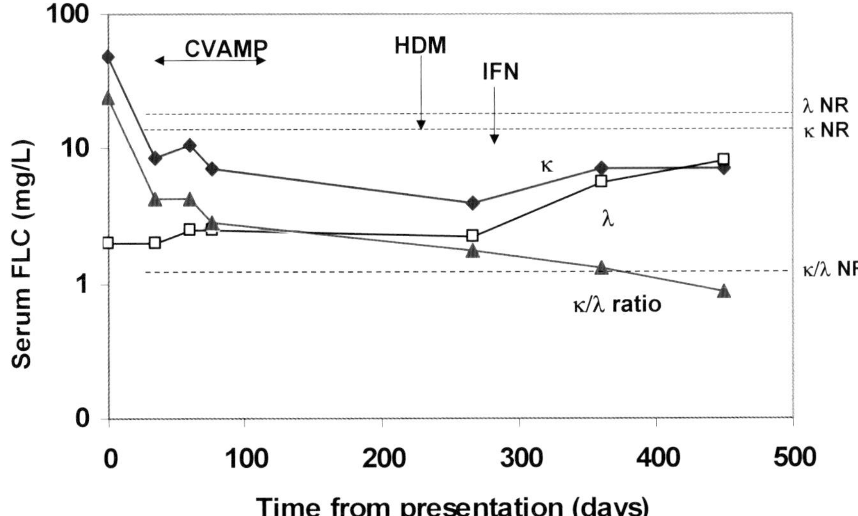

Figure 12.6. Changes in sFLC levels and κ/λ ratios during long-term tumour monitoring (same patient as *Figure 10.6*). IFN = interferon.

fluctuations in sFLC levels needs to be considered carefully *(see MM response criteria guidelines in Chapter 25).*

Summary: In MM patients in complete remission, sFLC concentrations:-

1. May be abnormal when other tests are normal.
2. Indicate residual disease and poor survival probability if they are abnormal.
3. Respond faster than intact immunoglobulin monoclonal proteins because of their shorter half-life.

References

1. **Blade J, Samson D, Reece D, Apperley J, Bjorkstrand B, Gahrton G, Gertz M, Giralt S, Jagannath S, Vesole D.** Criteria for evaluating disease response and progression in patients with multiple myeloma treated by high-dose therapy and haemopoietic stem cell transplantation. Br J Haematol 1998; **102**: 1115-1123.

2. **Sirohi B, Powles R, Kulkarni S, Carr-Smith HD, Patel G, Das M, Iqbal J, Bradwell AR, Dearden C, Mehta J.** Serum free light chain assessment in myeloma patients who are in complete remission (CR) by immunofixation predicts early relapse. Blood 2003; **102** (11): A5195.

3. **Reid SD, Drayson MT, Mead GP, Augustson B, Roberts S, Bradwell AR.** Serum free light chain assays for determining complete remission in multiple myeloma patients. Clin Chem 2004; **50** (6): Suppl, A79: C-34.

4. **Augustson BM, Reid SD, Cohen D, Hawkins K, Mead G, Drayson M, Child JA, Bradwell AR.** Normalisation Of Serum Free Light Chains and Negative Immunofixation Electrophoresis May Be Predictive Of Progression Free Survival And Overall Survival Following High Dose Melphalan. Haematologica 2005; **90** (1): 107: PO403.

5. **Moesbauer U, Schieder H, Renges H, Ayuk F, Zander A, Kröger N.** Serum Free Light Chain [FLC] Assay in Multiple Myeloma Patients Who Achieved Negative Immunofixation after Allogeneic Stem Cell

Transplantation. Blood 2005; **106** (11): 2023: 572a.

6. Hassoun H, Reich L, Klimek VM, Dhodapkar M, Cohen A, Kewalramani T, Zimman R, Drake L, Riedel ER, Hedvat CV, Teruya-Feldstein J, Filippa DA, Fleisher M, Nimer SD, Comenzo RL. Doxorubicin and dexamethosone followed by thalidomide and dexamethasone is an effective well tolerated initial therapy for multiple myeloma. Br J Haem 2005; **132**: 155-161.

7. Cavallo F, Rasmussen E, Zangari M, Tricot G, Fender B, Fox M, Burns M, Barlogie B. Serum Free-Lite Chain (sFLC) Assay in Multiple Myeloma (MM): Clinical Correlates and Prognostic Implications in Newly Diagnosed MM Patients Treated with Total Therapy 2 or 3 (TT2/3). Blood 2005; **106** (11) 3490: P974a.

Test questions

1. Can serum FLC measurements help when assessing residual disease in MM?

2. Can serum FLC tests be normal when IFE is abnormal in patients going into complete remission?

Answers

1. Some patients are normal by serum and urine electrophoretic tests but have abnormal sFLC concentrations. Statistically, these patients are more likely to have residual disease and shorter survival (page 97-98).

2. Yes. Because of the short serum half-life of serum FLCs they nomalise earlier than serum IFE for intact immunoglobulin monoclonal proteins (page 97-99).

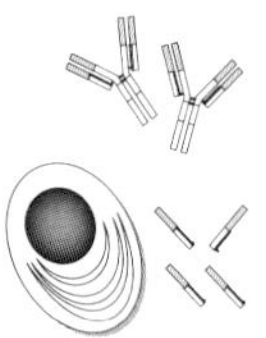

Chapter 13

Free light chain kinetics and disease management

13.1. Introduction

Only a few serum markers are helpful in the diagnosis of cancer but many play a critical role in monitoring patients. As a general rule, markers that are useful for diagnosis, such as sFLCs, are likely to be of particular benefit in patient follow-up.[1] Features that make a tumour marker useful include short half-life, clinical range, specificity, etc. This section is concerned first, with the theoretical aspects of sFLC kinetics and second, their application to tumour management using patient data. Potential applications in disease monitoring are discussed.[2,3]

13.2. Normal half-life of serum immunoglobulins

As indicated in Chapter 3, the dominating clearance mechanism for sFLCs is filtration through the renal glomerular fenestrations. At 25kDa, monomeric FLC molecules (usually κ) have a half-life of approximately 2 hours while dimeric molecules (usually λ) have a half-life of 4-6 hours (*Figure 13.1*). Serum FLCs that are more highly polymerised presumably have even longer half-lives.

In patients with renal failure sFLC half-life lengthens to a maximum of 2-3 days. Under such circumstances, clearance is by general pinocytotic mechanisms that account for the removal of many serum proteins, including albumin. In contrast, IgG molecules have a half-life of 20-25 days. This is because they are recycled from the pinocytotic vesicles, back into the circulation. This process is dependent upon FcBr receptors that bind IgG inside the vesicles and protect it from acid digestion (*Chapter 10*).

The 200-to 300-fold shorter serum half-life of FLCs compared with IgG allows a much more sensitive evaluation of changing monoclonal protein production during treatment. Figures 13.2 and 13.3 have been constructed using half-life equations to illustrate the effects of the various interacting factors on serum immunoglobulin concentrations.

The other influence on sFLC concentrations is the rate of production. In normal individuals this is thought to be approximately 500 mg per day, a similar amount to IgG. Production is largely by bone marrow plasma cells with a survival time of many days but some live for several weeks. Other cells of the B-cell lineage also produce FLC molecules and may have similar survival times but accurate data are not available.

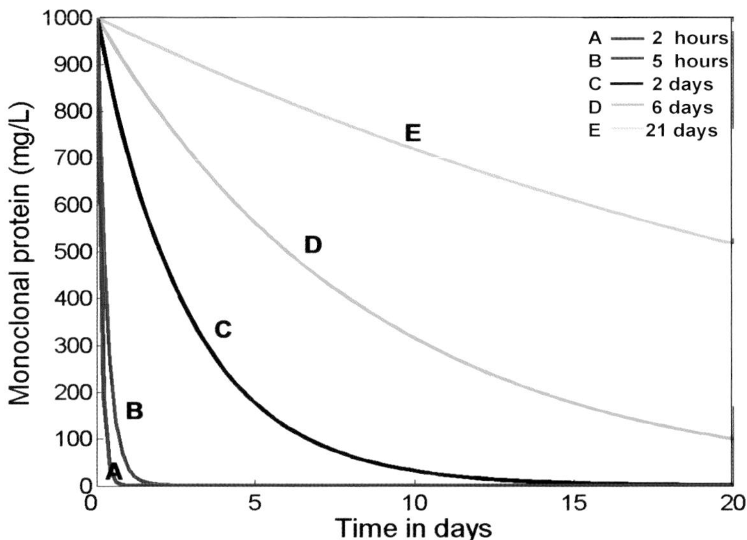

Figure 13.1. Calculated serum half-life curves for different immunoglobulin molecules. (A) monomeric κ; (B) dimeric λ; (C) monomeric κ with renal failure; (D) IgA and (E) IgG. (Courtesy of N Evans and M Chappell, Warwick University).

13.3. Tumour killing rates and half-life of immunoglobulins

During chemotherapy, tumour cells are destroyed at rates depending upon the killing mechanisms. Thus, dexamethasone causes apoptotic cell death, melphalan DNA disruption and vincristine cell-cycle related killing. The production of FLCs is switched off at a rate dependent upon the amount of tumour killed (which relates to the killing mechanism) and/or the rate of tumour cell division.

Figure 13.2 shows calculated half-life curves for serum monomeric κ and serum IgG when the tumour cells are killed at different rates. The half-life of sFLCs adds only a few hours to the actual tumour cell killing rate. Hence, tumour responses and complete remission can be rapidly identified. In contrast, the 21-day serum half-life of IgG is so long that it largely obscures differences in rates of tumour destruction. Furthermore, complete remission is identified many months later using IgG levels compared with FLCs. For the first time in MM, a short half-life marker allows reliable assessments of tumour cell killing rates and earlier identification of tumour remission.[3]

Production of both FLCs and intact immunoglobulins usually return when MM relapses *(Chapter 10)*. When tumour recurrence is associated with synthesis of both types of molecule then they, typically, become re-detectable at the same time. (In practice, re-synthesis is not always synchronous so one molecule may return before the other). If tumour re-growth occurs before all the monoclonal IgG has disappeared, then FLC measurements will be more sensitive for detecting tumour recurrence (*Figure*

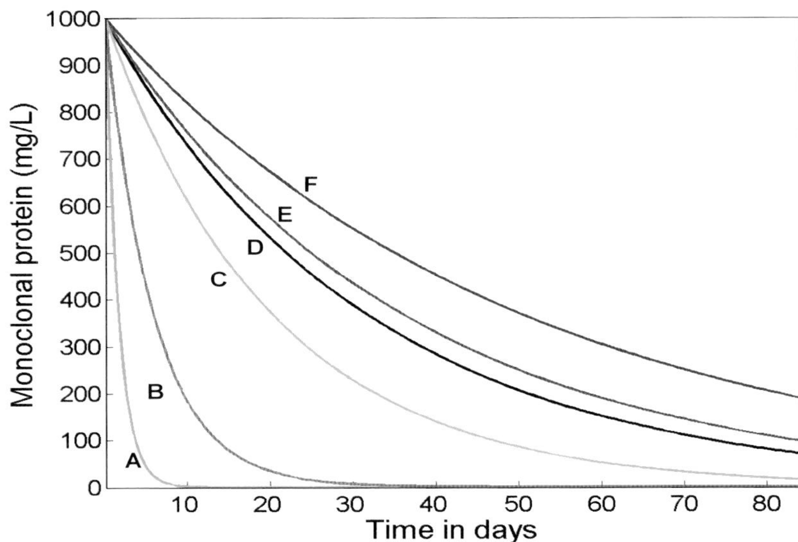

Figure 13.2. Calculated serum half-life curves for monomeric κ (A,B,C) and IgGκ (D,E,F) when the tumour cells are killed at: 50% per day (A, D); 50% in 4 days (B, E) and 50% in 2 weeks (C, F). (Courtesy of N Evans and M Chappell, Warwick University).[3]

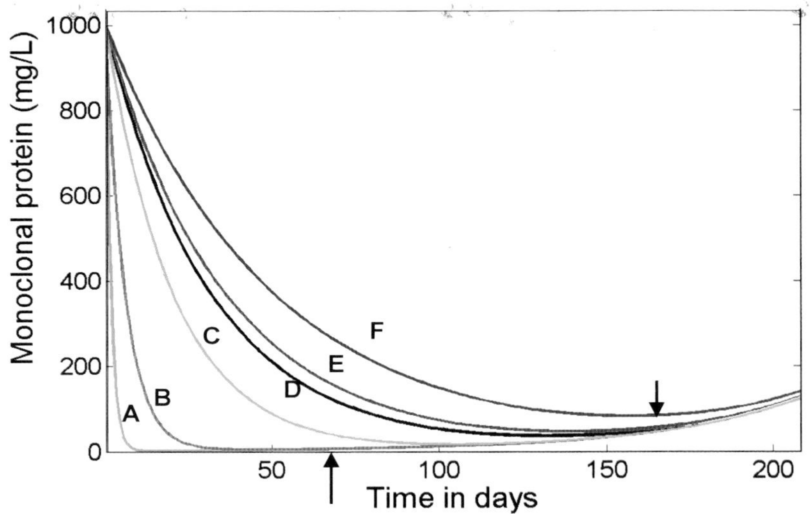

Figure 13.3. Calculated changes in κ FLCs and IgG during tumour relapse following chemotherapy. An increase in κ is seen many months before an increase in IgG (arrows). Tumour kill rate of: 50% per day for κ (A) and IgG (D); 50% in 4 days for κ (B) and IgG (E); 50% in 2 weeks for κ (C) and IgG (F). 0.1% residual tumour with a doubling time of 30 days after the initial chemotherapy, has been assumed. (Courtesy of N Evans and M Chappell, Warwick University).[3]

13.3). This is because the rising concentrations of monoclonal IgG from tumour relapse are superimposed upon falling concentrations from the initial tumour response, thereby obscuring an early IgG increase. In contrast, sFLCs normalise early so increasing production by the relapsing tumour is not hidden by residual levels.

Factors affecting the rate of return of monoclonal proteins include: residual tumour production rates, length of time of complete remission, tumour doubling times and renal function. The interplay of these factors is complex and is different for each patient. The following results, obtained while closely monitoring patients during high dose treatment, illustrate many of the key features discussed above and was recently published.[3]

Figures 13.4 and 13.5 compare sFLCs and intact immunoglobulin levels in patients treated with three courses of VAD followed by high dose melphalan (200mg/m^2) on day zero, prior to PBSCT. In Figure 13.4, serum λ levels fell with a half-life of 1 day while the monoclonal IgAλ concentrations showed only a slight fall over a week. In Figure 13.5 the half-life of tumour destruction was approximately 3 days. In Figures 13.6 and 13.7, FLCs were still high after initial induction chemotherapy and there was incomplete tumour killing at 14 days.

Figure 13.7 shows a patient treated with chemotherapy in whom there was an incomplete tumour response. This was was evident earlier from the failure of λ concentrations to normalise quickly, compared with the slow reduction of IgG levels (*also see Figure 13.3*).

Figures 13.8 and 13.9 illustrate bone marrow engraftment with functioning plasma cells after high-dose melphalan and PBSCT. In Figure 13.8, concentrations of both FLCs fell until day 10 and then increased rapidly. Three days later, total IgG began to

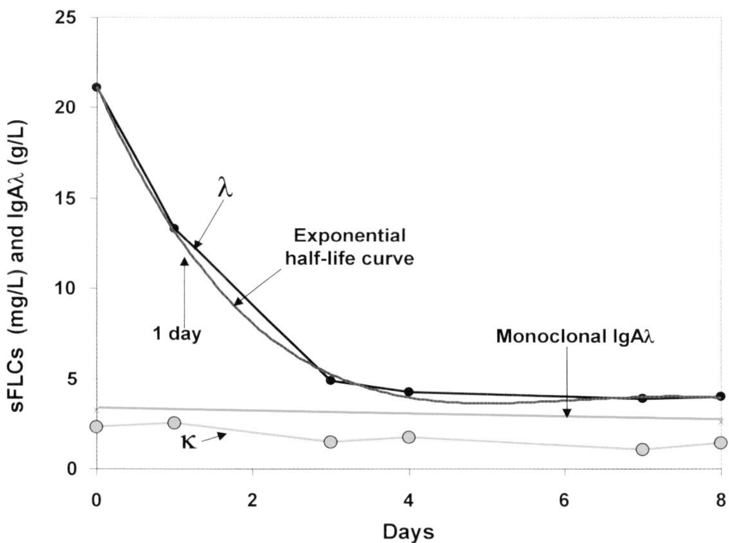

Figure 13.4. Serum IgAλ and λ FLC following high-dose melphalan and PBSCT. A half-life curve has been fitted to the λ concentrations. (Courtesy of G Pratt, Heartlands Hospital, Birmingham).[3]

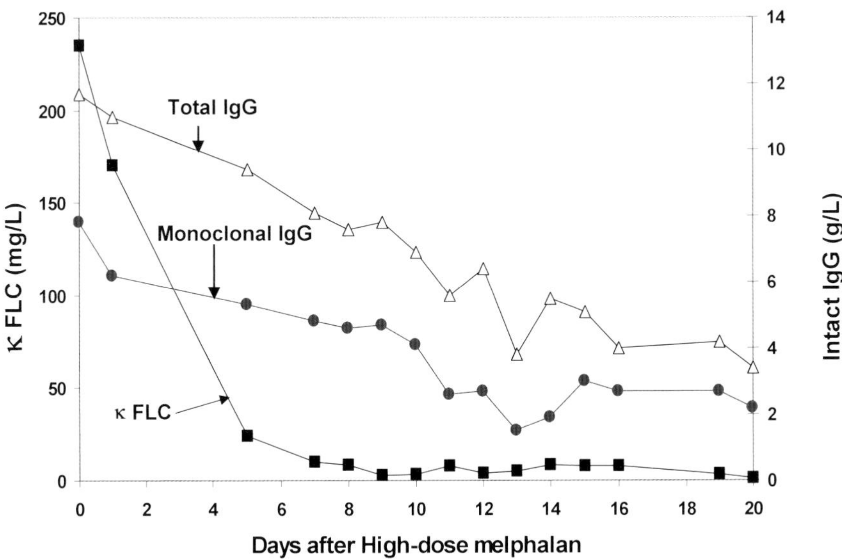

Figure 13.5. Concentrations of sFLC, total IgG and monoclonal IgGκ after high-dose melphalan. (Courtesy of G Pratt, Heartlands Hospital, Birmingham).[3]

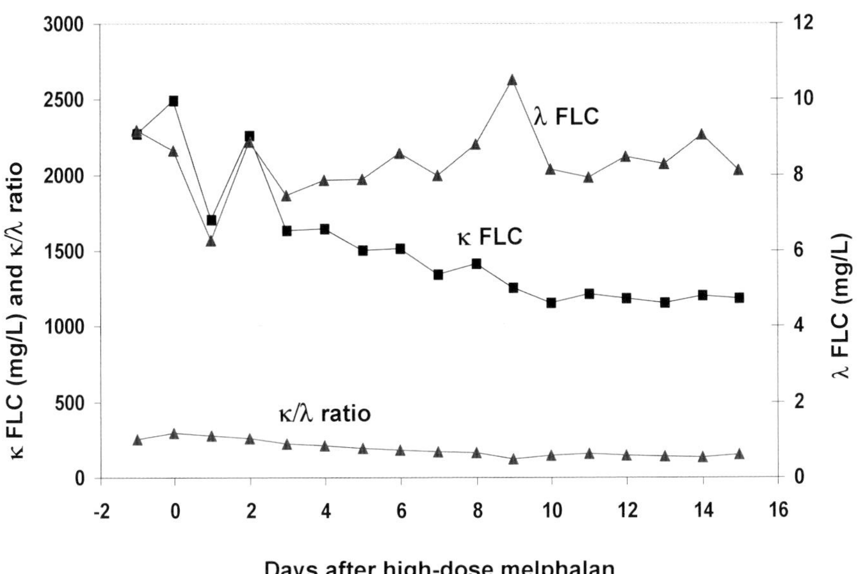

Figure 13.6. Concentrations of sFLC after high dose melphalan identifying a poor treatment response. (Courtesy of G Pratt, Heartlands Hospital, Birmingham).[3]

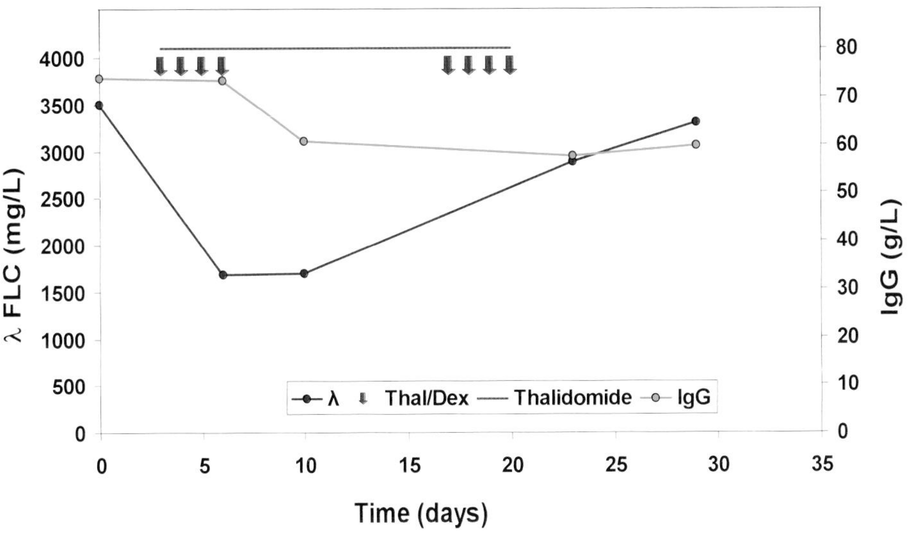

Figure 13.7. Early tumour recurrence identified from rising λ FLC levels while IgGλ continued to fall. Tumour relapse occurred before IgGλ had stabilised.

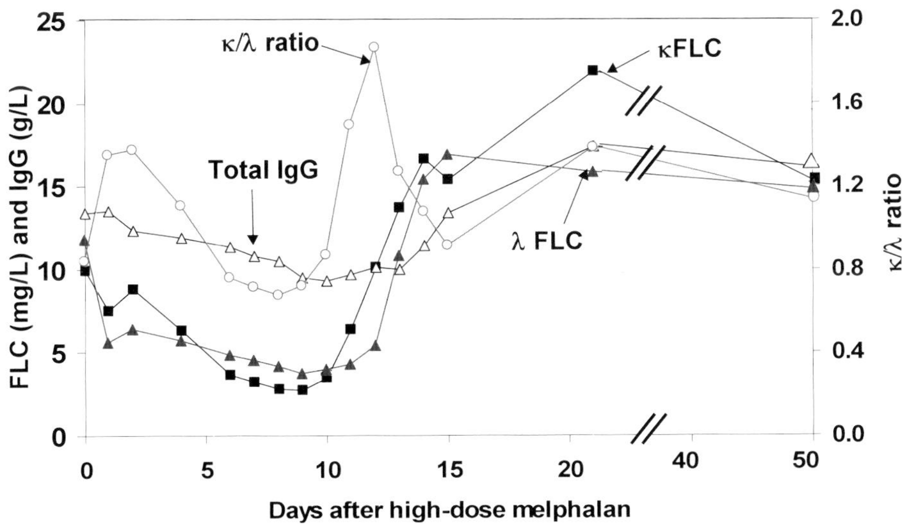

Figure 13.8. Changing immunoglobulin concentrations in a MM patient with IgGκ and FLC κ after high-dose melphalan treatment (day 0) and PBSCT. (Courtesy of G Pratt, Heartlands Hospital, Birmingham).[3]

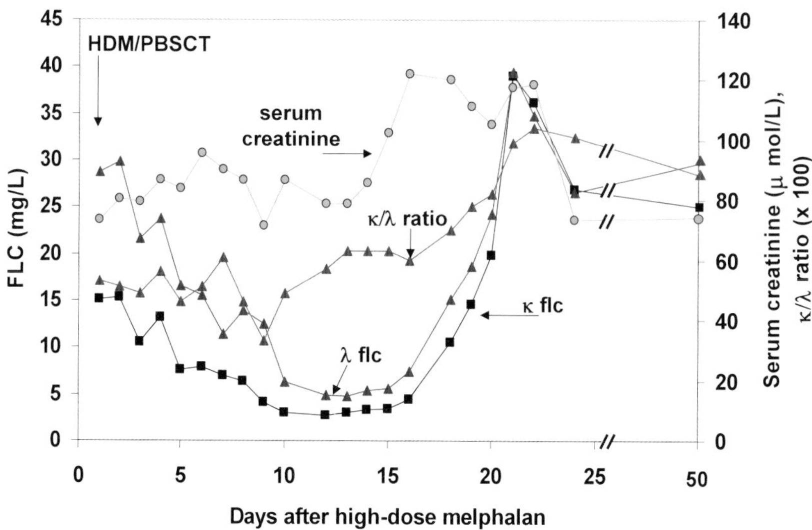

Figure 13.9. Changes in FLCs and creatinine while monitoring a patient with MM after high-dose melphalan and PBSCT. (Courtesy of G Pratt, Heartlands Hospital, Birmingham).[3]

rise. This indicated bone marrow engraftment and occurred a few days after the return of platelet and neutrophil production. This appears to be the normal pattern of FLC response as engraftment takes place.

Minimum levels of FLCs during treatment were 3-5mg/L. This indicated that some FLC production remained. Presumably, there were long-lived plasma cells that were resistant to the drugs. Since κ/λ ratios were normal, the producing cells were probably polyclonal rather than monoclonal tumour cells. In the early stages of engraftment, greater numbers of κ plasma cells were generated. This produced a 'spike' in the κ/λ ratio around day 12. Total IgG concentrations fell more slowly after treatment and increased later than FLCs during engraftment. By day 50, FLCs and immunoglobulins were within their normal concentration ranges.

Figure 13.9 illustrates similar features to Figure 13.8 but there is the added complication of renal impairment from gastrointestinal bleeding at day 14. This markedly affected the concentrations of sFLCs. Initially, after high-dose melphalan, serum λ half-life was 3 days, compared with 20 days for IgG. FLC concentrations increased from day 15 and exceeded normal levels by day 21. They returned to normal, alongside serum creatinine levels on day 24 when normal renal function was restored.

FLC recovery occurred either after or around the time of neutrophil engraftment in all the patients *(Figures 13.8 and 13.9)*. Since early lymphocyte recovery is associated with a more favourable outcome, the time to FLC normalisation may be a useful prognostic marker. Overall, FLC measurements provided a sensitive monitor of changes in the numbers of tumour cells after PBSCT and predicted the intact immunoglobulin response. Further follow-up is required to ascertain whether differences in the kinetics of the FLC responses have any prognostic value.

Several patients have been followed up for a year since the transplantation *(Figure 13.10)*. It should be noted that concentrations may not normalise for a considerable period but it is, as yet, unclear whether this is indicative of adverse outcome *(Chapter 12.3)*.

As discussed in Chapter 5, serum creatinine is not ideal for monitoring renal function changes since production is dependent upon muscle mass. Patients undergoing high dose chemotherapy are bed-bound and eat little so their muscle mass reduces during hospitalisation. Thus any changes in renal clearance of creatinine will be superimposed upon changing production rates in the muscles. Under such circumstances, serum cystatin C concentrations may provide a more accurate assessment of renal function.[4-6] Serum κ/λ ratios inherently compensate for changing renal function and must be used for assessing changing tumour mass rather than individual FLC concentrations.

The importance of these observations in terms of mortality and remission times is currently under investigation. FLC parameters of interest include:-

1. The reduction from levels at clinical presentation to minimum levels - indicative of the amount of tumour destroyed.
2. The rate of fall - relates to drug sensitivity and tumour cell-cycle time. Rapid reductions may indicate rapid tumour cell turnover and rapid tumour regrowth.
3. The lowest attained concentrations - relates to residual tumour mass.
4. Time to bone marrow engraftment - an indication of normal bone marrow function, tumour destruction and subsequent response rates (see below).

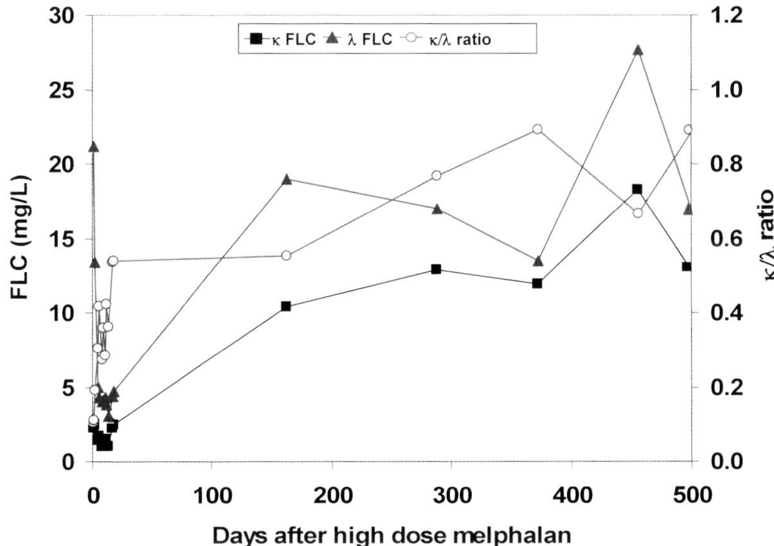

Figure 13.10. Long term evaluation of sFLC concentrations in a patient following high dose melphalan and PBSCT.

13.4. Drug selection using rapid responses in serum free light chains

The short half-life of sFLCs may be important for identifying effective drugs, and equally, ineffective drugs, particularly during the later stages of the disease. With each relapse, and as the disease becomes more refractory to treatment, patients are given more drugs, with many toxic side effects. The selection of a drug or drug combinations and the necessary doses can be based upon short-term responses in sFLC concentrations. When using IgG levels for such purposes it may be several weeks before it is appreciated which drug is effective.

An example of rapid response to drugs, identified using FLCs, is shown in Figure 13.11. The patient was diagnosed with LCMM and given dexamathasone 24 hours before vincristine and adriamycin and monitored frequently for sFLCs. 10-12 hours after the first dose of dexamethasone (apoptosis time), sFLC concentrations fell by 40%. Further falls followed subsequent doses. In contrast there was no clear evidence of the effect of vincristine or adriamycin. These observations suggests that serial monitoring of FLCs, whilst introducing drugs one-by-one, may allow the active component(s) to be rapidly identified.

In a study by Patten et al., the short serum half-life of FLCs was used to assess early treatment responses in relapsed, refractory MM.[7] 12 patients were treated with Actimid, (a new thalidomide analogue) while being observed for changes in monoclonal immunoglobulins *(Table 13.1)*. A beneficial change in the sFLC κ/λ ratio of greater than 50% by day 7 or 28 predicted clinically responding or stable disease. Changes of less than 25% by day 28 predicted clinical progression or stable disease. There was a relatively poor correlation between parameters but in responding patients reductions in sFLC concentrations predicted outcome earlier than intact immunoglobulin

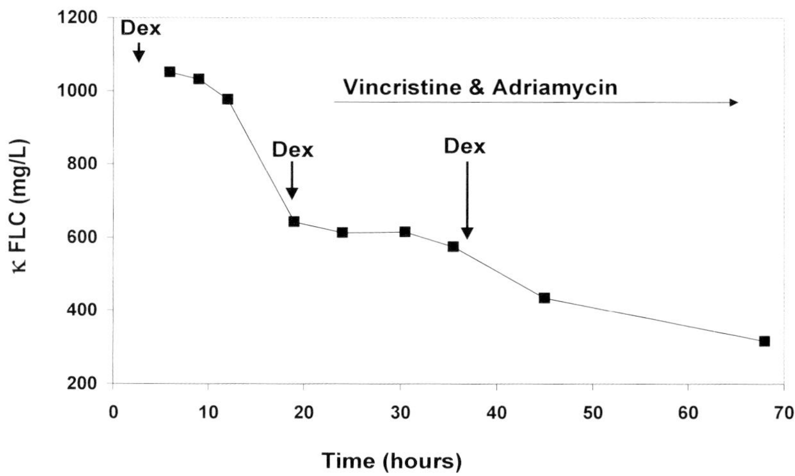

Figure 13.11. Changes in κ sFLC concentrations in a patient with LCMM at initial treatment. The effect of dexamethasone is clearly detectable within 24 hours. Dex = dexamethasone. (Courtesy of G Galvin, Walsall Manor Hospital, UK).[2]

Patient	Actimid	Immunoglobulin (g/L)		Free light chain κ/λ ratios		
	mg	pre	day 28	pre	day 7	day 28
&1	1	87	90	115	75	150
*2	1	30	22	38	5	5
&3	1	0	3	7	10	-
*4	1	22	22	50	35	28
*5	5	25	12	53	1	0.9
*6	10	69	52	157	50	-
&7	5	42	39	0.6	1	0.8
&8	5	37	31	8	6	7
&9	2	30	24	17	7	8
*10	2	3	3	1283	1547	1360
*11	2	69	60	37	27	7
*12	2	28	23	6	4	3

Table.13.1. Serum FLCs and monoclonal intact immunoglobulin concentrations in 12 patients treated with the thalidomide analogue, Actimid. *Early response seen in sFLCs. [&]FLC response at 7 or 28 days confirmed by relapsing or stable disease. (Courtesy of S Schey, Guys Hospital).[7]

measurements. The study concluded that sFLC κ/λ ratios allow early risk stratification and should allow tailoring of therapy in this difficult group of patients. In addition, faster dose escalation studies for drugs with serious side-effect profiles might be possible when using sFLC measurements.

Pratt et al. analysed the changes in sFLC concentrations after autologous peripheral blood stem cell transplantation in 19 patients.[3] Before transplant (but after induction chemotherapy), 11 of the patients had elevated levels of the tumour-produced FLC with abnormal κ/λ ratios. In all patients with associated intact monoclonal immunoglobulins, tumour-produced FLC concentrations fell within 48 hours (median half-life 4.3 days) and faster than the monoclonal paraprotein (median half-life 14 days). The rate of fall and range of reduction of FLCs varied between individual patients indicating different tumour killing rates/chemosensitivity *(Figures 13.4 - 13.9).*

Several studies have reported similar observations in patients during induction chemotherapy. Hassoun et al.,[8,9] assessed the usefulness of FLCs as an early predictor of final responses in patients with symptomatic MM. 37 patients had abnormal FLC k/λ ratios at baseline (i.e. < 0.26 or > 1.65). Normalization of the FLC ratio after cycle 1 or 2 occurred in 7 out of 15 patients who achieved near complete remission or complete remission, and only in one of 22 patients who achieved partial remission, stable disease, or progression of disease (p=0.003). They concluded that, ***"assessment of the free light chain ratio after two cycles may become an important milestone in the decision-making for patients with MM undergoing initial therapy"***. Since the aim of therapy is to achieve near complete remission or complete remission, the addition of alternative drugs might be advisable at an early stage of treatment in patients whose FLC k/λ ratios remain abnormal.

Cavallo et al.,[10] studied 140 patients, comparing early sFLCs responses with subsequent outcome. They found that normalization of sFLCs increased the probability of subsequent complete remission when assessed both at 30 days (p=0.002) and prior to PBSCT (p=0.001) *(Figure 13.12).* They also observed that sFLCs were highly correlated with cytogenetic abnormalities and MM staging - the 2 most important prognostic factors for event-free survival and overall survival. They concluded that ***"sFLCs can be expected to have a major independent predictive power for outcome with longer follow-up".*** Comparison was also made between sFLC responses and functional positron emission tomography (PET). There was a high correlation between the two measurements for predicting outcome (p<0.002) but the PET scans normalised faster.[11]

Das et al.[12] studied sFLC concentration kinetics in patients receiving Bortezomib (Velcade). Six of 8 patients showed a response to treatment by EBMT/Blade criteria (>25% fall in paraprotein). In 3 of these patients the tumour sFLC showed a fall and rapid recovery within 10-20 days of a treatment cycle. These patients were monitored over multiple treatment cycles and showed repeated falls and rises in sFLC co-incident with treatment *(Figure 13.13).* When seen, the relapse of sFLC was rapid with a doubling time of less than 10 days. This may correspond to the biological half-life of proteosome inhibition and recovery rather than tumour killing and regrowth. Such patterns of tumour response can only be observed with frequent sampling and the use of tumour markers that are rapidly cleared from the serum. In comparison, intact immunoglobulin monoclonal proteins did not show the same peaks and troughs. Generally the sFLC levels indicated disease response earlier than the immunoglobulin assays. They concluded that monitoring patients with sFLC provided an opportunity to

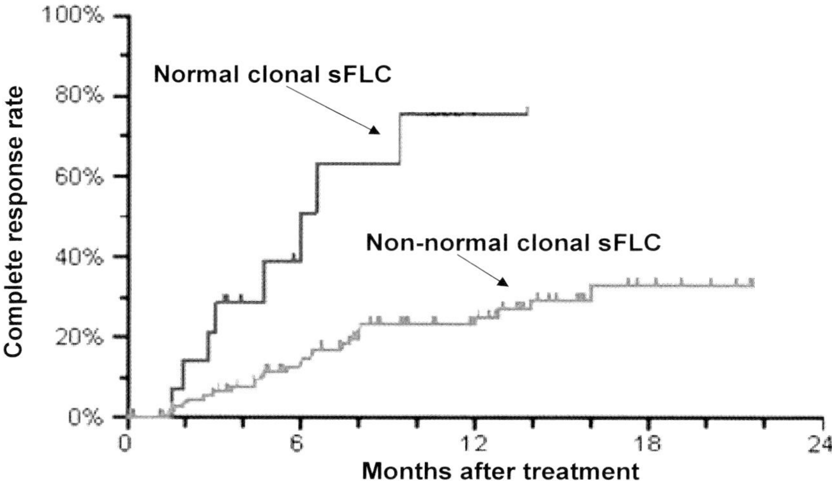

Figure 13.12. Normalisation of sFLCs prior to PBSCT in MM is a good indication of subsequent complete response after treatment. (Courtesy of G Tricot).[10]

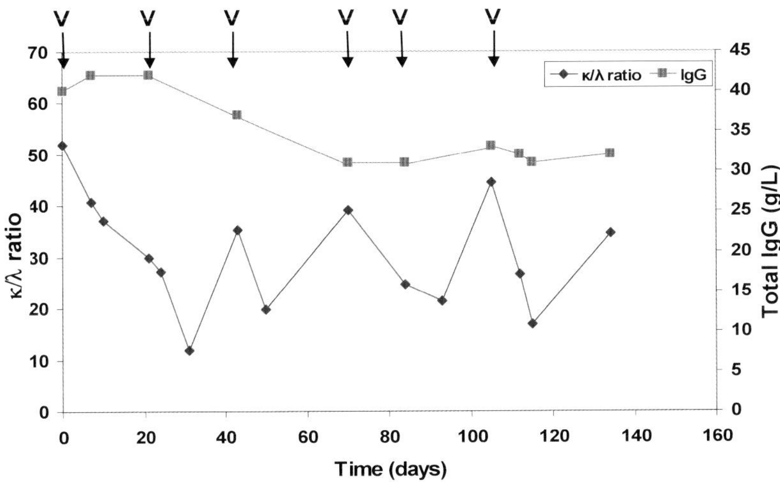

Figure 13.13. Changes in sFLC concentrations during 6 cycles of Bortezomib showing rapid responses to treatment and subsequent relapses. (Courtesy of GP Mead).

follow the kinetics of tumour kill, which is obscured by the slow clearance of intact immunoglobulin monoclonal proteins. They added that sFLC measurements indicated early tumour responses that could allow relevant changes of treatment strategy. This may have major bearing on cost of treatment and utilisation of resources. Similar observations have been made by others using Bortezomib.[13]

Summary:

1. The half-life of sFLCs is dominated by the glomerular filtration rate.
2. The 2-6 hour half-life allows tumour cell killing rates, residual disease and early tumour relapse to be observed during treatment.
3. sFLC responses following chemotherapy might allow rapid selection of effective drugs or drug combinations in refractory patients.
4. Early changes in sFLCs are indicative of long-term outcome in MM.

References

1. **Bidart J-M, Thuillier F, Augereau C, Chalas J, Daver A, Jacob N, Labrousse F, Voitot H.** Kinetics of Serum Tumor Marker Concentrations and Usefulness in Clinical Monitoring. Clin Chem 1999; **45**: 1695-1707.

2. **Bradwell AR, Mead G, Carr-Smith H, Galvin G, Pratt G.** Efficacy of high dose myeloma treatment and response to individual chemotherapy agents in myeloma is indicated by changes in serum free light chain concentrations. Blood 2003; **102** (11): A2547.

3. **Pratt G, Mead GP, Godfrey KR, Ying H, Evans ND, Chappell MJ, Lovell R, Bradwell AR.** The tumour kinetics of multiple myeloma following autologous stem cell transplantation as assessed by measuring serum-free light chains. Leukaemia and Lymphoma 2006; **47** (1): 21-28.

4. **Randers E, Erlandsen EJ.** Serum Cystatin C as an Endogenous Marker of Renal Function - a Review. Clin Chem Lab Med 1999; **37** (4): 389-395

5. **Keevil BG, Kilpatrick ES, Nichols SP, Mayor PW.** Biological variation of cystatin C: implications for the assessment of glomerular filtration. Clin Chem 1998; **44** (7): 1535-1539.

6. **Coll E, Botey A, Alvarez. L, Poch E, Quintó L, Saurina A, Vera M, Piera C, Darnell A.** Serum Cystatin C as a New Marker for Noninvasive Estimation of Glomerular Filtration Rate and as a Marker for Early Renal Impairment. Am J Kid Dis 2000; **36** (1): 29-34.

7. **Patten PE, Ahsan G, Kazmi M, Fields PA, Chick GW, Jones RR, Bradwell AR, Schey SA.** The early use of the serum free light chain assay in patients with relapsed refractory myeloma receiving treatment with thalidomide analogue (CC-4047). Blood 2003; **102** (11): A1640.

8. **Hassoun H, Reich L, Klimek VM, Dhodapkar M, Cohen A, Kewalramani T, Riedel ER, Hedvat CV, Teruya-Feldstein J, Filippa DA, Fleisher M, Nimer SD, Comenzo RL.** The Serum Free Light Chain Ratio after One or Two Cycles of Treatment Is Highly Predictive of the Magnitude of Final Response in Patients Undergoing Initial Treatment for Multiple Myeloma. Blood 2005; **106** (11): 3481: 972a.

9. **Hassoun H, Reich L, Klimek VM, Dhodapkar M, Cohen A, Kewalramani T, Zimman R, Drake L, Riedel ER, Hedvat CV, Teruya-Feldstein J, Filippa DA, Fleisher M, Nimer SD, Comenzo RL.** Doxorubicin and dexamethosone followed by thalidomide and dexamethasone is an effective well tolerated initial therapy for multiple myeloma. Br J Haem 2006; **132**: 155-161.

10. **Cavallo F, Rasmussen E, Zangari M, Tricot G, Fender B, Fox M, Burns M, Barlogie B.** Serum Free-Lite Chain (sFLC) Assay in Multiple Myeloma (MM): Clinical Correlates and Prognostic Implications in Newly Diagnosed MM Patients Treated with Total Therapy 2 or 3 (TT2/3). Blood 2005; **106** (11): 3490: 974a.

11. **Walker R, Rasmussen E, Cavallo F, Jones-Jackson L, Anaissie E, Alpe T, Epstein J, an Rhee F, Zangari M, Tricot G, Shaughnessy J, Barlogie B.** Correlation of Suppression of FDG PET Uptake with Serum Free Light Chain Levels - Both FDG PET-CT and Serum Clonal Free Light Chain Response Precede and Predict the Likelihood of Subsequent Complete Remission in Newly Diagnosed Multiple Myeloma. Blood 2005; **106** (11): 3493: 975a.

12. **Das M, Mead GP, Sreekanth V, Anderson J, Blair S, Howe T, Cavet J, Liakopoulou E.** Serum Free Light Chain (SFLC) Concentration Kinetics in Patients Receiving Bortezomib: Temporary Inhibition of Protein Synthesis and Early Biomarker for Disease Response. Blood 2005; **106** (11): 5094: 355b.

13. **Kyrtsonis M-C, Sachanas S, Vassilakopoulos TP, Kafassi N, Tzenou T, Papadogiannis A, Kalpadakis C, Antoniadis AG, Dimopoulou MN, Angelopoulou MK, Siakantaris MP, Dimitriadou EM, Kokoris SI, Plata E, Tsaftaridis P, Panayiotidis P, Pangalis GA.** Bortezomib in Patients with Relapsed-Refractory Multiple Myeloma (MM). Clinical Observations. Blood 2005; **106** (11): 5193: 382b.

Test questions

1. What is the ideal serum half-life of a tumour marker?
2. Will sFLC assays help with drug selection decisions in MM?
3. Do early falls in sFLCs after induction therapy relate to response rates?

Answers

1. The shorter the half-life the better, provided sufficient amounts remain for accurate detection (page 104).
2. While this has yet to be evaluated, failure to respond to a drug is apparent earlier using sFLC measurements. More appropriate drugs can then be selected (page 112).
3. Yes (page 113-114).

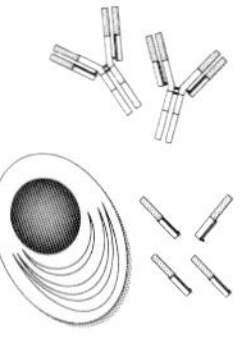

Chapter 14

Free light chains and nephrotoxicity in myeloma

14.1. Introduction

30% of MM patients at disease presentation have significant renal impairment (serum creatinine >1.5mg/dL or >130μmol/L).[1,2] In most of these cases the renal failure is reversible but in >30% permanent dialysis is required. In 75% of this group the renal failure and MM present within a month of each other. While other factors such as dehydration, hypercalcaemia and medication are involved, FLCs remain the most potent cause of complete renal failure in these patients. Furthermore, there is a 30% mortality within 2 months of diagnosis.

This chapter discusses the normal renal handling of FLCs, their role in renal failure, clinical case studies and current management strategies such as plasma exchange. Finally, the role of serum FLC measurements is discussed and the potential use of 'protein-leaking' dialysers to reduce long term renal damage.

14.2. Free light chain clearance and metabolism

In normal individuals, sFLCs are rapidly cleared by the kidneys depending upon their molecular size *(Figure 14.1 and Chapter 3)*. Monomeric FLCs, characteristically κ, are cleared in 2-4 hours at 40% of the glomerular filtration rate. Dimeric FLCs, typically λ, are cleared in 3-6 hours at 20% of the glomerular filtration rate, while larger polymers are cleared more slowly. Removal is prolonged to 2-3 days in MM patients who are in complete renal failure when FLCs are removed by the liver and other tissues.[3-7] In contrast, IgG has a normal serum half-life of 21 days that is not affected by renal impairment.

After filtration by the glomeruli, FLCs enter the proximal tubules and bind to brush-border membranes via low-affinity, high-capacity receptors called cubulins (gp280).[8] Binding provokes internalisation of the FLCs and their subsequent metabolism. The concentration of FLCs leaving the proximal tubules, therefore, depends upon the amounts in the glomerular filtrate, competition for binding uptake from other proteins and the absorptive capacity of the tubular cells. A reduction in the glomerular filtration rate increases serum FLC concentrations so that more is filtered by the remaining functioning nephrons. Subsequently, and with increasing renal failure, hyperfiltering

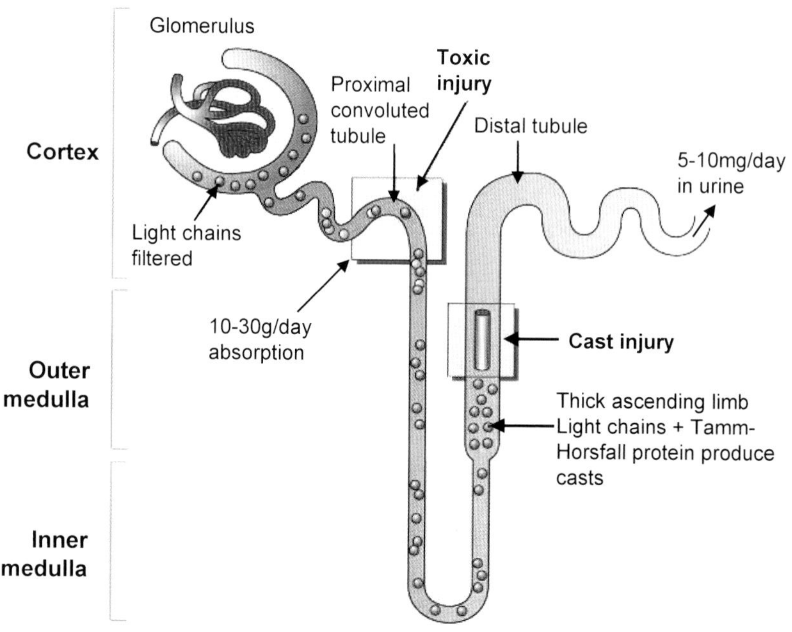

Figure 14.1. Renal injury caused by FLCs. (Courtesy of R Johnson and J Feehally).[8]

glomeruli leak albumin and other proteins which compete with FLCs for absorption thereby causing more to enter the distal tubules.

FLCs entering the distal tubule usually bind to uromucoid (Tamm-Horsfall protein). This is the dominant protein in normal urine and is thought to be important in preventing ascending urinary infections. It is a glycoprotein (85kDa) that aggregates into high molecular weight polymers of 20-30 units. Interestingly, it contains a short peptide motif that has a high affinity for FLCs.[9] Together, the two proteins form waxy casts that are characteristically found in acute renal failure associated with LCMM *(Figure 14.2)*.[10-12] The casts obstruct tubular fluid flow, leading to disruption of the basement membrane and interstitial damage. Rising concentrations of sFLCs are filtered by the remaining functioning nephrons leading to a vicious cycle of accelerating renal damage with further increases in sFLCs. This may explain why some MM patients, without apparent pre-existing renal impairment, suddenly develop catastrophic and irreversible renal injury and renal failure. The process is aggrevated by other factors such as dehydration, diuretics, hypercalcaemia, infections and nephrotoxic drugs.

Monoclonal FLCs can also cause renal impairment by other mechanisms. Chapters 15 and 17 describe monoclonal FLCs in AL amyloidosis and LCDD. In addition, FLCs may be found in the proximal tubular cells as crystalline inclusions when associated with acquired Fanconi's syndrome.[2,14] These additional mechanisms may contribute to both acute myeloma kidney and chronic renal failure *(Chapter 20)*.

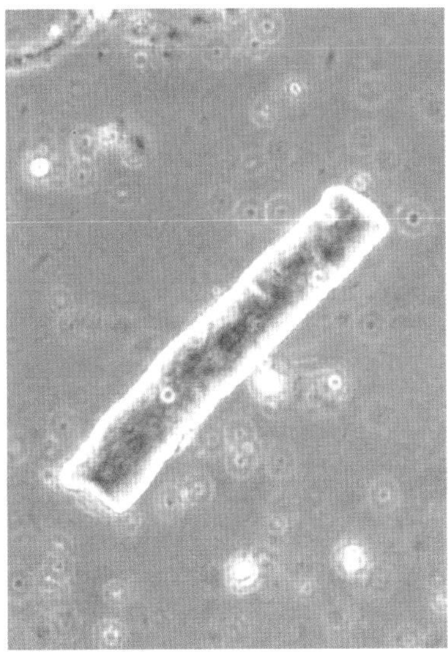

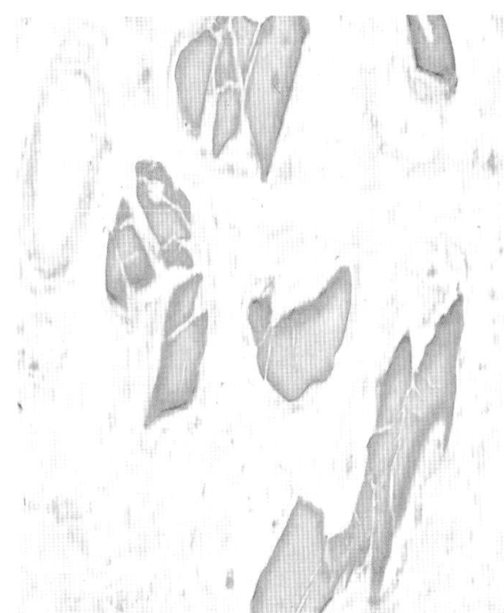

Figure 14.2. (A). A waxy cast in urine. **(B).** Classic fractured casts in the distal tubules in a patient with acute renal failure from LCMM, stained with an immunoperoxidase labelled antibody. (Courtesy of R Johnson and J Feehally).[8]

14.3. Nephrotoxicity of free light chains

Serum FLC concentrations are abnormal in >95% of patients with MM *(Figure 10.3)* and have a wide range of concentrations, but their inherent toxicity also varies considerably. This was elegantly shown by Sanders and Brooker using isolated rat nephrons. The toxicity is in part related to binding with Tamm-Horsfall protein.[10-13]

In spite of much effort to show otherwise, particular molecular charge and/or κ or λ type are not now considered relevant to FLC toxicity. Furthermore, highly polymerised FLCs (a frequent finding in MM - *Chapter 9*) are probably not nephrotoxic because they cannot readily pass through the glomeruli. This may partly account for the lack of renal damage in some patients who have very high serum FLC concentrations.

The amounts of serum FLCs necessary to cause renal impairment was recently studied by Nowrousian et al.[15]. They showed that the median serum concentrations associated with overflow proteinuria (and hence potential for tubular damage) was 113mg/L for κ and for 278mg/L for λ. These are approximately 5-to 10-fold above the normal serum concentrations and presumably relate to the maximum tubular reabsorption capacity of the proximal tubules. Since the normal daily production is ~500mg, increases to ~5g/day are likely to be nephrotoxic in many patients.

As renal impairment develops, progressive increases occur in both the tumour FLCs and the polyclonal non-tumour FLCs (*Figures 8.2, 10.1-10.2 and 10.4).* Concentrations of monoclonal FLCs below 300mg/L are rarely associated with apparent renal impairment as judged by normal levels of the non-tumour FLC *(Figure 10.4).* These concentrations are somewhat higher than those observed by Nowrousian et al. in patients with renal impairment, but are in the same general range.

There have been several urine studies that have related urine FLC excretion rates to renal impairment. Typically, the associated renal impairment rises with increasing urine FLCs. One study showed that 7%, 17% and 39% of patients had renal impairment with excretions rates of <0.005g/day, 0.005-2.0g/day, and >2g/day, respectively.[2] However, FLC excretion is a indicator of renal damage in addition to its cause.

The causal relationship between serum FLC concentrations and renal impairment is illustrated in 3 patients below *(Figures 14.3 to 14.5)*. In each case, urine FLC concentrations were low and not indicative of the underlying renal deterioration.

The patient shown in Figure 14.3 had developed MM expressing IgAλ and λ FLCs, 3 years earlier. She had a good initial response to VAD but was frail. Over a 7-month period, her serum λ FLC levels increased from 1,500 to 2,800 mg/L, then 4,500 mg/L and finally 15,000mg/L, while serum creatinine increased slightly to 120 μmol/L. Her medication was not changed from thalidomide, cyclophosphamide and pulsed dexamethasone on account of her frailty. Unfortunately, the sharp rise in serum FLCs led to acute renal failure which was apparent one month later. She failed to respond to therapy and died shortly after.

Figure 14.4 illustrates a patient who developed acute renal failure that responded to chemotherapy and haemodialysis. As in Figure 14.3, the serum FLC concentrations were a sensitive indicator of impending renal failure and concentrations appeared to reach a threshold before acute renal failure developed. Although renal function was deteriorating at the 4th month, the patient felt well and declined treatment, only to present in renal failure one month later. The potential seriousness of the high FLC concentrations had not been fully appreciated. She was given VAD and put on haemodialysis for 6 weeks. This produced a good response of the MM but only partial renal recovery.

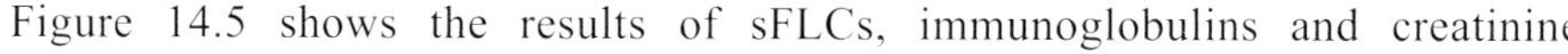

Figure 14.5 shows the results of sFLCs, immunoglobulins and creatinine

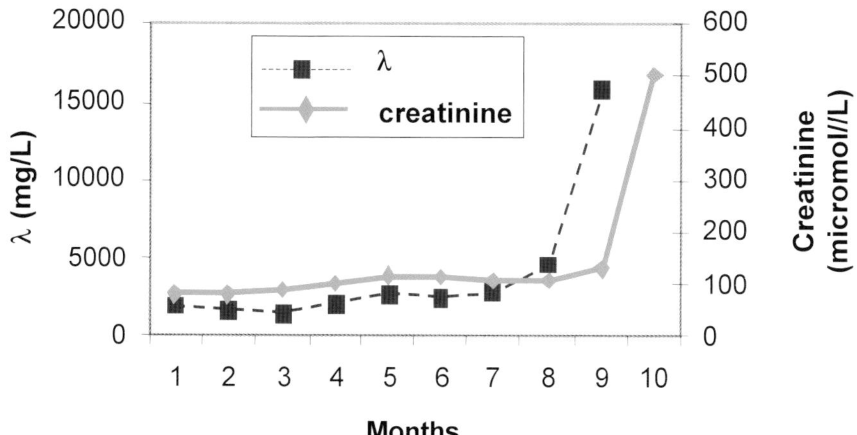

Figure 14.3. Serum FLC concentrations in a patient with IgAλ and λ FLCs during development of acute renal failure. (Courtesy of S Abdalla, St Mary's Hospital, London).

measurements in another patient over a 30-week period. Total protein and IgG tests indicated stable disease during the first 18 weeks of monitoring. However, the serum creatinine increased from 12 to 30mg/L (130 to 240 μmol/L). sFLCs measurements showed unexpectedly high κ concentrations at 500 mg/L with a κ/λ ratio of 4.04, in spite of no FLCs in the urine. It was considered that the high FLC concentrations might be causing renal damage so chemotherapy was commenced (VED: vincristine, epirubicin and dexamethasone). Over the ensuing two months the serum κ and serum creatinine almost returned to normal concentrations.

14.4. Removal of free light chains by plasma exchange

Results from these 3 patients indicate that the pre-renal load of FLCs is an important factor in renal toxicity. It seems logical that renal recovery might occur if serum FLC levels were rapidly lowered. Assessment of the pre-renal load of FLCs and, if present, their removal by, plasma exchange or haemodialysis might improve the current poor outcome of these patients.

Several early studies indicated renal function improvement using plasma exchange. For example, in 1988, Zucchelli et al., compared MM patients on peritoneal dialysis (control group) with plasma exchange (and haemodialysis in some patients).[16] Only 2 of 14 in the control group had improved renal function compared with 13 of 15 in the plasma exchange arm, and survival was better ($P<0.01$). However, peritoneal dialysis is less effective than haemodialysis for removing FLCs *(Chapter 20)* so selection of the patients for plasma exchange was not ideal.

These early successes were not repeated in subsequent controlled trials. Johnson et al., in 1990, compared 10 patients on forced diuresis with 11 who had additional plasma

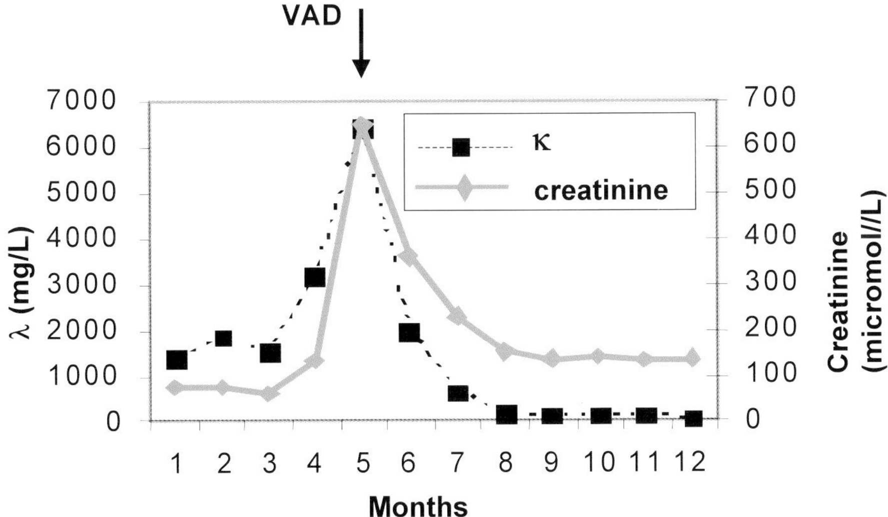

Figure 14.4. Serum FLC concentrations in a patient with LCMM during development of acute renal failure and subsequent response to VAD. (Courtesy of S Abdalla, London).

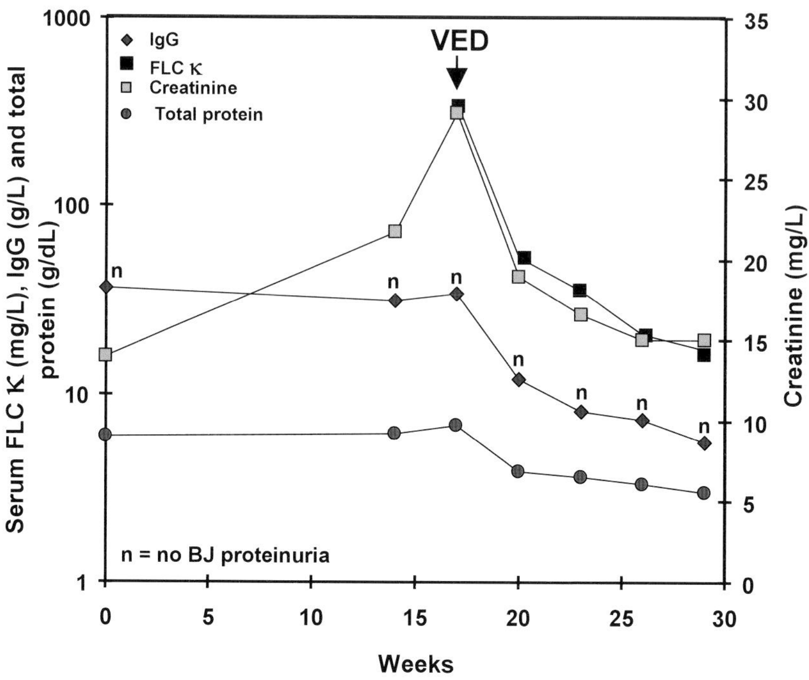

Figure 14.5. λ FLCs causing renal impairment in a patient who appeared to have stable disease from IgGλ measurements. Satisfactory improvement in renal function followed chemotherapy. VED: vincristine, epirubicin and dexamethasone. (Courtesy of MR Nowrousian).

exchange and found no difference in outcome.[17] Most recently, a large series was reported by Clark et al.[18] Half of 97 patients who were on chemotherapy, haemodialysis or a combination of the two, were randomly allocated to receive plasma exchange. Again, there was no statistically significant benefit from plasma exchange. Currently, the MERIT trial in the UK is recruiting patients in another attempt to determine the role of plasma exchange.

14.5. Model of FLC removal by plasma exchange and haemodialysis

In order to try and understand the potential effectiveness of plasma exchange we developed a compartmental mathematical model that was applicable to patients being treated for MM and renal failure.[19] The following parameters were considered:- sFLC concentrations in MM at clinical presentation; normal monomeric κ and dimeric λ clearance rates; partition of sFLC between vascular and extravascular compartments (including oedema fluid); flow of FLCs between compartments; half-life of sFLC in renal failure, sFLC production rates, and tumour killing rates with chemotherapy. The model was interrogated for various treatment strategies including a plasma exchange protocol of 3 litres x6 over a 2-week period, and haemodialysis using different time periods and different protein-leaking dialyzers *(Chapter 20)*.

In renal failure the half-life of sFLCs is approximately 3 days. Assuming a starting concentration of 10g/L, it would take approximately 20 days for the FLCs to be metabolised assuming complete tumour killing with the first chemotherapy dose *(Figure 14.6: Baseline 100% kill)*. More realistically, 25% of the tumour might be destroyed per day by aggressive chemotherapy resulting in a slower FLC reduction *(Figure 14.6: red line)*. Addition of the plasma exchange procedure had a modest additional effect on the FLC removal rates compared with the 25% tumour kill rate per day *(Figure 14.6)*. The rapid reductions in serum FLC concentrations during the procedure and their subsequent re-entry from the extra-vascular to the intra-vascular compartment can be seen.

The results from the model calculations suggest that the procedure may not be very effective. Anecdotal reports on individual patients undergoing plasma exchange also indicate little reduction of FLC concentrations during plasma exchange. This can be explained by on-going high production rates and the re-entry of FLCs from extravascular compartments (including oedema fluid). Accurate measurements of sFLCs during plasma exchange should allow a proper assessment of clearance rates and amounts. This might help resolve the continuing doubt about the effectiveness of the procedure.

14.6. Removal of free light chains by haemodialysis

As an alternative to plasma exchange, sFLCs might be removed more effectively by haemodialysis provided the pore sizes of the membranes are large enough. Conventional

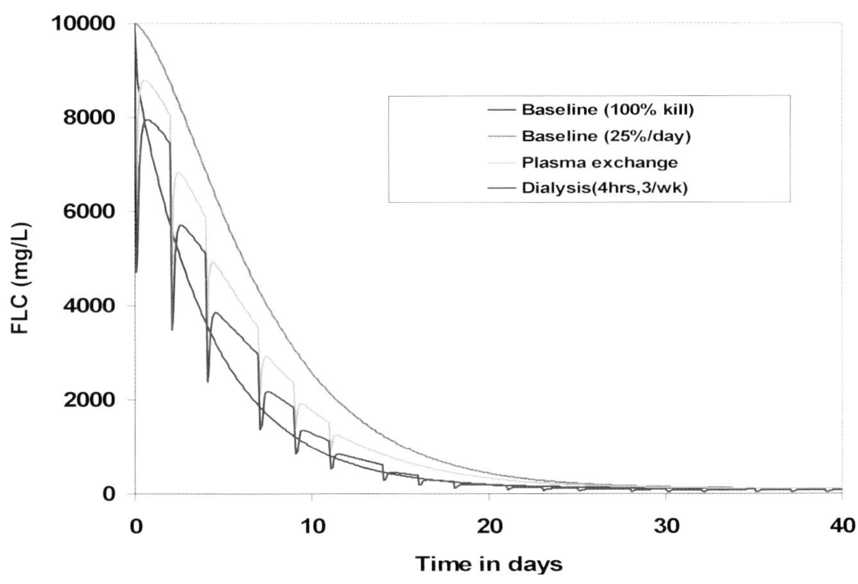

Figure 14.6. Calculated disappearance of κ sFLCs in a patient with LCMM by 100% (immediate) tumour killing and 25% per day. The effect of plasma exchange and of haemodialysis (4hr: x3/week) on FLC concentrations, using 'protein-leaking' dialysers, are shown (courtesy of N Evans and M Chappell).

dialysers have a molecular weight cut-off around 15-20kDa so the filtration efficiency for FLCs is very low. However, some of the new "protein-leaking" dialysers have much larger pores.[20] Furthermore, haemo-dialfiltration is more effective at removing small protein molecules than haemodialysis. Indeed, there is a report of a patient with AL amyloidosis and end-stage renal failure who appeared to have an improved survival when haemo-dialfiltration was instigated.[21] However, there is currently inadequate clinical data to provide a clear conclusion in amyloidosis patients.

There is some published data on the removal of polyclonal FLCs by dialysis. In a study of patients with chronic renal failure, Bradwell et al. found that over a 4-hour dialysis period using a polysulphonate membrane, 60% of κ and 37% of λ molecules were removed. *(Chapter 20, Figure 20.7).* While serum concentrations were much lower than in MM, the results suggested that haemodialysis may be more efficient for FLC removal than previously thought and possibly more effective than plasma exchange *(Figure 14.6)*.[20] Model calculations indicated that the prolonged use of 'protein-leaking' dialysers could reduce κ sFLC concentrations to less than 0.5g/L in 2-3 days with ~95% of the sFLC removed. Because dimeric λ molecules are considerably larger they are removed more slowly *(Figure 14.7)*.[19]

We have assessed the utility of various dialysers for serum FLC removal in a few patients with MM. Figure 14.8 compares the reduction in sFLC in a patient with κ LCMM over 4-hour haemodialysis periods using 3 different dialysers. The Toray BK-F 2.1 dialyser (super-flux) was more efficient than the BBraun HIPeS 1.8 dialyser (normal, high-flux membrane) while the Gambro dialyser was the most efficient. Figure 14.9 shows the very rapid removal of λ FLCs in another MM patient using the Gambro HCO dialyser. Provided concurrent chemotherapy is effective, such procedures might quickly

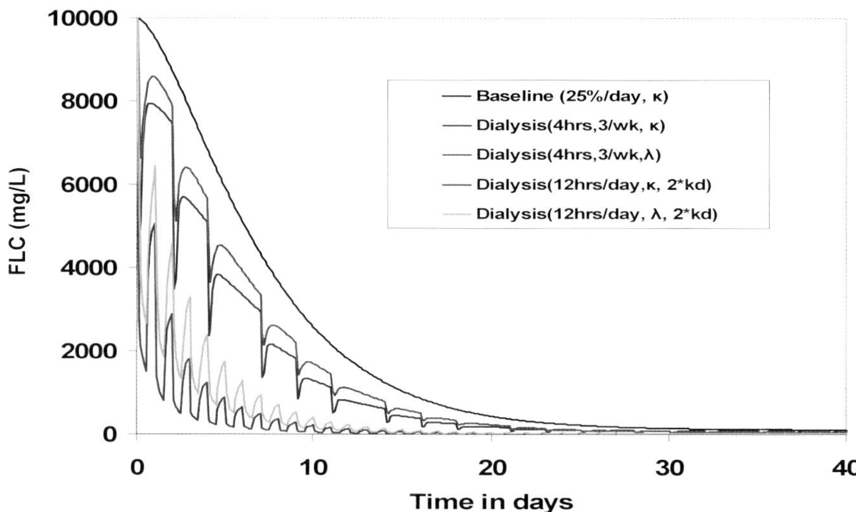

Figure 14.7. Calculated clearance of serum FLCs with 25%/day tumour killing, κ and λ removal using protein-leaking membranes for 4 hours, x3 per week and 12 hours/day (courtesy of N Evans and M Chappell).

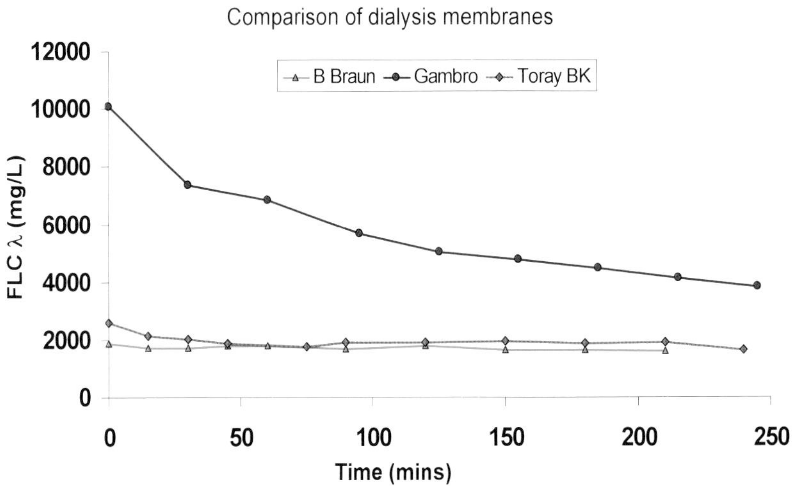

Figure 14.8. Reductions of serum FLC concentrations during 4-hour dialysis periods using different dialysers in 3 patients. Routine high-flux (BBraun 1.8); super-flux (Toray BK-F 2.1) and a 'protein-leaking' dialyser (Gambro HCO 1100).

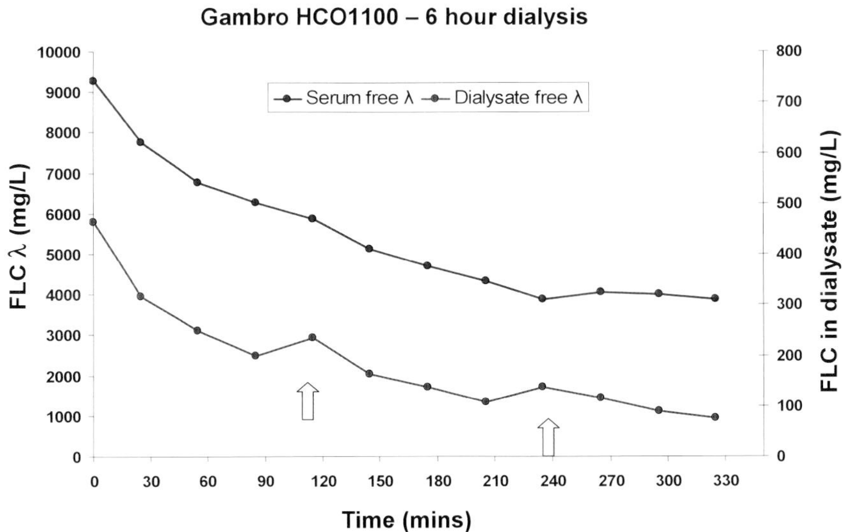

Figure 14.9. Concentrations of λ FLCs in the serum and dialysate fluid of a patient with acute renal failure due to LCMM undergoing dialysis with the Gambro HCO 1100 'protein-leaking' dialyser. The dialyser was renewed (arrows) as FLC leakage slowed.

prevent further FLC renal damage and allow renal recovery. These and other 'protein-leaking' dialysers need to be assessed in a clinical trial of patients with acute myeloma kidney since renal recovery is possible in the long term.[22]

It should be noted that peritoneal dialysis does not remove FLCs efficiently *(Chapter 20).* Presumably, this is because the volume of exchanged fluid is much lower than in haemodialysis.

Summary: Serum free light chains:-

1. Cause renal impairment in approximately 30% of patients with MM.
2. Should be measured in all MM patients to identify those at risk of renal damage.
3. Are not adequately removed by plasma exchange.
4. Can be removed by haemodialysis using "protein-leaking" dialysers.

References

1. **Knudsen LM, Hjorth M, Hippe E**. Renal failure in multiple myeloma: reversibility and impact on prognosis. European Jounal of Haematology 2000; **65**: 175-181.

2. **Blade J.** Management of Renal, Hematologic, and Infectious Complications. In: Myeloma: Biology and Management 3rd Edition. Eds: Malpas JS, Bergsagel DE, Kyle RA, Anderson KC. Pubs Saunders. 2004.

3. **Waldmann TA, Strober WS, Mogielnicki RP**. The Renal Handling of Low Molecular Weight Proteins II. Disorders of Serum Protein Catabolism in Patients with Tubular Proteinuria, the Nephrotic Syndrome or Uraemia. J Clin Invest 1972; **51**: 2162-2174.

4. **Wochner RD, Strober W, Waldmann TA.** The role of the kidney in the catabolism of Bence Jones proteins and immunoglobulin fragments. J Exp Med 1967; **126**: 207-221.

5. **Miettinen TA, Kekki M.** Effect of impaired hepatic and renal function on Bence Jones protein catabolism in human subjects. Clin Chim Acta, 1967; **18**: 395-407.

6. **Abraham GN, Waterhouse C.** Evidence for defective immunoglobulin metabolism in severe renal insufficiency. Amer J Med Sci 1974; **268**: 227-233.

7. **Russo L, Bakris GL, Comper WD.** Renal handling of Albumin: A Critical Review of Basic Concepts and Perspective. Am J Kidney Dis 2002; **39**: 899-919.

8. **Winearls CG**. Myeloma kidney. In Comprehensive Clinical Nephrology; 2nd Edition Chapt 17. Eds Johnson RJ, Feehally J. Pub: Mosby 2003.

9. **Ying W-Z, Sanders PW.** Mapping the Binding Domain of Immunoglobulin Light Chains for Tamm-Horsfall Protein. Am J Path 2001; **158**: 1859-1866.

10. **Kyle RA.** Monoclonal Proteins and Renal Disease. Ann Rev Med 1994; **45**: 71-77.

11. **Winearls CG**. Acute myeloma kidney. Kidney Int 1995; **48**: 1347-1361.

12. **Alexanian R, Barlogie B, Dixon D.** Renal failure in multiple myeloma. Pathogenesis and prognostic implications. Arch Intern Med 1990; **150**: 1693-1695.

13. **Sanders PW, Brooker BB.** Pathobiology of Cast Nephropathy from Human Bence Jones Proteins. J Clin Invest 1992; **89**: 630-639.

14. **Sanders PW, Brooker BB, Bishop JB, Cheung HC.** Mechanism of intranephronal proteinaceous cast formation by low molecular weight proteins. J Clin Invest 1990; **85**: 570-576.

15. **Nowrousian MR, Brandhorst D, Sammet C, Kellert M, Daniels R, Schuett P, Poser M, Mueller S, Ebeling P, Welt A, Bradwell AR, Buttkereit U, Opalka B, Flasshove M, Moritz T, Seeber S.** Serum Free Light Chain Analysis and Urine Immunofixation Electrophoresis in Patients with Multiple Myeloma. Clin Cancer Res 2005; **11** (24): 8706-8714.

16. **Zucchelli P, Pasquali S, Cagnoli L, Ferrari G.** Controlled plasma exchange trial in acute renal failure due to multiple myeloma. Kidney Int 1988; **33**: 1175-1180.

17. **Johnson WJ, Kyle RA, Pineda AA, O'Brian PC, Holly KE.** Treatment of multiple myeloma associated with renal failure. Arch Intern Med 1990; **150**: 863-869.

18. Clarke WF, Stewart AK, Rock GA, Sternbach M, Sutton DM, Barrett BJ, Heidenheim AP, Garg AX, Churchill DN. Plasma Exchange when myeloma presents as acute renal failure. Anals of Int Med 2005; **143**: 777-785.

19. Bradwell AR, Evans ND, Chappell MJ, Cockwell P, Reid SD, Harrison J, Hutchinson C, Mead GP. Rapid removal of free light chains from serum by hemodialysis for patients with myeloma kidney. Blood 2005; **106** (11): 3482: 972a.

20. Ward RA. Protein-Leaking Membranes for Hemodialysis: A New Class of Membranes in Search of an Application. J Am Soc Nephrol 2005; **16**: 2421-2430.

21. Machiguchi T, Tamura T, Yoshida H. Efficacy of haemodiafiltration treatment with PEPA dialysis membranes in plasma free light chain removal in a patient with primary amyloidosis. Nephrol Dial Transplant 2002; **17**: 1689-1691.

22. Tauro S, Clark FJ, Duncan N, Lipkin G, Richards N, Mahendra P. Recovery of renal function after autologous stem cell transplantation in myeloma patients with end-stage renal failure. Bone Marrow Trans 2002; **30**: 471-473.

Test questions

1. *What percentage of patients with MM have renal impairment at presentation?*
2. *What protein binds FLCs in the distal tubules?*
3. *What is the benefit of plasma exchange in acute myeloma kidney?*
4. *Are haemodialysis membranes porous to free light chains?*

Answers

1. *30% (page 117).*
2. *Uromucoid or Tamm-Horsfall protein (page 118).*
3. *Clinical trials suggest there is minimal benefit (page 122).*
4. *Yes, particularly the protein-leaking dialysers (page 124).*

Section 2B. Diseases with monoclonal light chain deposition

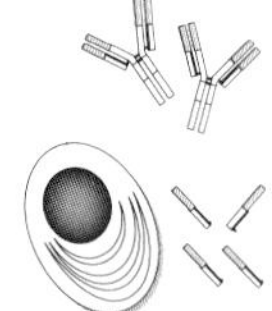

Chapter 15

AL Amyloidosis

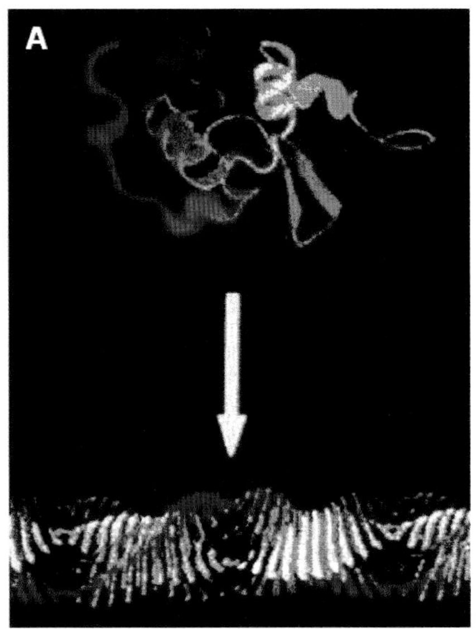

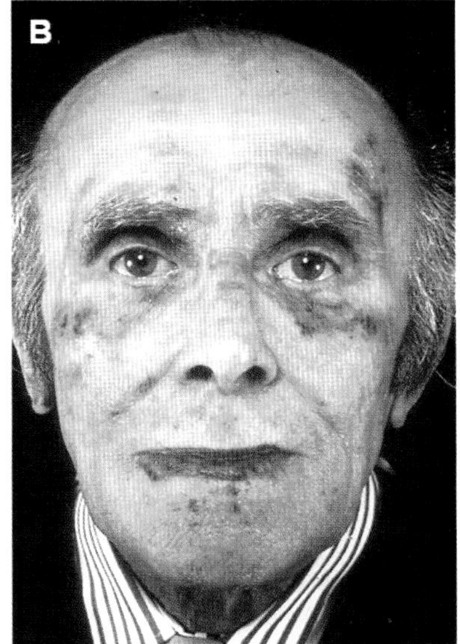

Figure 15.1. AL amyloidosis showing (A) formation of amyloid fibrils from FLC domains and (B) classic facial features with periorbital purpura. (Courtesy of PN Hawkins).

15.1. Introduction

AL amyloidosis (primary systemic amyloidosis) is a protein conformation disorder characterized by the accumulation of monoclonal FLCs, or their fragments, as amyloid deposits (*Figure 15.1*). Typically, these patients present with heart or renal failure but the skin, peripheral nerves and other organs may be involved (*Figures 15.2 - 15.3*).[1-4]

Median survival is little more than 12 months although patients who respond well to chemotherapy may live many years. A slowly growing clone of plasma cells secretes the monoclonal FLCs that are typically λ type (κ to λ frequency: 1:2). It is of interest that clonal plasma cells from patients with renal deposits more commonly have the *6α Vλ*

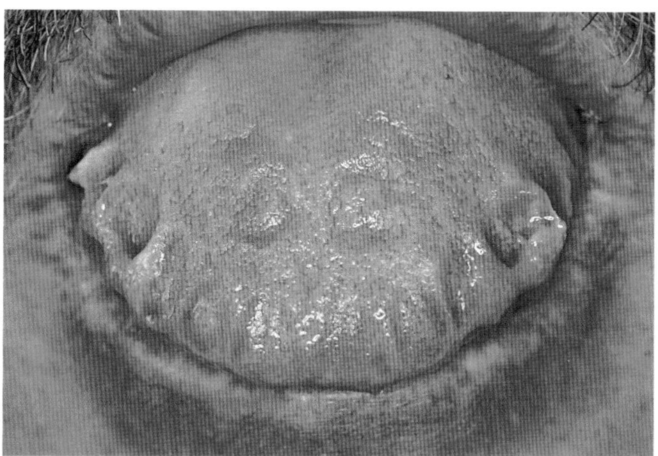

Figure 15.2. AL amyloidosis showing macroglossia that occurs in 20% of patients. (Courtesy of PN Hawkins).

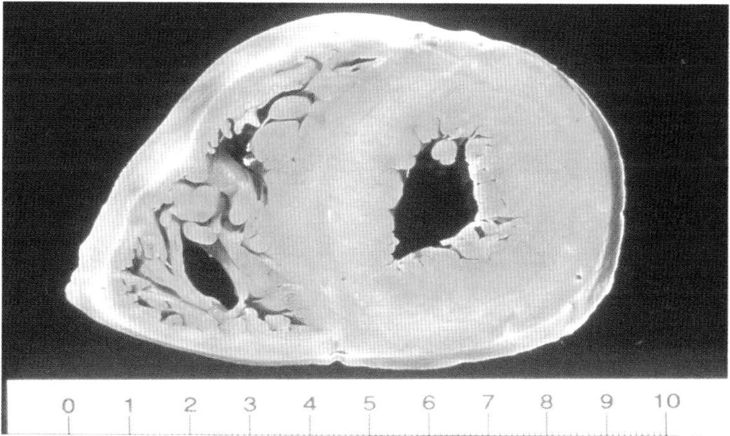

Figure 15.3. AL amyloidosis in the heart showing thickening of the left ventricular walls leading to heart failure. (Courtesy of PN Hawkins).

light chain, variable region genes, while those with cardiac and multisystem disease have the *1c, 2α2 and 3r Vλ* genes, although associations with other genes may be found.[5]

AL amyloidosis is one-fifth as common as MM with an annual incidence of 9 per million, ie., there are approximately 600 new patients per year in the UK and 2,500 in the USA. The median age of presentation is 70 years of age and it is rare before 40. Men represent between 60% and 65% of patients and less than 10% have MM.

The presence of a monoclonal protein in the serum and urine of patients is an important diagnostic feature and is a common finding. However, the underlying monoclonal gammopathies can be subtle and are undetectable in 5-20% of patients, depending upon the sensitivity of the electrophoretic method. Figure 15.4 shows the serum abnormalities in a patient with AL amyloidosis. SPE indicates a typical nephrotic pattern (low albumin, elevated α2 and low γ fraction), but there is no observable monoclonal spike. sIFE shows some polyclonal immunoglobulin in the γ fraction and a small monoclonal λ protein that migrates in the β/γ region. This band is too small to be quantified by scanning densitometry of the SPE gel since it is undetectable against the background proteins.

Figure 15.5 shows the UPE from the same patient. It contains a considerable amount of protein, particularly albumin and there is a small monoclonal spike. IFE indicates a monoclonal λ protein against a background of polyclonal κ and λ FLCs. The monoclonal band is difficult to quantify by UPE and is of modest use for the purpose of disease monitoring.

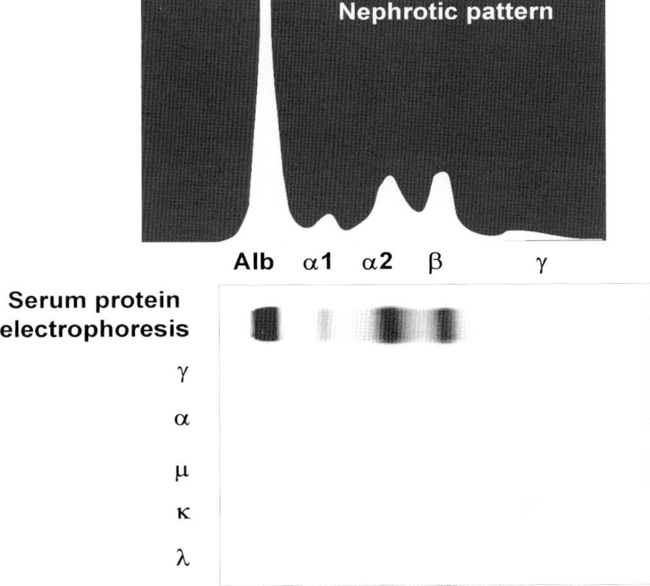

Figure 15.4. Serum from a patient with AL amyloidosis showing a nephrotic pattern on SPE (top) and a small (non-quantifiable) monoclonal λ protein in the β/γ region by IFE (below). (Courtesy of RA Kyle and JA Katzmann).

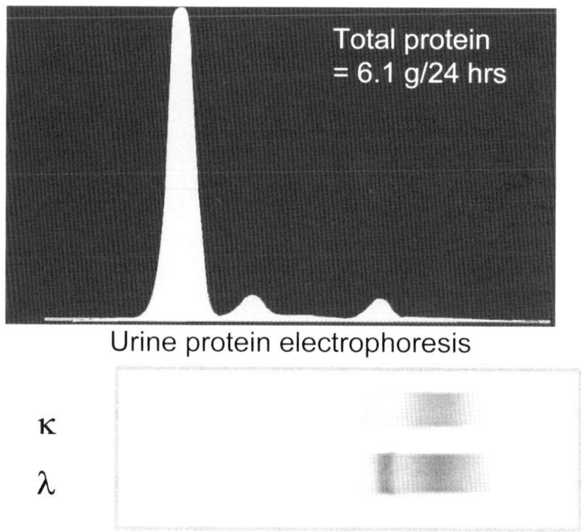

Figure 15.5. UPE and IFE from the same patient as in Figure 15.4, showing a monoclonal λ protein band. (Courtesy of RA Kyle and JA Katzmann).

15.2. Diagnosis of AL amyloidosis

The role of FLC assays has been assessed for diagnostic utility in a large series of patients with AL amyloidosis at the National Amyloidosis Centre in London, UK. In a retrospective analysis of stored serum, 98% of 262 patients had abnormal FLC concentrations at the time of clinical presentation.[6] In contrast, only 3% of patients had sufficient serum concentrations of monoclonal FLCs to be quantitated by SPE. Many patients had elevated FLCs in the urine but as discussed in Chapter 3, serum measurements are preferable. Comparison of the results with electrophoretic tests is shown in Figures 15.6 and 15.7.

Comparison of the FLC results from individual patients with normal serum samples is shown in Figure 15.8. Concentrations of FLCs in the AL amyloidosis patients are similar to those observed in NSMM but lower than those found in LCMM. Classification into κ or λ types by FLC immunoassays agreed fully with IFE and bone marrow phenotyping (in 207 samples that were available from the total 262). In most patients, the concentrations of monoclonal FLCs were within the range of 30-500 mg/L. There was no correlation with the concentrations of intact monoclonal immunoglobulins, when present, and sFLCs.

The diagnostic accuracy of traditional serum and urine tests has been compared with sFLC assays in a study from The Mayo Clinic.[8] Samples from 95 patients with AL were selected, based upon whether serum or urine tested positive or negative for monoclonal proteins by IFE and bone marrow immunohistochemistry. For samples that were serum and urine positive by IFE, the sensitivity of sFLC immunoassays was marginally lower (*Figures 15.9 and 15.10*). In patients whose serum was IFE negative for κ or λ, the sFLC results showed a sensitivity of 95% and 100% respectively. In patients who were

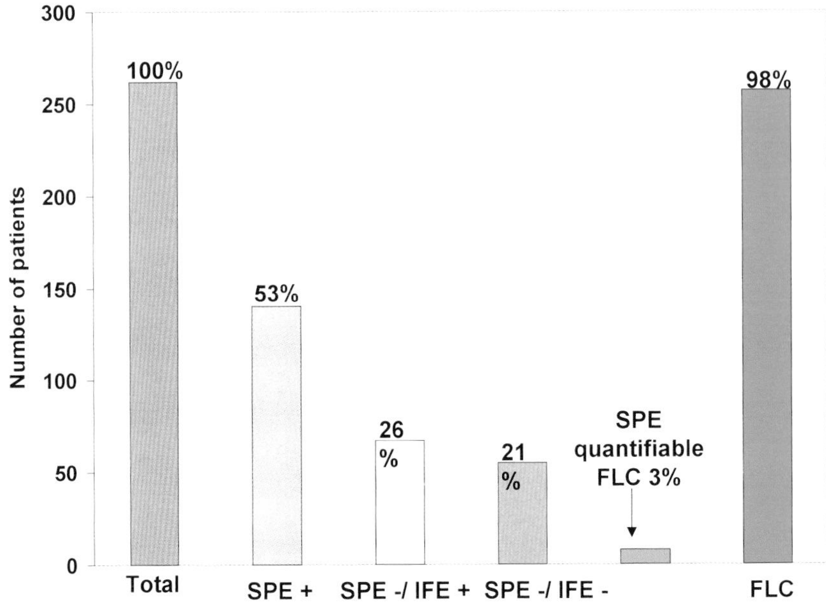

Figure 15.6. Comparison of electrophoretic tests and serum FLC immunoassays in 262 patients with AL amyloidosis studied at the UK National Amyloidosis Centre.[6] Only 3% were quantifiable by SPE.

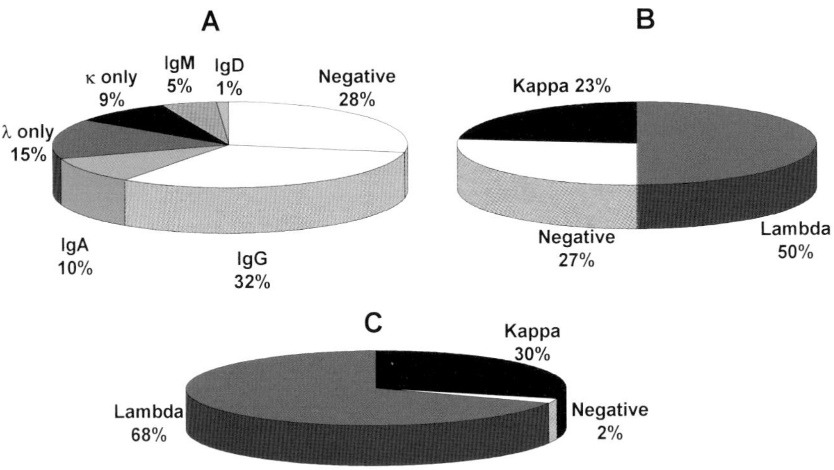

Figure 15.7. Diagnostic accuracy of different assays in AL amyloidosis. Electrophoretic test results in serum (A) and urine (B) were based on 430 patients studied at The Mayo Clinic.[4] Serum FLCs (C) are from 262 patients studied at The UK National Amyloidosis Centre.[6]

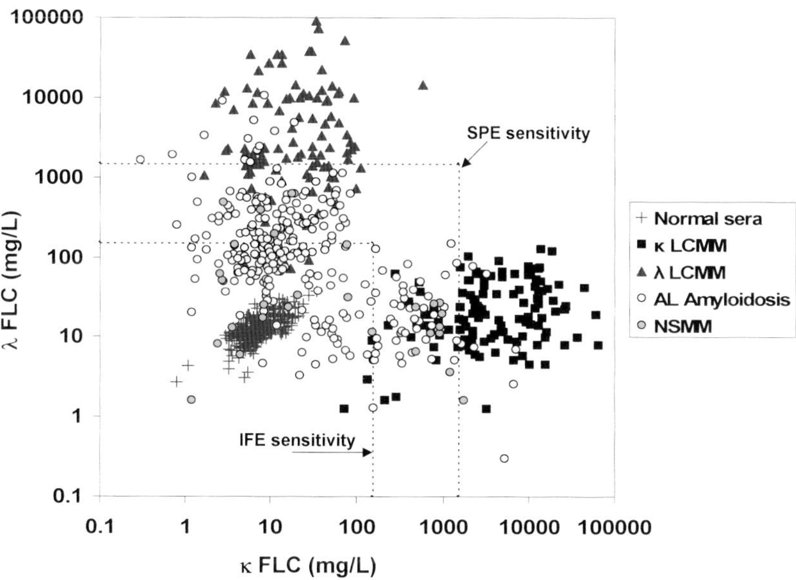

Figure 15.8. Serum FLCs in 262 patients with AL amyloidosis at diagnosis, 282 normal sera, 224 patients with LCMM and 28 patients with NSMM.

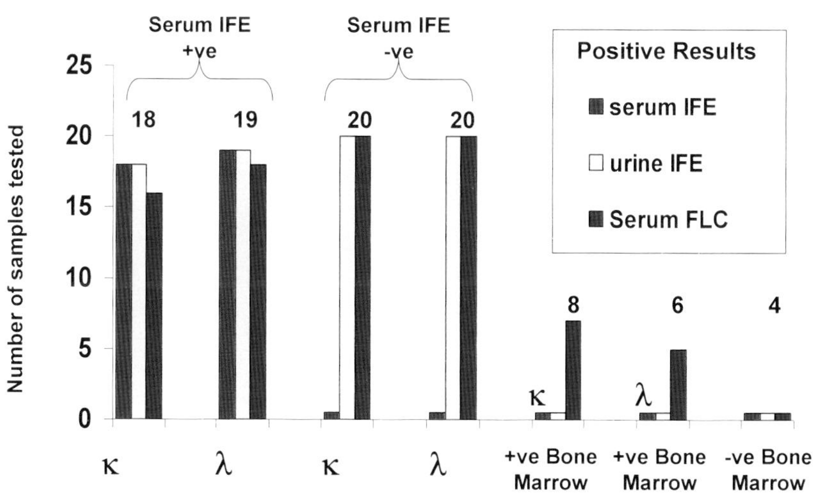

Figure 15.9. Diagnostic sensitivity of serum FLCs and IFE in 95 patients with AL amyloidosis. Numbers refer to the samples in each category. (Courtesy of RA Kyle and JA Katzmann).

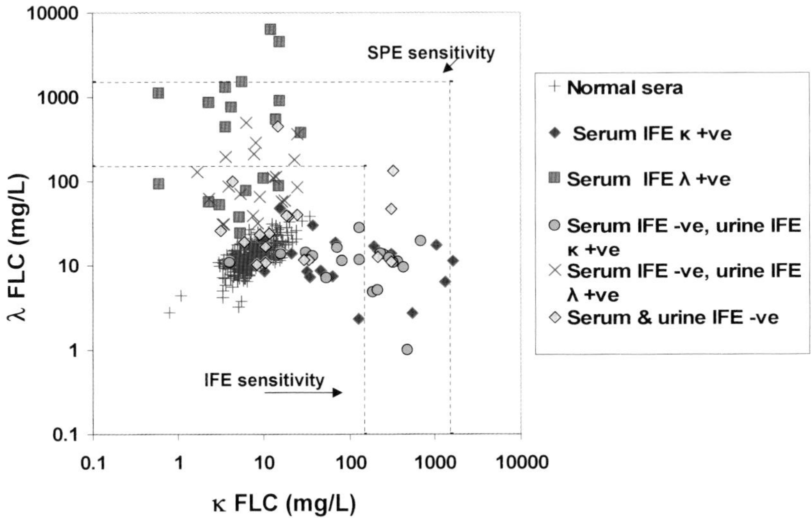

Figure 15.10. Serum FLCs in 95 patients with AL amyloidosis and 282 normal serum samples. The patients are divided into the diagnostic categories shown in Figure 15.9. (Courtesy of RA Kyle and JA Katzmann).

negative by serum and urine IFE (but confirmed by bone marrow tests), sFLCs had a sensitivity of 86%. In the indeterminate group of 4 patients, sFLCs were not diagnostic.

The study above was based on samples from highly selected diagnostic groups. A further study was undertaken to evaluate FLC assays in 34 unselected patients with AL amyloidosis who had undergone PBSCT.[8] Of the 34 patients at the time of transplantation, 26 were abnormal by serum IFE, 28 by urine IFE and 24 by both serum and urine IFE. However, only 19 patients had a monoclonal serum and 17 a monoclonal urine protein that could be quantified by electrophoretic tests. Overall, only about half of the patients who had undergone transplantation could be evaluated by serum or urine monoclonal proteins. In contrast, changes in sFLCs could be used for assessing all 34 patients although, in four, the concentrations were within the normal range.

Similar results were found by Akar et al.,[9,10] in 169 patients with AL amyloidosis that were evaluated for the utility of sFLC immunoassays. Elevated concentrations of κ or λ FLCs were found in 96% and 94% respectively, higher than any other individual test. However, monoclonality, as defined by κ/λ ratios was less sensitive - 89% for κ patients and 73% for λ patients. For the κ patients, sensitivity was higher than other tests but for λ patients serum and urine IFE were more sensitive (79% and 92% respectively). The conclusions were similar to those from Katzmann et al.[7] described above: 1) sFLC measurements are a useful screening test and supplement other tests: 2) The quantitative nature of the FLC immunoassays have value in monitoring patients: 3) FLC tests are complementary to IFE and other tests used in AL amyloidosis.

Test	Sensitivity
FLC κ/λ ratio	91%
Serum IFE	69%
Urine IFE	83%
FLC κ/λ ratio and urine IFE	91%
FLC κ/λ ratio and serum IFE	99%
Serum IFE and urine IFE	95%
All three tests	99%

Table 15.1. Sensitivity of different diagnostic tests and their combinations in 110 patients with AL amyloidosis at the time of disease diagnosis.[11]

Recently, an audit of the utility of different diagnostic tests in AL amyloidosis, during the year 2003, was published by Katzmann et al., *(Table 15.1)*.[11] In 110 new patients, the FLC κ/λ ratio was the most sensitive test and in combination with serum IFE identified 109 of the patients. Urine tests failed to identify the remaining patient that was negative by serum tests.

In the studies described above, there was little correlation between the concentrations of sFLCs detected by immunoassays and the electrophoretic results *(Figure 15.10)*. Some patients had surprisingly high concentrations of FLCs by immunoassay but IFE was normal. It is possible that the FLCs were polymerised in some of the samples and this may have inhibited the formation of narrow bands on the electrophoretic gels. This has been observed in sera from patients with NSMM (*see Figure 9.2*).

In 5-10% of patients, serum FLCs are normal by immunoassay but detectable by serum IFE. Explanations include:-

- The FLCs may be missing epitopes that are the target for the FLC antibodies. (Modest truncation of FLCs in AL amyloidosis has been reported but these particular FLC molecules were detectable by the antisera).[11,12]
- The FLCs may be truncated so that they pass quickly into the urine. Accumulation cannot occur in the serum so concentrations are in the normal range, but FLCs may be detectable in the urine. (Very rare patients produce monoclonal proteins that comprise only the variable domains of the light chains).
- Structurally aberrant molecules occasionally produce antigen excess conditions even at low concentrations and produce normal FLC results. (Dilution of the samples might allow the molecules to be detected accurately and thereby produce more reliable assessments of their concentrations).

In rare patients both serum FLCs and serum IFE are normal. Explanations include:-

- Some FLC molecules may have a high affinity for the amyloid deposits so any circulating FLCs would be rapidly removed. Possibly, these patients are particularly resistant to treatment.
- In a similar manner, patients with extensive amyloid deposits might have a huge capacity for FLC removal. Any newly synthesised molecules would be cleared

rapidly by a combination of binding to the amyloid mass and glomerular filtration, thereby, preventing the accumulation of FLCs in serum.

- The amyloid may be due to the deposition of a different protein.
- The reference range for serum FLCs includes some borderline abnormal results because it has been made too wide *(Chapter 5).*

Whatever the reason for normal sFLC results in some AL amyloidosis patients, in the vast majority these assays provide an important diagnostic tool.

Clinical case history No 5. AL amyloidosis identified by FLC analysis when electrophoretic tests were doubtful.[13]

A 40-year-old woman, with spontaneous bruises, asthenia, abdominal pains and a possible cardiomyopathy, was investigated for suspicion of AL amyloidosis. Abdominal fat biopsy showed Congo Red positivity. SPE showed hypogammaglobulinaemia but no monoclonal proteins.

IFE showed a weak λ band without a corresponding intact immunoglobulin (*Figure 15.11*). A weak λ arc was also visible by serum immunoelectrophoresis. Quantitative immunoglobulin measurements were: IgG 4.9g/L; IgA 1.02g/L; IgM 0.32g/L indicating hypogammaglobulinaemia. sFLC analysis showed: κ 7.8mg/L; λ 210 mg/L; κ/λ ratio 0.04.

Nephelometric FLC quantification was, thus, clearly abnormal and provided a measurable parameter for subsequent disease monitoring. In contrast, FLCs were barely detectable by conventional electrophoretic assays.

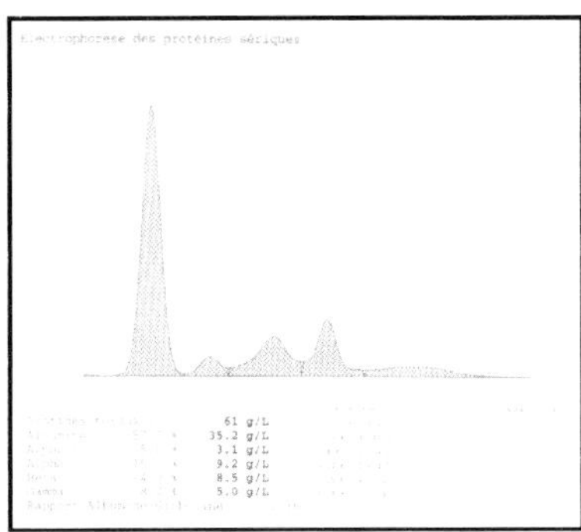

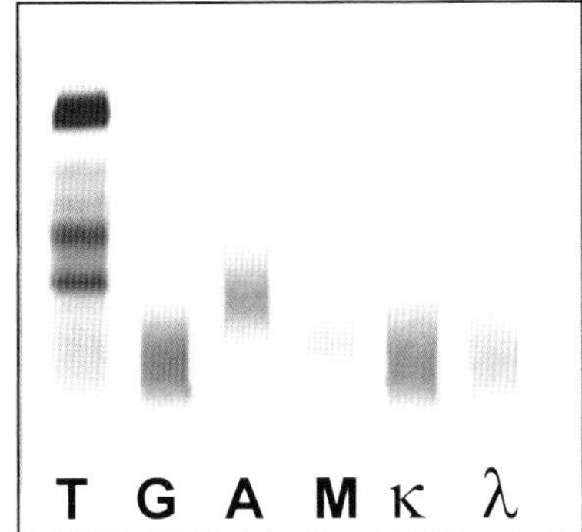

Figure 15.11. Clinical Case history No 5.[13] SPE scan and IFE of the patient's serum. A weak λ band is visible. (Courtesy of L Guis).

15.3. Monitoring patients with AL amyloidosis

"The introduction of the serum immunoglobulin free light chain assay has revolutionized our ability to access hematological responses in patients with low tumour burden......." Dispenzieri A, Gertz MA, Kyle RA. Blood 2004.[14]

The aim of therapy in AL amyloidosis is to suppress the monoclonal plasma cell clone that produces the amyloidogenic FLC. When the supply of amyloid-forming protein is reduced, the balance between amyloid deposition and clearance may be favourably altered. Although complete suppression of the clonal plasma cells is desirable, reduction in the amyloidogenic sFLC concentrations by 50-70% is often sufficient to lead to stabilisation or regression of the amyloid deposits.

Using SPE, the depositing monoclonal FLCs can rarely be quantified in serum. In the study by Lachmann et al.,[6] only 3% of patients had sufficiently high concentrations of monoclonal sFLCs to be quantitated by SPE (*Figure 15.6*). While intact monoclonal immunoglobulins are more readily measured, changes in their concentrations during treatment are clinically unreliable (*e.g., Figure 15.14*). This has led to the use of I^{123} labelled serum amyloid P scans (SAP scans) as an alternative method of assessment. Uptake of the radiolabelled protein into amyloid deposits allows identification of the affected organs and the amounts deposited. Furthermore, uptake varies with time, in parallel with changes in clinical status. This is shown in a patient during treatment with

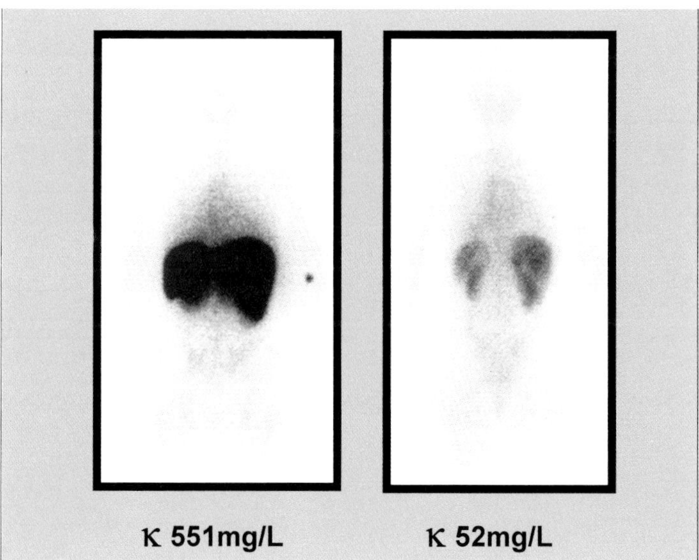

Figure 15.12. I^{123} labelled serum amyloid P scans in a 52-year-old woman, viewed posteriorly. Reduction of AL deposits in the liver and spleen after one year of chemotherapy can be seen. Serum κ FLCs reduced from 551mg/L to 52mg/L over the same period . (Courtesy of PN Hawkins).

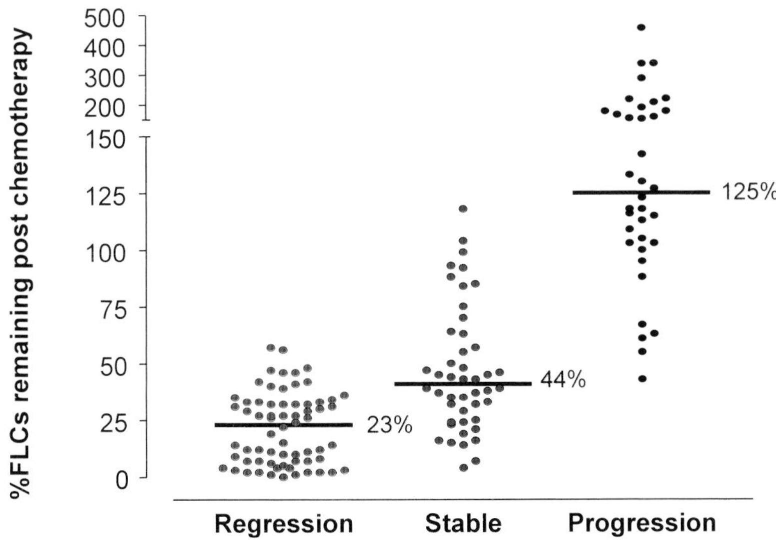

Figure 15.13. Comparison of disease status from serum amyloid P scans and serum FLCs in 127 patients with AL amyloidosis before and 12 months after commencing chemotherapy. The mean percentage of remaining FLCs in each group are indicated (Kruskal-Wallis test: $P<0.0001$). (Courtesy of PN Hawkins).

chemotherapy and is compared with the concentrations of sFLCs (*Figure 15.12*).

Similar investigations on stored serum samples were extended to 137 patients with AL amyloidosis who survived more than 6 months after chemotherapy. Patients were divided into three groups dependent upon whether the SAP scans of the amyloid deposits showed regression, no change, or progression following chemotherapy. There was a good correlation with changes in sFLC concentrations during the same period (*Figure 15.13*).[6] This indicates that sFLC measurements can provide a simple measure of changes in disease status in patients with AL amyloidosis.

Clinical case history No 6. Use of sFLCs to monitor a patient with AL amyloidosis.

A 49 year old man presented, with congestive cardiac failure. After establishing a diagnosis of AL amyloidosis, he was given a heart transplant. He was subsequently treated with melphalan and prednisolone for a year, but then gradually developed increasing autonomic neuropathy with gastrointestinal symptoms, weight loss, hypotension and proteinuria. A cardiac biopsy showed evidence of amyloid in the graft. Two years after his initial presentation, he was given high dose melphalan and a PBSCT. This was successful as judged by diminishing proteinuria from 5.5g to 2.3g per day over the following months and more stable blood pressure. The patient regained some weight, returned to jogging and was relatively well for the following few years.

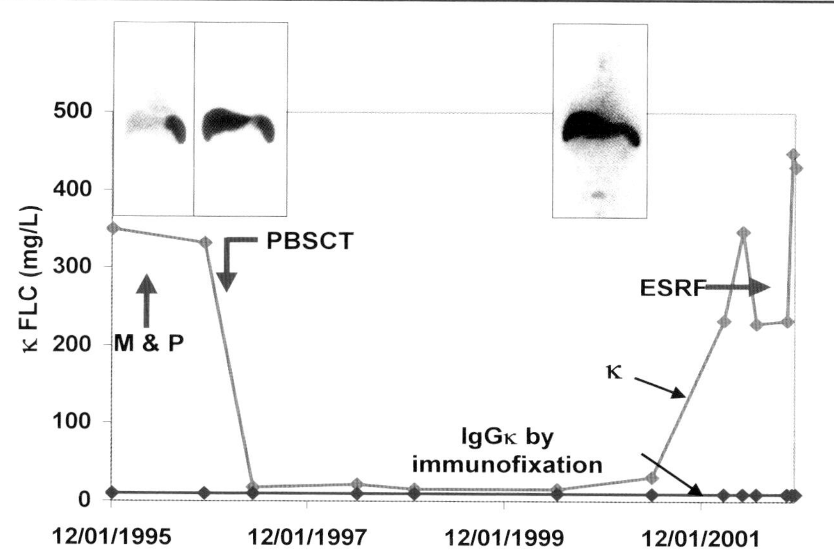

Figure 15.14. Changes in SAP scans and serum monoclonal proteins during the disease course of a patient with AL amyloidosis. M&P: melphalan and prednisolone; ESRF: end stage renal failure. (Courtesy of PN Hawkins).

During his 6th year of illness, he gradually became short of breath, lost weight and renal function worsened. Deterioration continued during the year 2001, with an episode of aspiration pneumonia followed by syncopal episodes. End-stage renal failure finally developed and he died seven and a half years after the initial presentation. Throughout his illness, he had a low level of monoclonal IgGκ protein in his serum, detectable only by IFE. Changes in its concentration had not been sufficient to act as a useful clinical marker (*Figure 15.14*).

Retrospective analysis of serum samples showed that a monoclonal free κ protein had been present at different stages of his disease. It was present in greatly elevated concentrations at presentation but fell following the PBSCT and was undetectable for several years. It then recurred in August 2000, as minor symptoms developed. Investigations at that time were normal and it was considered that the amyloidosis remained under control. In retrospect, rising FLC concentrations indicated otherwise. Subsequently, symptoms progressed in parallel with rising κ sFLC levels but the monoclonal IgGκ, detectable by IFE, remained unchanged. Development of progressive renal and cardiac failure indicated the terminal phase of the illness and he became too ill to be treated with chemotherapy. Perhaps, if FLC results had been available before the final illness, earlier treatment with chemotherapy could have produced a more favourable outcome.

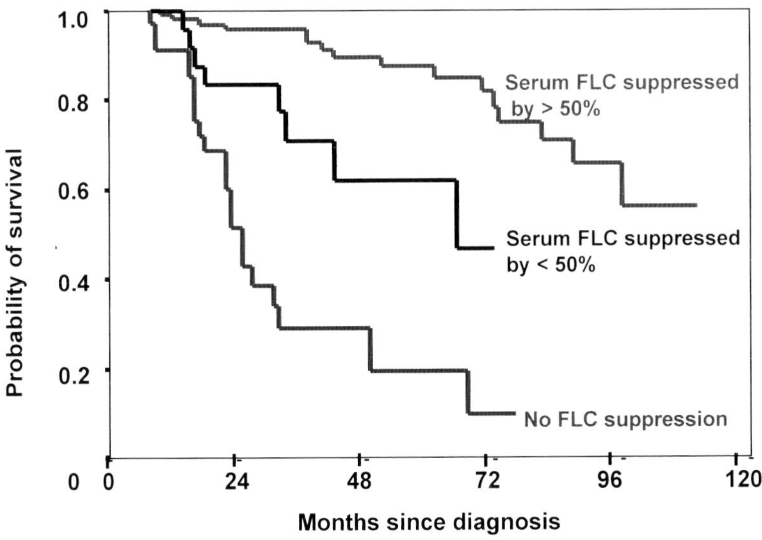

Figure 15.15. Kaplan-Meier probability of survival in 137 patients with AL amyloidosis showing that a reduction of sFLCs by greater than 50% following chemotherapy was associated with increased survival. (Courtesy of PN Hawkins).

15.4. Assessing responses to chemotherapy

The potential utility of sFLC measurements for assessing chemotherapy in AL amyloidosis was studied in a retrospective analysis of 164 patients.[6] Each patient received high-dose melphalan, intermediate or low-dose therapy and all were monitored with SAP scans and blood tests on a six-monthly basis. Stored blood samples were analysed for sFLCs in the 137 patients who survived at least six months. Results showed that a reduction in the amyloidogenic FLCs by 50% or more, following chemotherapy, was associated with a 10-fold survival advantage. There was an 88% probability of survival for five years if the sFLCs had fallen by more than 50%, compared with 39% if the sFLCs had reduced by less than 50% ($P < 0.001$) (*Figure 15.15*). Median survival was 15 months in the 27 patients whose sFLCs showed no response ($P < 0.0001$). A greater than 50% fall in sFLC was more significantly related to good outcome than any other clinical or biochemical measure while reductions by >90% were associated with the best survival. As a result of these and many other studies, chemotherapy is altered to take into account favourable or unfavourable responses in sFLC concentrations.[11,14,16-30]

While complete suppression of the clonal plasma cells is desirable, reduction in the amyloidogenic sFLC concentrations by 50-70% is often sufficient to lead to stabilisation or regression of amyloid deposits. Continuation of toxic chemotherapy when FLC concentrations have responded may be unnecessary or even harmful. Risk-adapted therapy, based upon early changes in FLCs, may become common practice.[21,29]

Lachmann et al., made several recommendations on the use of sFLC measurements, many of which are in the new UK guidelines *(Chapter 25)*.[6,15]

1. In order to minimise the toxicity associated with chemotherapy, measurements of the sFLC should be made approximately 2 weeks after each course of chemotherapy. This should assist with decision-making about continuation of treatment.
2. It may be appropriate to discontinue chemotherapy at an early stage if the amyloidogenic FLC concentrations have:-
   a. Fallen to within the normal range.
   b. Fallen to a plateau level for at least a month.
   c. Fallen by 50-70% and toxicity or adverse effects are deemed to render further chemotherapy undesirable.
   d. Not fallen significantly after three courses of treatment, suggesting that an alternative regimen should be considered.

15.5. Using free light chains to monitor stem cell transplantation

The first study was from The Mayo Clinic.[8] 34 patients with AL amyloidosis were assessed following PBSCT and 4 different serological responses were identified (*Figure 15.16*):- 10 patients showed a good correlation between changes in sFLCs and urine monoclonal proteins; 13 patients showed decreased sFLCs levels before changes in

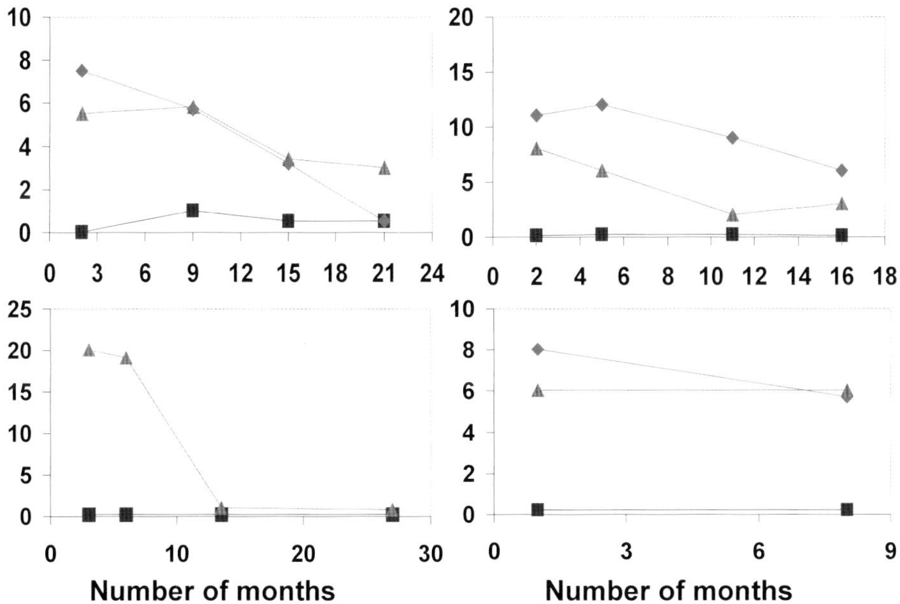

Figure 15.16. Evaluation of haematologic responses in 4 patients with AL amyloidosis after PBSCT. The urine protein concentration is expressed in g/24h; the serum M protein in g/L, and serum FLCs in mg/dL. Diamonds indicate urine protein; squares, serum M-protein and triangles, sFLCs.

serum and urine monoclonal proteins; 8 patients had sFLCs as the only marker that could be evaluated; 3 patients had decreased urine protein concentrations that preceded falls in sFLCs or serum monoclonal proteins measured by electrophoretic tests.

Of the 34 patients, 75% could be evaluated for clinical responses by serum or urine electrophoretic tests, whereas all could be assessed using sFLC concentrations. sFLCs were either the only marker for measurement, or decreased before the other tests in 21 of the 34 patients. Overall, changes in FLC concentrations showed a better correlation with changes in organ function than changes in electrophoretic tests.

A subsequent study by the same authors showed that high sFLC concentrations prior to PBSCT were an adverse risk factor (upper quartile median FLCs: 382mg/L) with a 5.4-fold greater risk of death than the lowest quartile.[31] Furthermore, reduction to <20mg/L (81%) post-transplant was a more powerful predictor of survival than complete haematological responses.

The conclusion was that FLC quantification would become a standard technique for monitoring AL amyloidosis patients undergoing PBSCT.

15.6. Other recent studies using serum free light chains in AL amyloidosis

Myers et al. used sFLCs to assess responses to the combination therapy of cyclophosphamide, thalidomide and dexamethasone in 6 patients with κ and 2 patients with λ AL amyloidosis.[18] All patients showed a prompt sFLC response to therapy and 6 of the 8 patients achieved a maximum of >77% reduction in concentrations. Two patients who did not respond clinically had <42% reduction. Even when the dosage was minimised to avoid excessive side effects, satisfactory FLC responses occurred. This would suggest that dose escalation while monitoring for early FLC responses might reduce drug toxicity in many patients. As with the other studies, it was clear that sFLC concentrations were a sensitive indicator of treatment responses.

Cohen et al.,[19] reported the association between a persistently abnormal κ/λ ratio 3 months after treatment and an increased risk of death (p=0.02). Indeed, all recently reported studies on AL amyloidosis include sFLC measurements,[20-25] including in the context of cardiac transplantation,[26] second PBSCT,[27] IgM associated AL amyloidosis,[28] and novel combinations of chemotherapeutic agents.[29,30]

An important link between cardiac dysfunction in AL amyloidosis and falling sFLC concentrations was observed by Merlini and colleagues.[3,24,25] 21 AL amyloidosis patients with symptomatic myocardial involvement were given chemotherapy and monitored for sFLCs and the amino-terminal fragment of naturetic peptide type B (NT-proBNP), a sensitive marker of myocardial dysfunction in AL amyloidosis. During treatment, 11 of the patients had a reduction of sFLCs by more than 50% and 7 patients had disappearance of monoclonal immunoglobulins by IFE. In all of the 11 patients, there was a corresponding reduction of NT-proBNP levels (p = 0.02) and in 6 patients the heart failure resolved without concommitant reduction of wall thickness at echocardiography. Thus, cardiac function rapidly improved due to a reduction in circulating FLCs. These important observations are to be published, in full, shortly.[25]

These observations suggest that the amyloidogenic precursors equate to the circulating monoclonal FLCs and seem to have a direct toxic effect on cardiac muscle cells. It also emphasises the utility of the FLC assays and the importance of rapidly reducing their concentrations, by treatment, in order to help control heart failure.

15.7. Free light chains in renal failure complicating AL amyloidosis

Renal failure frequently complicates AL amyloidosis and inevitably leads to increased serum concentrations of the amyloidogenic FLC even if the amyloidosis is not progressing. However, increases also occur in the concentrations of the non-depositing FLC (*Chapter 20.1*) so the κ/λ ratio is a good determinant of disease progression. Furthermore, changes in the alternate FLC can be used to assess changes in renal function. This is illustrated in a patient with AL amyloidosis caused by a κ-secreting plasma cell clone (*Figure 15.17*).

The accuracy of the κ/λ ratio is poorer in patients with renal failure, particularly if the ratio is close to the normal range. As renal function deteriorates, less FLCs are cleared through the glomeruli and more are removed by pinocytosis in other tissues. This reduces the clearance rate of κ more than λ, so the median value for a normal κ/λ ratio increases slightly. A correction factor for the κ/λ ratio, in those patients who have reduced glomerular clearance, can be calculated from serum concentrations of cystatin C *(Chapter 20.3)*. Subtraction of the tumour from the non-tumour FLC concentrations may also be used.[32]

Clinical case history No 7. Use of the κ/λ ratio to assess AL amyloidosis in a patient with renal impairment.

After chemotherapy with C-VAMP, serum κ FLC concentrations increased and then remained stable for six months before increasing further. Serum creatinine concentrations changed in a similar manner suggesting that a reduction in renal clearance could account for the rise in κ concentrations. However, the κ/λ ratio steadily increased over the same period, indicating a clonal increase in κ concentrations. The κ/λ ratio then increased sharply which suggested that the deteriorating renal function was due to increased amyloid deposition. A renal transplant was then successfully performed.

These results illustrate a typical dilemma facing the clinician managing these patients. The deteriorating renal function could be due to one or more factors. However, the steadily rising κ/λ ratio indicated a recurrence of the FLC clone leading to renal deposition of amyloid.

Clearly, the κ/λ ratio should be carefully monitored, but it is not clear whether this is the only consideration. As renal function deteriorates, a greater proportion of the sFLC are due to failure of renal clearance rather than de-novo synthesis. The additional circulating amounts of depositing FLCs might accelerate amyloid formation. The depositing FLC concentrations can be estimated by subtraction of the non-depositing FLC concentrations (polyclonal). Indeed, it has been suggested that this should replace κ/λ ratios when monitoring patients with MM.[32] Guidelines for the diagnosis and monitoring of AL amyloidosis are described in Chapter 25.

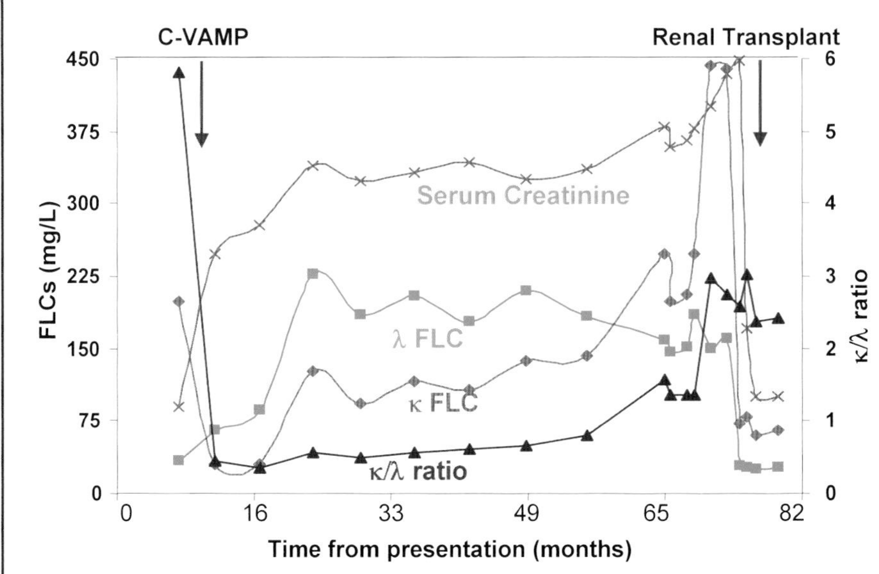

Figure 15.17. Changes in serum FLCs and renal function in a patient with monoclonal κ AL amyloidosis. (Courtesy of PN Hawkins).

Summary: In patients with AL amyloidosis, sFLC concentrations:-

1. Are elevated in over 95% of patients at disease presentation.
2. Provide a quantitative assessment of circulating fibril precursors.
3. Correlate with changes in amyloid load during treatment and are predictive of clinical outcome.
4. Are helpful in measuring early responses to treatment and identifying disease relapses because of their short serum half-life.
5. Are useful for monitoring patients undergoing bone marrow transplantation.
6. Increase during renal failure, independently of FLC synthesis.
7. May be directly cardiotoxic in some patients.

References

1. **Gertz MA, Lacy MQ, Dispenzieri A, Hayman SR.** Amyloidosis: Diagnosis and Management. Clin Lymph & Myeloma 2005; **6** (3): 208-219.

2. **Palladini G, Perfetti V, Merlini G.** AL amyloidosis. Haematologica 2004; **89**: 30-36.

3. **Merlini G**. Sharpening therapeutic strategy in AL amyloidisis. Blood 2004; **104**: 1593-1594.

4. **Kyle RA, Gertz MA.** Primary systemic amyloidosis: Clinical and laboratory features in 474 cases. Seminars in Hematology 1995; **32**: 45-59.

5. **Commenzo RL, Gertz MA.** Autologous stem cell transplantation for primary systemic amyloidosis. Blood 2002; **99**: 4276-4282.

6. **Lachmann HJ, Gallimore R, Gillmore JD, Carr-Smith HD, Bradwell AR, Pepys MB, Hawkins PN.** Outcome in systemic AL amyloidosis in relation to changes in concentration of circulating free

immunoglobulin light chains following chemotherapy. Brit J Haematol 2003; **122**: 78-84.

7. Katzmann JA, Clark RJ, Abraham RS, Bryant S, Lymp JF, Bradwell AR, Kyle RA. Serum Reference Intervals and Diagnostic Ranges for Free κ and Free λ Immunoglobulin Light Chains: Relative Sensitivity for Detection of Monoclonal Light Chains. Clin Chem 2002; **48**: 1437-1444.

8. Abraham RS, Katzmann JA, Clark RC, Bradwell AR, Kyle RA, Gertz MA. Quantitative analysis of serum free light chains. A new marker for the diagnostic evaluation of primary systemic amyloidosis. Am J Clin Pathol 2003; **119**: 274-278.

9. Akar H, Seldin DC, Magnani B, O'Hara C, Berk JL, Schoonmaker C, Cabral H, Dember LM, Sanchorawala V, Connors LH, Falk RH, Skinner M. Quantitative serum free light-chain assay in the diagnostic evaluation of AL amyloidosis. In: Amyloid and Amyloidosis; Eds Grateau G, Kyle RA, Skinner M: CRC Press: 2005: 90-92.

10. Akar H, Seldin DC, Magnani B, O'Hara C, Berk JL, Schoonmaker C, Cabral H, Dember LM, Sanchorwala V, Connors LH, Falk RH, Skinner M. Quantitative serum free light chain assay in the diagnostic evaluation of AL amyloidosis. Amyloid 2005; **12** (4): 210-215

11. Katzmann J, Abraham RS, Dispenzieri A, Lust JA, Kyle RA. Diagnostic performance of Quantitative Kappa and Lambda Free Light Chain Assays in Clinical Practice. Clin Chem 2005; **51** (5); 878-881.

11. Abraham RS, Bergen RH, Naylor S, Katzmann JA, Bradwell AR, Kyle RA, Fonseca R. Characterisation of Free Immunoglobulin Light Chains (LC) by Mass Spectrometry in Light Chain-Associated (AL) Amyloidosis. Blood 2001; **98** (11): 3722.

12. Solomon A, Weiss DT, Murphy CL, Hrncic R, Wall JS. Light chain-associated amyloid deposits comprised of a novel kappa constant domain. Proc Nat Acad Sci 1998; **95**: 9547-9551.

13. Guis L, Diemert MC, Ghillani P ,Choquet S, Leblond V, Vernant JP, Musset L. The quantitation of serum free light chains: Three case reports. Clin Chem 2004; **50** (6): Suppl, A183; F-38.

14. Dispenzieri A, Gertz MA, Kyle RA. Determining appropriate treatment options for patients with primary systemic amyloidosis. Blood 2004; **104**: 2992: letter.

15. Bird JM, Cavenagh J, Samson D, Mehta A, Hawkins P, Lachmann H. Guidelines on the diagnosis and management of AL amyloidosis. Br J Haematol 2004; **125**: 681-700.

16. Jaccard A, Moreau P, Aucouturier P, Ronco P, Fermand J-P, Hermine O. Amylose immunoglobulinique. Hematologie. 2003; **9** (6): 485-495.

17. Gertz MA, Comenzo R, Falk RH, Fermand JP, Hazenberg BP, Hawkins PN, Merlini G, Moreau P, Ronco P, Sanchorawala V, Sezer O, Solomon Al, Grateau G. Definition of Organ Involvement and Treatment Response in Immunoglobulin Light Chain Amyloidosis (AL): A Consensus Opinion From the 10th International Symposium on Amyloid and Amyloidosis. Am J Hematology 2005; **79**: 319-328.

18. Myers B, Russell NH, McMillan AK. Use of a novel combination chemotherapy for AL-Amyloidosis: cyclophosphamide, thalidomide and dexamethasone - serum free light chain (SFLC) and serum amyloid protein P (SAP) scan results. Blood 2003; **102** (11): A5249.

19. Cohen AD, Zhou P, Reich L, Quinn A, Fircanis S, Drake L, Hedvat C, Teruya-Feldstein J, Filippa DA, Fleisher M, Comenzo RL. Risk-adapted intravenous melphalan followed by adjuvant dexamethazone (D) and Thalidomide (T) for newly diagnosed patients with systemic AL amyloidosis (AL): Interim results of a phase II study. Blood 2004: **104** (11): 542.

20. Sanchorawala V, Seldin DC, Wright DG, Skinner M, Finn KT, Falk RH. Pulsed Low Dose Intravenous Melphalan in Patients with AL Amyloidosis, Ineligible for Aggressive Treatment with High-Dose Melphalan and Stem Cell Transplantation. Blood 2004; **104** (11): 2393.

21. Sanchorawala V, Seldin DC, Magnani B, Skinner M, Wright DG. Serum free light chain responses after high-dose intravenous melphalan and autologous stem cell transplantation for AL (primary) amyloidosis. Bone Marrow Transplantation 2005; **36**: 597-600.

22. Goodman HJB, Lachmann HJ, Bradwell AR, Hawkins PN. Intermediate dose intravenous melphalan and dexamethasone treatment in 144 patients with AL amyloidosis. Blood 2004: **104** (11): 755.

23. Commenzo R, Zhou P, Reich L, Costello S, Quinn A, Fircanis S, Drake L, Hedvat C, Teruya-Feldstein J, Filippa D, Fleisher M. Prospective evaluation of the utility of the serum free light chain assay (FLC), clonal IgV_L gene identification and troponin levels in a phase II trial of risk-adapted intravenous melphalan with adjuvant thalidomide and dexamethasone for newly diagnosed untreated patients with systemic AL amyloidosis. In: Amyloid and Amyloidosis; Eds Grateau G, Kyle RA, Skinner M: CRC Press: 2005: 112-115.

24. Palladini G, Perlini S, Vezzoli M, Perfetti V, Lavatelli F, Ferrero I, Obici L, Caccialanza R, Bradwell AR, Merlini G. The reduction of the serum concentration of the amyloidogenic light-chain in cardiac AL results in prompt improvement of myocardial function and prolonged survival despite unaltered amount of myocardial amyloid deposits. In: Amyloid and Amyloidosis; Eds Grateau G, Kyle RA, Skinner M: CRC Press: 2005: 73-75.

25. Palladini G, Lavatelli F, Rosso P, Perlini S, Perfetti V, Vezzoli M, Bosoni T, Obici L, Bradwell AR, Melzi D'Eril G, Fogari R, Moratti R, Merlini G. Circulating amyloidogenic free light chains and serum N-terminal natruiretic peptide type B decrease simultaneously in association with improvement of survival in AL amyloidosis. Blood 2006; *In Press.*

26. Gillmore JD, Wechalekar AD, Goodman HJB, Lachmann HJ, Offer M, Joshi J, Hawkins PN. Cardiac Followed by Autologous Stem Cell Transplantation for Systemic AL Amyloidosis. Blood 2005; **106** (11): 1158: 338a.

27. Gertz MA, Lacy MQ, Dispenzieri A, Hayman SR, Kumar SK, Ansell SM, Elliott MA, Gastineau DA, Inwards DJ, Johnston PB, Micallef IN, Porrata LF, Litzow MR. Role of Second Stem Cell Transplant in Patients with Amyloidosis Who Are Refractory or Relapsing. Blood 2005; **106** (11): 5469: 455b.

28. Wechalekar AD, Goodman HJB, Gillmore JD, Lachmann HJ, Offer M, Bradwell AR, Hawkins PN. Clinical Profile and Treatment Outcome in 92 Patients with AL Amyloidosis Associated with IgM Paraproteinaemia. Blood 2005; **106** (11): 3498: 977a.

29. Wechalekar AD, Goodman HJB, Gillmore JD, Lachmann HJ, Offer M, Bradwell AR, Hawkins PN. Efficacy of Risk Adapted Cyclophosphamide, Thalidomide and Dexamethasone in Systemic AL Amyloidosis. Blood 2005; **106 (**11): 3496: 976a.

30. Matsuda M, Yamada T, Gono T, Shimojima Y, Ishii W, Fushimi T, Sakashita K, Koike K, Ikeda S. Serum levels of free light chain before and after chemotherapy in primary systemic AL Amyloidosis. Internal Medicine 2005; **44** (5): 428-433.

31. Dispenzieri A, Lacy MQ, Katzmann JA, Rajkumar VS, Abraham RS, Hayman SR, Kumar SK, Clark R, Kyle RA, Litzow MR, Inwards DJ, Ansell SM, Micallef IM, Porrata LF, Elliott MA, Johnston P, Greipp PR, Witzig TE, Zeldenrust SR, Russell SR, Gastineau D, Gertz MA. Absolute Values of Serum Immunoglobulin Free Light Chains Predict for Survival in Patients with Primary Systemic Amyloidosis Undergoing Peripheral Blood Stem Cell Transplant. Blood 2006; *In Press.*

32. Kumar S, Gertz MA, Hayman SR, Lacy MQ, Dispenzieri A, Zeldenrust SR, Lust JA, Greipp PR, Kyle RA, Fonseca RS, Rajkumar VS. Use of the Serum Free Light Chain Assay in Assessment of Response to Therapy in Multiple Myeloma: Validation of Recently Proposed Response Criteria in a Prospective Clinical Trial of Lenalidomide Plus Dexamethasone for Newly Diagnosed Multiple Myeloma. Blood 2005; **106 (**11): 3479: 971a.

Test questions

1. What is the best, first-line diagnostic test for suspected AL amyloidosis?

2. Why are some patients with AL amyloidosis negative for sFLCs?

3. How frequently should patients undergoing treatment for AL amyloidosis be assessed for sFLCs?

Answers

1. sFLCs (page 131).

2. There is no clear explanation but possibly the sFLCs are being cleared very quickly into the amyloid deposits (page 136).

3. Response or lack of response to treatment can be detected within 1-2 weeks using sFLC measurements (page 140).

Chapter 16

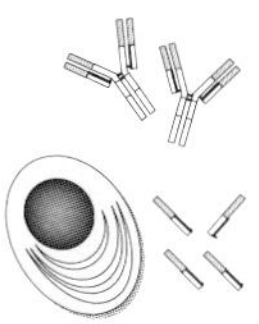

Localised amyloid disease

Rather than being a systemic disease, amyloid deposition may be limited to single organs. The distribution depends upon the biochemical nature of the amyloid fibril protein and as in AL amyloidosis, light chain fragments may be involved. Serum FLCs have been evaluated in a variety of such patients attending the UK National Amyloidosis Centre and are shown in Table 16.1. An enlarged series of 235 cases was recently reported by Goodman et al.[1]

Overall, elevated serum FLCs are less commonly observed than in AL amyloidosis and even when present, the concentrations are lower. Serum FLC concentrations may, therefore, assist in distinguishing the different types of amyloid disease and systemic from localised light chain amyloid disease.

Site of amyloid deposits	Number of patients	Monoclonal proteins*	κ or λ free light chain excess
Bone	7	3 (43%)	6 (88%)
Bladder	25	1 (4%)	3 (12%)
Bowel	10	4 (40%)	3 (30%)
Bronchial	13	2 (15%)	1 (8.0%)
Nodular pulmonary	13	3 (23%)	3 (23%)
Laryngeal	22	0	1 (4.5%)
Nasopharynx	16	1 (6%)	2 (13%)
Skin	18	2 (11%)	2 (11%)
Occular	10	2 (20%)	2 (20%)
Lymph node	16	3 (19%)	5 (31%)
Miscellaneous	6	0	1 (17%)

Table 16.1. Frequency of monoclonal proteins in patients with localised amyloid disease. *Serum monoclonal proteins or light chain proteinuria identified by electrophoretic tests. (Courtesy of PN Hawkins).

Reference

1. **Goodman H, Bridoux F, Lachmann HJ, Gilbertson JA, Gallimore R, Joshi J, Gopaul D, Hawkins PN.** Localised amyloidosis: clinical features and outcome in 235 cases. Haematologica 2005; **90** (s1): PO1413: p203.

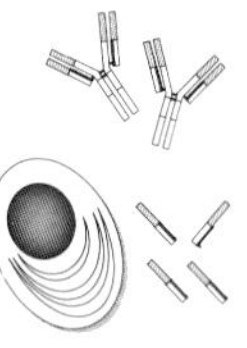

Chapter 17

Light chain deposition disease (LCDD)

17.1. Introduction

In LCDD, monoclonal sFLCs are precipitated on the basement membranes of cells in the kidneys and other organs. As with AL amyloidosis, the disease is progressive and leads to organ failure of the kidneys, heart or liver and has a poor prognosis.[1-3] This rare disease differs from AL amyloidosis by being more frequent in younger women (30-50 years) and renal failure is a common presenting feature. The deposits usually contain κ FLCs (*V*κ1 *and V*κ*4*) without amyloid P component. Some of the patients have serum and urine monoclonal proteins detectable by electrophoretic tests.

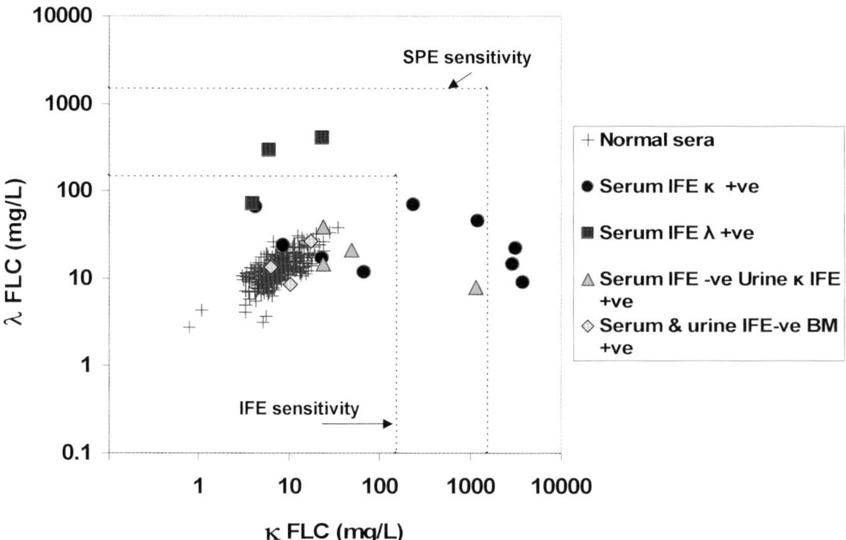

Figure 17.1. Serum FLCs and serum and urine electrophoretic tests in 19 patients with LCDD. BM = bone marrow. (Courtesy of RA Kyle and JA Katzmann).

17.2. Diagnosis and monitoring using serum free light chain assays

Serum FLC concentrations were measured in 19 patients with LCDD by Katzmann et al.,[4] and were abnormal in 17 (*Table 17.1 and Figure 17.1*). One sample was falsely negative by serum FLC analysis but positive by serum IFE. It is possible that the FLC epitopes were truncated or aberrant in this sample. In a subsequent publication by the same authors, 7 further patients were studied and all had raised serum FLC concentrations.[5] Clinical case history No 8 illustrates the clinical sensitivity of the FLC tests compared with electrophoretic assays *(Figure 17.2)*.[6]

It is logical to monitor these patients using serum FLC assays and initial reports indicate that changes in concentrations are as helpful as in patients with AL amyloidosis. Case history 9 illustrates the utility of serum FLC analyses in a patient who was difficult to monitor by other methods.[7]

Classification	**Elevated FLC**	**FLC κ/λ ratio**
Serum: IFE κ +ve	8/9	8/9
Serum: IFE λ +ve	2/3	3/3
Serum: IFE -ve; Urine: IFE κ +ve	4/4	4/4
Serum and urine: IFE -ve. BM: κ +ve	1/3	2/3
Total abnormal for serum FLCs	**15**	**17**

Table 17.1. Detection rates by sFLCs in 19 LCDD patients.[4] BM: bone marrow.

Clinical case history No. 8. Light chain deposition disease undetectable by conventional electrophoretic assays.[6]

A 66-year-old man suffering from asthenia and anaemia was investigated for serum protein abnormalities. SPE and IFE tests showed no evidence of monoclonal

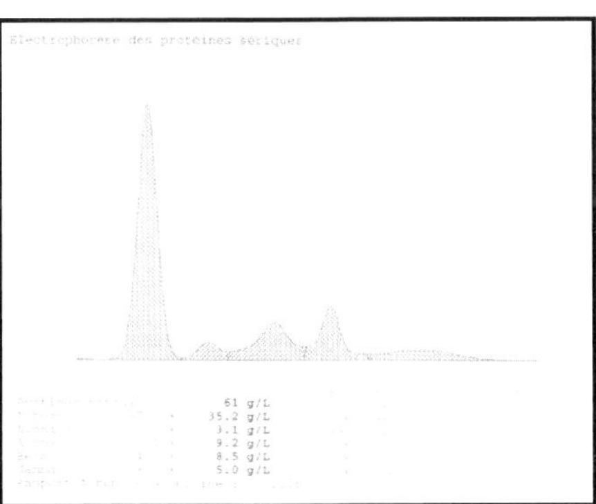

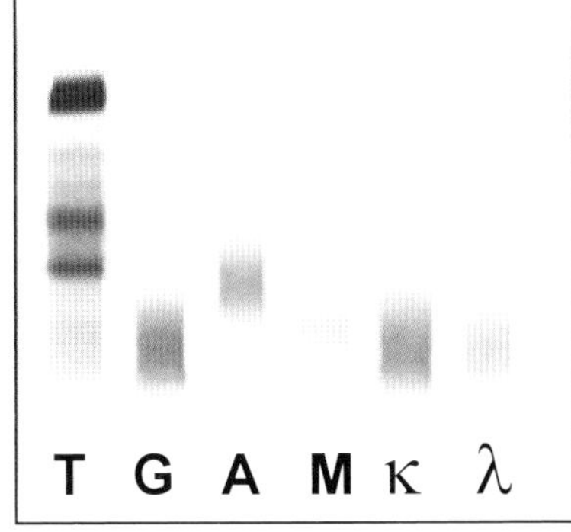

Figure 17.2. LCDD showing normal SPE (scanning densitometry) and IFE, but highly abnormal sFLCs (κ 294mg/L: λ 71.6mg/L and κ/λ ratio: 4.1). T: Protein stain. (Courtesy of L Guis[6]).

immunoglobulins *(Figure 17.2)*. Serum immunoglobulins were normal/low: IgG 8.5g/L; IgA 0.4g/L and IgM 0.2g/L. However, serum FLC concentrations were highly abnormal: κ 294mg/L; λ 71.6mg/L and κ/λ ratio: 4.1. These results indicated a monoclonal gammopathy and renal impairment. FLC quantification allowed the depositing FLC to be easily identified and supported the clinical diagnosis of LCDD obtained by renal biopsy.

Clinical case history No 9. Light chain deposition disease monitored with FLC assays. (Courtesy of I Brockhurst, Leicester, UK).[7]

A 49-year-old Caucasian male presented to the nephrologists with flu-like symptoms, hypertension and face, hand and leg swelling. Serum electrolytes were normal, creatinine clearance was 140mL/min and urinary protein quantification was 2.4g/24 hours. A renal biopsy demonstrated normal histology and immunofluorescence tests. He was managed with a 120mg daily dose of frusemide and antihypertensives. Follow-up was initially uneventful with renal function remaining stable.

10 years later he presented with nephrotic syndrome. Serum biochemistry showed: creatinine 165μmol/L (NR 60-120μmol/L), albumin 33g/L (NR >40g/L), cholesterol 8.7mmol/L (NR <5.5mmol/L) and urinalysis revealed 3+ proteinuria. A further renal biopsy showed nodular glomerulosclerosis with evidence of LCDD on electron microscopy. Congo red staining was negative. SPE, immunoglobulin levels and urinary Bence Jones protein assays were all normal.

He was referred to the Haematology department to rule out an underlying B cell

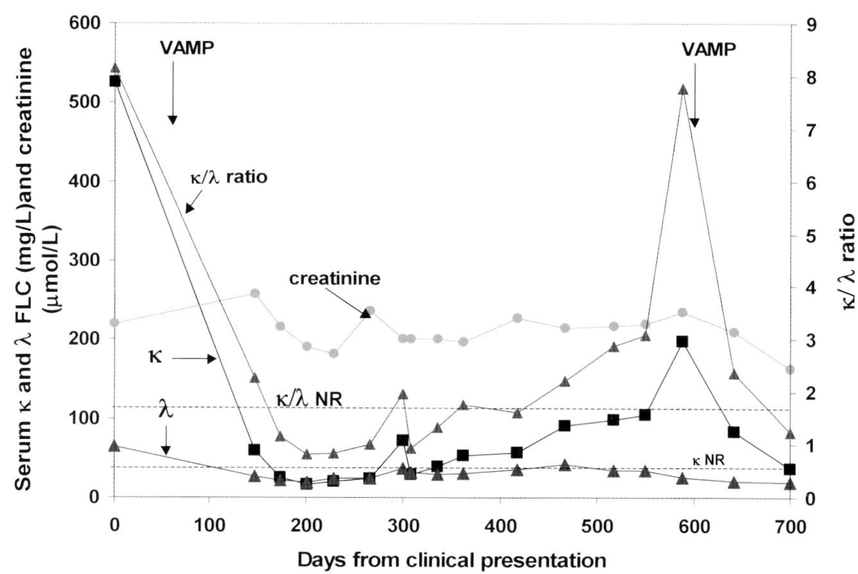

Figure 17.3. Monitoring of a patient with LCDD using sFLC assays (Courtesy of Ian Brockhurst, Leicester, UK).[7]

clonal disorder. Bone marrow aspirate and trephine revealed normal cellular marrow with no morphological or immunophenotypic evidence of MM and, again, Congo Red staining was negative. An iodine[123] labelled, serum amyloid P scan showed no evidence of amyloid deposition. Serum was tested for sFLCs with the following results: κ 526.0mg/L (normal range 3.3 - 19.4mg/L), λ 64.6 mg/L (normal range 12.7 - 26.3mg/L) and κ/λ ratio 8.14 (normal range 0.26 - 1.65). (*Figure 17.3*)

Subsequently he developed atrial fibrillation. A 24-hour tape showed irregularities in the atrial chamber and intermittent disruption of AV node conduction. He had a dual chamber pacemaker fitted and cardiac biopsy performed, which showed no evidence of amyloid or light chain deposition.

Within 2 months his renal function had deteriorated further with a serum creatinine of 210 μmol/L, creatinine clearance of 67mL/min and a 24 hour urine protein leakage of 13.8g. In order to delay the need for dialysis he was treated with 3 cycles of VAMP chemotherapy (vincristine 0.4mg/day for 4 days, doxorubicin 9mg/m^2/day for 4 days and methylprednisolone 1g/m^2 for 5 days per cycle). Subsequent to the chemotherapy, renal function improved and this was also observed in the sFLC levels and κ/λ ratio. 3 months after the chemotherapy, 24 hour urinary protein excretion was 0.1/L.

For the following year renal function remained stable but then the κ/λ ratio and serum creatinine rise began to increase again. He was treated with a further 3 cycles of VAMP and similar improvements in renal function and sFLC levels were seen. The patient has remained reasonably well since.

A series of 17 patients with biopsy-proven LCDD has recently been studied by Wechalekar et al.[8] sFLCs were abnormal with a clonal bias in 15 (88%). 11 (64%) had κ excess, 4 (23%) had λ excess while 2 (11%) had polyclonal increased FLCs. The median κ levels were 317mg/L (range 8.5-2,260) while the median λ levels were 64mg/L (range 17-10,700).

A total of 10 patients received systemic chemotherapy for the underlying plasma cell dyscrasias as follows:- VAD - 4, C-VAMP - 1, VAD followed by autologous stem cell transplant - 2, melphalan and prednisone - 1 and intermediate dose melphalan - 2. 8 (80%) patients had sFLC responses with a median decrease of 63% (range 31 - 95%) compared with pre-treatment values. One had no change in sFLC levels (which did not show clonal bias pre-treatment) but had a very good partial response of the intact monoclonal immunoglobulin. Only two patients had complete normalization of FLC levels. Renal function improved in 2, remained unchanged in 5 (including 3 patients with end-stage renal failure) and worsened in 1 patient. Both patients with abnormal liver function and cardiac involvement showed improvement. The median overall survival was 59 months.

The authors concluded that measurement of sFLCs detected 33% more patients with LCDD than standard electrophoretic methods. The assay was also useful for monitoring response to treatment. Detection of abnormal sFLCs may shorten time to diagnosis in patients without monoclonal intact immunoglobulins. Measurements of sFLCs can be recommended as a useful addition to the screening tests for patients with suspected

LCDD and also for monitoring responses to chemotherapy.

It is important to note that patients with chronic kidney disease due to renal deposition of monoclonal light chains are difficult to identify and monitor.[9,10] It is likely that many of these patients have detectable monoclonal FLCs in serum but not in urine and remain undiagnosed. This issue is discussed in detail in Chapter 20.5.

Summary: sFLC measurements are important in LCDD because:-

1. They are abnormal in 90% of patients at the time of diagnosis.
2. They are important for monitoring disease progress.
3. They may identify patients that were previously unrecognised.

References

1. **Solomon A, Weiss DT, Herrera GA.** Chapt. 29; Light-chain deposition disease. In: Myeloma. Eds. J Mehta & S Singhal; Pub. Martin Dunitz Ltd., London, UK. 2002; **29**: 507-518.

2. **Buxbaum JN, Chuba JV, Hellman GC, Solomon A, Gallo GR.** Monoclonal Immunoglobulin Deposition Disease: Light Chain and Light and Heavy Chain Deposition Diseases and Their Relation to Light Chain Amyloidosis. Ann Int Med 1990; **112**: 455-464.

3. **Buxbaum JN, Gallo G.** Nonamyloidotic Monoclonal Immunoglobulin Deposition Disease: Light-chain, Heavy-chain, and Light- and Heavy-chain Deposition Diseases. In: Hematology/Oncology Clinics of North America: Monoclonal Gammopathies & related disorders. Eds. RA Kyle & MA Gertz; Pub: W B Saunders Co. Philadelphia; 1999; **13** (6): 1235-1248.

4. **Katzmann JA, Clark RJ, Abraham RS, Bryant S, Lymp JF, Bradwell AR, Kyle RA.** Serum Reference Intervals and Diagnostic Ranges for Free κ and Free λ Immunoglobulin Light Chains: Relative Sensitivity for Detection of Monoclonal Light Chains. Clin Chem 2002; **48**: 1437-1444.

5. **Katzmann J, Abraham RS, Dispenzieri A, Lust JA, Kyle RA.** Diagnostic performance of Quantitative Kappa and Lambda Free Light Chain Assays in Clinical Practice. Clin Chem 2005; **51** (5): 878-881.

6. **Guis L, Diemert MC, Ghillani P, Choquet S, Leblond V, Vernant JP, Musset L.** The quantitation of serum free light chains: Three case reports. Clin Chem 2004; **50** (6): Suppl. A183: F-38.

7. **Brockhurst I, Harris KPG, Chapman CS.** Diagnosis and monitoring a case of light-chain deposition disease in the kidney using a new, sensitive immunoassay. Nephrol Dial Transplant 2005; **20**: 1251-1253.

8. **Wechalekar AD, Lachman HJ, Goodman HJB, Bradwell AR, Hawkins PN.** Role of serum free light chains in diagnosis and monitoring response to treatment in light chain deposition disease. Haematologica 2005; **90** (s1): PO1414.

9. **Sanders PW, Herrera GA, Kirk KA, Old CW, Galla JH.** Spectrum of Glomerular and Tubulointerstitial Renal Lesions Associated with Monotypical Immunoglobulin Light Chain Deposition. Lab Invest 1991; **64** (4): 527-537.

10. **Possi C, D'Amico M, Fogazzi GB, Curioni S, Ferrario F, Pasquali S, Quattrocchio G, Rollino C, Segagni S, Locatelli F.** Light chain deposition disease with renal involvement: clinical characteristics and prognostic factors. Am J Kidney Dis 2003; **42** (6): 1154-1163.

Test question

1. What proportion of patients with LCDD have raised serum FLCs?

Answer

1.~90% (page 149).

Section 2C. Other diseases with monoclonal free light chains

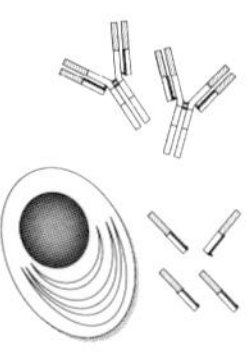

Chapter 18

Other malignancies with monoclonal proteins

18.1. Solitary plasmacytoma of bone

These bone tumours represent 3-5% of plasma cell neoplasms and are twice as common in women than men. Approximately 50% progress to MM over 3-4 years while 30-50% are alive at 10 years. The criteria for the disease are shown below.[1]

Criteria for the diagnosis of solitary plasmacytoma of bone

- Low concentration or no M-protein in serum and/or urine
- Single area of bone destruction due to clonal plasma cells
- Bone marrow not consistent with MM
- Normal skeletal survey (and MRI of spine and pelvis if done)
- No related organ or tissue impairment (no end organ damage other than a solitary bone lesion)

IFE of serum and/or concentrated urine shows a small monoclonal protein in approximately 50% of patients. When present, this is useful for guiding therapy and persistence is associated with worse outcome.

The potential use of sFLCs has recently been investigated in two studies.[2,3] In the first report, 13 patients with solitary plasmacytoma were assessed at diagnosis and during progression to MM. By conventional electrophoretic tests, 5 patients had IgG, 2 IgA and 3 FLC only monoclonal proteins, while 2 were nonsecretory. In total, 5 of the 13 had monoclonal κ FLCs detectable by electrophoretic methods. However, using the

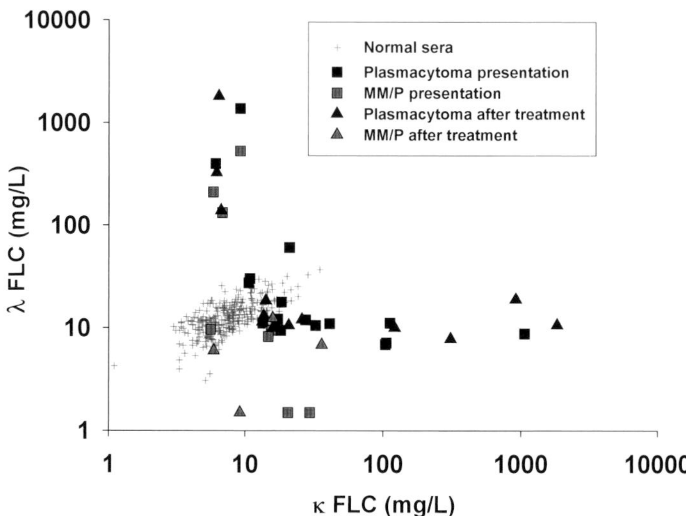

Figure 18.1. Serum FLC concentrations in 13 patients with solitary plasmacytoma of the bone at presentation and after treatment. 8 patients with MM and plasmacytomas are shown for comparison.[2]

more sensitive sFLC immunoassays, 7 patients had κ and 2 λ monoclonal proteins, *(Figure 18.1),* including one of the nonsecretory plasmacytomas that was serum κ positive. There was complete concordance between the κ and λ types identified by the FLC assays and the bound light chain type on the intact immunoglobulin molecules identified by IFE. After radiotherapy, 7 patients showed reductions in sFLC concentrations. Three patients who progressed to MM showed no reductions in FLC levels.

In the second and larger study from the Mayo Clinic, 126 patients were retrospectively investigated using stored sera.[3] At the time of the study, 48 had progressed to MM with a median time of 1.9 years. On univariate analysis, abnormal sFLC ratio at diagnosis (p=0.009) and persistence of serum or urine M-protein after therapy (p=0.007) were associated with a shorter overall survival and time to progression. The presence of serum and urine M-proteins were also associated with poorer outcome but were detectable in fewer patients. They concluded that serum FLC levels at the time of diagnosis were a powerful predictor of outcome and a useful aid to management.

These two studies indicate that sFLCs can be used to detect and monitor most patients with solitary plasmacytomas of the bone. In many patients, sFLCs provide a more accurate identification of progression and response to radiotherapy than other markers.

References

1. **Kyle RA et al. The International Myeloma Working Group.** Criteria for the classification of monoclonal gammopathies, multiple myeloma and related disorders: a report of the International Myeloma Working Group. Br J Haem 2003; **121**: 749-757.

2. **Leleu X, Moreau AS, Hennache B, Dupire S, Faucompret JL, Facon T, Bradwell AR, Reid S, Mead G.** Serum Free Light Chain Immunoassays Measurements for Monitoring Solitary Bone Plasmacytomas. Haematologica 2005; **90** (1): 110: PO410.

3. **Dingli D, Kyle RA, Rajkumar VS, Nowakowski GS, Larson DR, Bida JP, Gertz MA, Dispenzieri A, Melton III LJ, Therneau TM, Katzmann JA.** Immunoglobulin Free Light Chains at Diagnosis: Predictors of Progression and Survival in Solitary Plasmacytoma of Bone. Blood 2005; **106** (11): 5080.

18.2. Extramedullary plasmacytoma

This is a plasma cell tumour that arises outside the bone marrow and can occur in any organ although it is found particularly in the upper respiratory tract. Local tumour irradiation is the treatment of choice and only 15% progress to MM. When present, the monoclonal protein is typically IgA.[1] As with solitary plasmacytomas, sFLC measurements may be helpful in managing some of these patients.

Criteria for the diagnosis of extramedullary plasmacytoma

- Low concentration or no M-protein in serum and/or urine
- Extramedullary tumour of clonal plasma cells
- Normal bone marrow
- Normal skeletal survey
- No related organ or tissue impairment (no end organ damage including bone lesions)

Reference

1. **Kyle RA et al. The International Myeloma Working Group.** Criteria for the classification of monoclonal gammopathies, multiple myeloma and related disorders: a report of the International Myeloma Working Group. Br J Haem 2003; **121**: 749-757.

18.3. Multiple solitary plasmacytomas (+/- recurrent)

Up to 5% of patients presenting with solitary plasmacytomas develop multiple lesions in the bone or elsewhere, without evidence of MM.[1] As with solitary plasmacytomas, sFLC measurements may be helpful in managing some of these patients.

Criteria for the diagnosis of multiple solitary plasmacytomas (± recurrent)

- Low concentration or no M-protein in serum and/or urine
- More than one localised area of bone destruction or extramedullary tumour of clonal plasma cells which may be recurrent
- Normal bone marrow
- Normal skeletal survey and MRI of spine and pelvis if done
- No related organ or tissue impairment (no end organ damage other than the localised bone lesions)

Reference

1. **Kyle RA et al. The International Myeloma Working Group.** Criteria for the classification of monoclonal gammopathies, multiple myeloma and related disorders: a report of the International Myeloma Working Group. Br J Haem 2003; **121**: 749-757.

18.4. Plasma cell leukaemia

High concentrations of plasma cells in the blood (>20% and >2.0 x 10^9/L) define plasma cell leukaemia. It may occur without evidence of MM or may develop from leukaemic transformation of pre-existing myeloma.[1] Monoclonal proteins are present in some patients but there is no data on the occurrence of monoclonal FLCs.

Reference

1. **Kyle RA et al. The International Myeloma Working Group.** Criteria for the classification of monoclonal gammopathies, multiple myeloma and related disorders: a report of the International Myeloma Working Group. Br J Haem 2003; **121**: 749-757.

18.5. Waldenström's macroglobulinaemia

Waldenström's macroglobulinaemia is a low-grade, lymphoproliferative disorder that is associated with the production of monoclonal IgM. The incidence is 5-10% of multiple myeloma with approximately 1,500 new cases per year in the USA and 300 in the UK. The median age of presentation is 65 years of age. The median survival is five years but over 20% of patients live for more than 10 years and many die from unrelated causes.

Typically, patients present with high concentrations of IgM and infiltration of the bone marrow, spleen and lymph nodes with plasmacytoid lymphocytes and mast cells. Patients may have suppression of bone marrow function, enlarged spleen, liver and lymph nodes, hyperviscosity syndrome, cryoglobulinaemia, neuropathy or AL amyloidosis. All aspects of Waldenström's macroglobulinaemia have been reviewed in the April 2003 edition of Seminars in Oncology.[1] The diagnostic criteria for Waldenström's macroglobulinaemia are shown below.

Proposed criteria for the diagnosis of Waldenström's macroglobulinaemia.[2]

- IgM monoclonal gammopathy of any concentration
- Bone marrow infiltration by small lymphocytes showing plasmacytoid/ plasma cell differentiation
- Inter-trabecular pattern of bone marrow infiltration
- Surface IgM+, CD10-, CD19+, CD20+, CD22+, CD23-, CD25+, CD27+, FMC7+, C D103-, CD138- immunophenotype (variations from this immunophenotypic profile can occur).

Serum IgM quantification is important for both diagnosis and monitoring. Unfortunately, nephelometric determinations may be unreliable because polymerisation of the IgM molecules distorts the results. At high concentrations in particular, accurate measurements require the use of SPE and scanning densitometry. At low concentrations no method is accurate because the inclusion of normal IgM leads to overestimation of the monoclonal IgM concentrations. IFE may be more sensitive than SPE for detecting low concentrations of IgM but is non-quantitative. In addition, the presence of cryoglobulins or cold agglutinins affects IgM measurements by all methods, so serum samples may need to be assessed under warm conditions.[3]

Another laboratory assessment criterion is the presence of FLC proteinuria. This occurs in approximately 50% of patients and may exceed 1g/day. However, the amounts excreted are usually low and do not relate particularly well to changes in tumour burden.[4]

Since FLC proteinuria occurs in many patients it is likely that concentrations of sFLCs are frequently abnormal. Figure 18.2 shows sFLC concentrations in 37 patients (21 IgMκ, 15 IgMλ and one biclonal) at the time of plasma exchange for hyperviscosity syndrome. All but one had abnormal FLC concentrations and/or abnormal κ/λ ratios. The non-tumour FLCs were not elevated in any of the patients, indicating no significant renal impairment, but occasionally renal failure does occur.[5]

Since sFLCs are elevated in nearly all patients this may be clinically useful. Their short half-life and the large clinical range should provide a sensitive marker for treatment responses. Also, FLCs do not cryoprecipitate and are not affected by other factors that can make IgM measurements difficult.

In Waldenström's macroglobulinaemia the current clinical response criteria include changes in serum IgM and urine FLC concentrations and are as follows:- [3,4]

1. **Complete response**: disappearance of serum IgM and urine FLCs by IFE.
2. **Partial response**: decrease of at least 50% in serum IgM. When considering the FLC half-life and its catabolism by the kidney, the required decrease in the urinary FLC protein excretion is >90% (because of improvement in renal function) or a reduction to <200mg/24 hours.

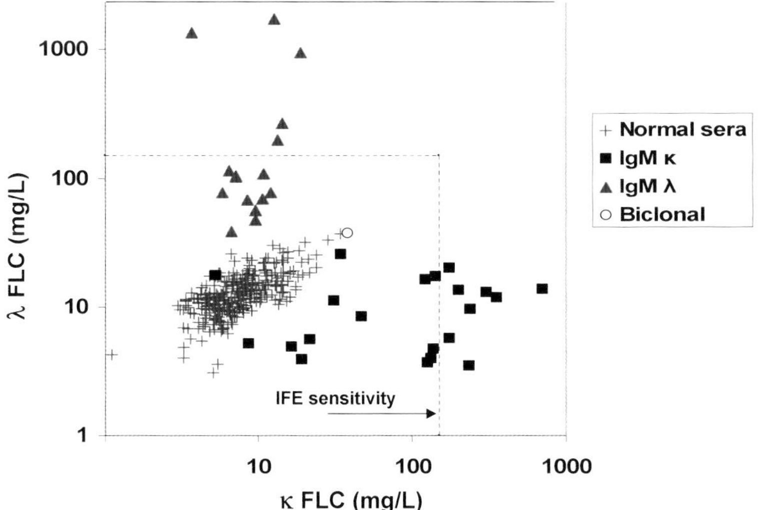

Figure 18.2. FLC concentrations in normal sera and 37 patients with Waldenström's macroglobulinaemia at the time of plasma exchange for hyperviscosity syndrome.

3. **Minimal response**: serum IgM reduction of 25% - 49% and a decrease in the 24-hour urine protein excretion of between 50% and 89% and exceeding 200mg/L.
4. **Minimum required period for confirming response:** 6 weeks.
5. **No change criteria**: patient does not meet the criteria for minimal response or progressive disease.
6. **Plateau phase:** stable IgM levels for >3 months after achieving the maximum serological response.
7. **Relapse from complete response**: reappearance of monoclonal proteins in serum or urine.
8. **Progressive disease**: in patients with an incomplete response an increase in serum IgM of >25% with an absolute increase of at least 5g/L; an increase in 24-hour urine FLC protein excretion of >25% with an absolute increase of at least 200mg.

Serum FLC measurements are likely to be helpful in several situations:

1. Re-evaluation of complete, partial and minimal responses because sFLC analysis is more sensitive than urine FLC analysis and technically superior to IgM measurements.
2 Minimum required period for confirming responses, stable disease and plateau phase may be less using sFLCs because of their short half-life.
3. Relapse and progression may be identified more accurately because sFLC concentrations more accurately reflect tumour burden than urine concentrations that are hugely influenced by renal catabolism.

Summary: Serum FLCs tests may be helpful in Waldenström's macroglobulinaemia:-

1. When IgM measurements are inaccurate.
2. To identify patients at risk of renal failure.
3. As an additional criteria for treatment responses or disease relapse.

References

1. **Proceedings of the 2nd International Workshop on Waldenström's Macroglobulinemia.** Athens, Greece, September 2002. Sem in Onc 2003; **30**: 107-335.

2. **Owen RG, Treon SP, Al-Katib A, Fonseca R, Greipp PR, McMaster ML, Morra E, Pangalis GA, San Miguel JF, Branagan AR, Dimopoulos MA.** Clinicopathological definition of Waldenström's Macroglobulinemia: Consensus panel recommendations from the second international workshop on Waldenström's Macroglobulinemia. Sem in Onc 2003; **30**: 110-115.

3. **Weber D, Treon SP, Emmanouilides C, Branagan AR, Bryd JC, Blade J, Kimby E.** Uniform response criteria in Waldenström's Macroglobulinemia: Consensus panel recommendations from the second international workshop on Waldenström's Macroglobulinemia. Sem in Onc 2003; **30**: 127-131.

4. **Blade J, Montoto S, Rosinol L, Montserrat E.** Appropriateness of Applying the Response Criteria for Multiple Myeloma to Waldenström's Macroglobulinemia? Sem in Onc 2003; **30**: 329-331.

5. **Bradwell AR, Mead GP, Drayson MT, Carr-Smith HD.** Serum immunoglobulin free light chain measurement in intact immunoglobulin multiple myeloma. Blood 2002; **100** (11): 5054.

18.6. B-cell, non-Hodgkin lymphomas

Non-Hodgkin lymphomas represent about 2.6% of all cancer deaths in the UK (approximately twice that of MM) and the incidence is rising by 3-4% per year in all age groups and both sexes. This is largely unexplained but immunosuppression is a well-defined causative factor, leading to a high excess risk. Approximately 80% of lymphoid malignancies are derived from B-lymphocytes at various stages of differentiation (*Table 18.1 and Figure 18.3*).

Monoclonal immunoglobulins can be identified in the serum of 10-15% of patients

Precursor B-lymphoblastic leukaemias/lymphomas	<1%
Chronic lymphocytic leukaemia/B-cell small lymphocytic leukaemia	7%
B-cell prolymphocytic leukaemia	<1%
Lymphoblastic lymphoma	1%
Splenic marginal zone B-cell lymphoma	<1%
Hairy cell leukaemia	<1%
Plasma cell myeloma/plasmacytoma	<1%
Extranodal marginal zone B-cell lymphoma (MALT lymphoma)	8%
Nodal marginal zone B-cell lymphoma	2%
Follicular lymphoma	22%
Mantle cell lymphoma	6%
Diffuse large B-cell lymphomas (DLC)	33%
Burkitt's lymphoma/leukaemia	2%

Table 18.1. The REAL/WHO classification of B-cell, non-Hodgkin lymphomas and their frequency in relation to all non-Hodgkin lymphomas.[1]

B-cell neoplasm	Number studied	FLC +ve	FLC +ve only	SPE/IFE +ve	SPE/IFE +ve only	Total +ve
Small lymphocytic	25	5 (20%)	3 (12%)	4 (16%)	2 (8%)	7 (28%)
Lymphoblastic	8	0	0	0	0	0
Lymphoplasmacytic	14	2 (14%)	0	4 (29%)	2 (14%)	4 (29%)
MALT lymphoma	19	3 (16%)	1 (5%)	7 (37%)	5 (26%)	8 (42%)
Follicular, stage I	25	0	0	4 (16%)	4 (16%)	4 (16%)
Follicular, stage II	25	2 (8%)	1 (4%)	5 (20%)	4 (16%)	6 (24%)
Follicular, stage III	25	1 (4%)	1 (4%)	3 (12%)	3 (12%)	4 (16%)
Mantle cell lymphoma	25	9 (36%)	5 (20%)	6 (24%)	2 (8%)	11(44%)
Diffuse large B-cell	25	2 (8%)	1 (4%)	2 (8%)	1 (4%)	3 (12%)
Burkitt's lymphoma	17	2 (12%)	1 (6%)	2 (12%)	1 (6%)	3 (18%)
Total	**202**	**26 (13%)**	**13 (6%)**	**37 (18%)**	**24 (12%)**	**50(25%)**

Table 18.2. Serum FLC concentrations in B-cell non-Hodgkin lymphoma.

using standard electrophoretic methods. The proteins may be IgG, IgA or IgM and are occasionally biclonal. Reports have indicated that monoclonal FLCs can be detected in the urine of 60-70% of patients with B-CLL if the urine is highly concentrated, but interpretation may be difficult if there is co-existing proteinuria.[2-4]

In order to determine the frequency of abnormal sFLC concentrations in B-cell non-Hodgkin lymphomas, frozen sera were studied from the Lymphoma SPORE serum bank at The Mayo Clinic by Martin et al.[5] For comparison, samples were also tested for monoclonal immunoglobulins by SPE and IFE. Of 206 patients with non-Hodgkin's lymphoma, a total of 13% (26/202) had abnormal sFLC concentrations (*Table 18.2 and Figures 18.4 and 18.5*). The highest incidence was in patients with B-cell small lymphocytic leukaemia (20%) and mantle cell lymphoma (36%). The concentrations of the FLCs were typically much lower than those found in patients with MM. Using SPE and IFE, 18% (37/202) of the patients had a detectable monoclonal protein. In 13 patients, monoclonal proteins were detected only by sFLC immunoassays.

References

1. **Evans LS, Hancock BW.** Non-Hodgkin lymphoma. Lancet 2003; **362**: 139-146.

2. **Deegan MJ, Abraham JP, Sawdyk M, Van Slyck EJ.** High Incidence of Monoclonal Proteins in the Serum and Urine of Chronic Lymphocytic Leukemia Patients. Blood 1984; **64**: 1207-1211.

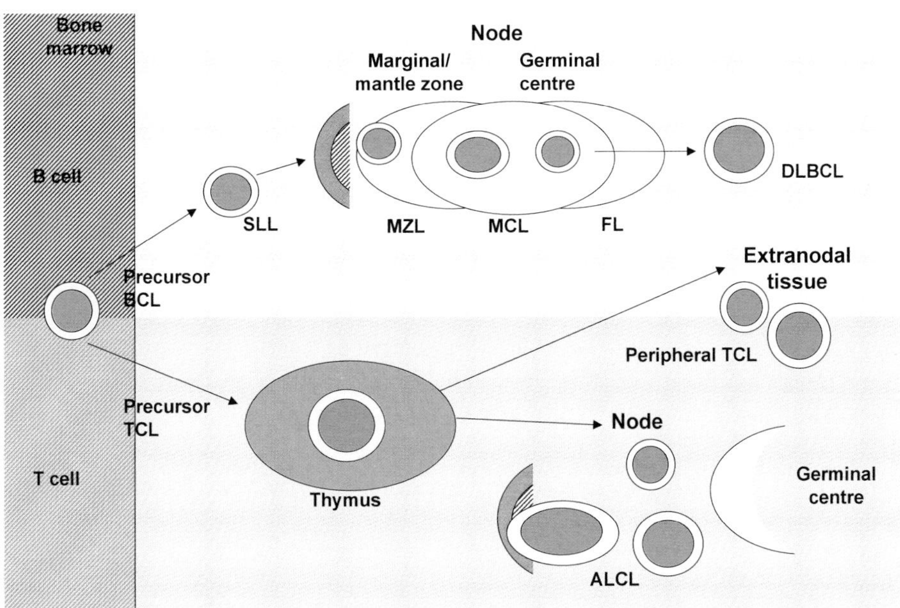

Figure 18.3. Cellular origins of representative non-Hodgkin lymphomas.[1] ALCL: anaplastic large-cell lymphoma. BCL: B-cell lymphoma. DLBCL: diffuse large B-cell lymphoma. FL: follicular lymphoma. MCL: mantle-cell lymphoma (pre-germinal centre). MZL: marginal zone (MALT) lymphoma (post-germinal centre). SLL: small lymphocytic lymphoma. TCL: T-cell lymphoma.

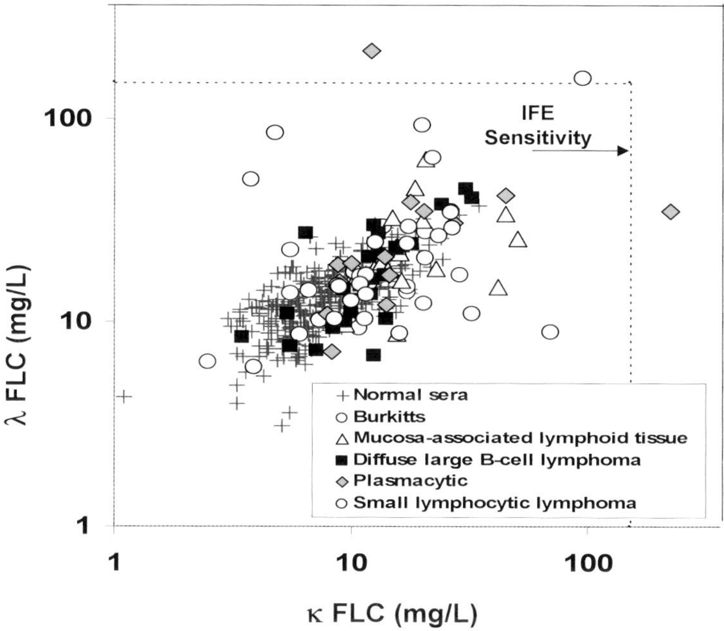

Figure 18.4. Serum FLC concentrations in non-Hodgkin B-cell lymphomas.

3. **Pezzoli A, Pascali E.** Monoclonal Bence Jones proteinuria in chronic lymphocytic leukaemia. Scand J Haematol 1986; **36**: 18-24.

4. **Pascali E.** Bence Jones Proteinuria in Chronic Lymphocytic Leukemia. Amer J Clin Pathol 1995; **103**: 665-666.

5. **Martin M, Clark RJ, Shanafelt T, Katzmann JA, Bradwell AR, Abraham R, Kay NE, Witzig TE.** Detection of Serum Free Light Chains in Patients with B-Cell Non-Hodgkin Lymphoma (NHL) and Chronic Lymphocytic Leukemia (CLL). Blood 2003; **102** (11): 4827.

B-cell, Non-Hodgkin Lymphoma complicated by AL amyloidosis

Rarely, AL amyloidosis is associated with non-Hodgkin lymphoma. Six patients with this pattern of disease were studied by Cohen et al.,[1] and comprised five patients with lymphoplasmacytic lymphoma and one with small lymphocytic lymphoma with plasmacytic features. Organ involvement with amyloid was characterised by bulky lymphadenopathy and visceral deposits but no cardiac disease. Measurements of sFLC concentrations showed elevations at diagnosis and responses to successful treatment. It was concluded that sFLCs were useful for monitoring these patients.

Reference

1. **Cohen AD, Zhou P, Xiao Q, Fleisher M, Kalakonda N, Akhurst T, Chitale DA, Moskowitz C, Dhodapkar MV, Teruya-Feldstein J, Filippa DA, Raymond L.** Systemic AL Amyloidosis due to Non-Hodgkin Lymphoma: An unusual clinicopathologic Association. Blood 2003; **102** (11): 4838.

18.7. B-cell chronic lymphocytic leukaemia

Several reports have suggested that a high percentage of patients with B-CLL may have urine monoclonal proteins.[1-3] These results are supported by the finding of raised sFLCs in many patients with B-CLL.[4] Of 20 sera studied, 7 patients (35%) had abnormal sFLCs alone (*Table 18.3*). Using SPE and IFE, only 2 additional patients (10%) had an intact immunoglobulin monoclonal protein. Monoclonal proteins were more commonly found in patients with germline chronic lymphocytic leukaemia (60%) than those with somatic hypermutation (30%). As in patients with B-cell lymphomas, the concentrations of the FLCs were typically much lower than those found in MM (*Figure 18.5*).

A prospective study that screened 1,003 serum samples from symptomatic patients identified five new patients with B-CLL/ lymphoma *(Chapter 23)*.[5] This surprisingly high number of positive samples perhaps reflects the relative frequency of lymphomas compared with MM. However, the concentrations of monoclonal FLCs were low, supporting the observations shown in Figures 18.4 and 18.5.

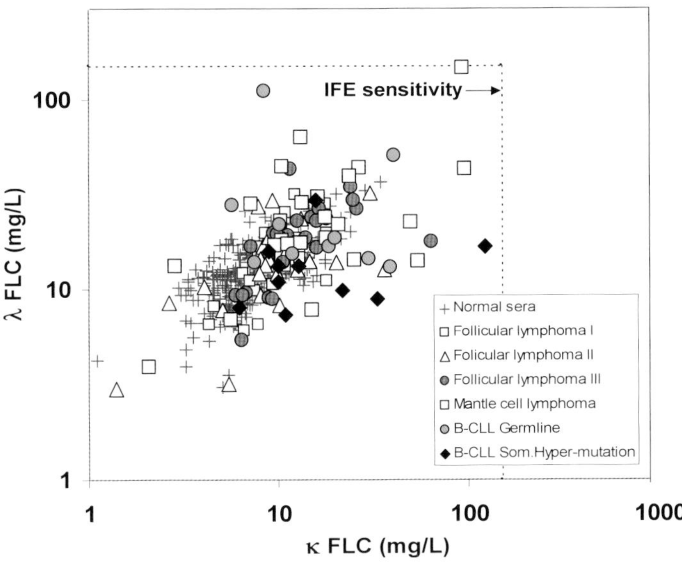

Figure 18.5. Serum FLC concentrations in non-Hodgkin lymphoma and B-cell chronic lymphocytic leukaemia.

B-cell CLL type	Number studied	FLC +ve	FLC +ve only	SPE/IFE +ve	SPE/IFE +ve only	Total +ve
Germline	10	4 (40%)	4 (40%)	2 (20%)	2 (20%)	6 (60%)
Som. Hyper-mutation	10	3 (30%)	3 (30%)	0	0	3 (30%)
Total	**20**	**7 (35%)**	**7 (35%)**	**2 (10%)**	**2 (10%)**	**9 (45%)**

Table 18.3. Serum FLC concentrations in B-cell chronic lymphocytic leukaemia.

Summary:

1. Abnormal sFLC concentrations can be detected in a substantial fraction of patients with B-cell, non-Hodgkin lymphoma and B-CLL.
2. Serum FLC analysis identifies additional patients to those detected by SPE and IFE.
3. Future studies are warranted to elucidate the role of sFLCs as markers of disease, for monitoring of residual disease and as a prognostic factor for response and survival.

References

1. **Deegan MJ, Abraham JP, Sawdyk M, Van Slyck EJ.** High Incidence of Monoclonal Proteins in the Serum and Urine of Chronic Lymphocytic Leukemia Patients. Blood 1984; **64**: 1207-1211.
2. **Pezzoli A, Pascali E.** Monoclonal Bence Jones proteinuria in chronic lymphocytic leukaemia. Scand J Haematol 1986; **36**: 18-24.
3. **Pascali E.** Bence Jones Proteinuria in Chronic Lymphocytic Leukemia. Amer J Clin Pathol 1995; **103**: 665-666.
4. **Martin M, Clark RJ, Shanafelt T, Katzmann JA, Bradwell AR, Abraham R, Kay NE, Witzig TE.** Detection of Serum Free Light Chains in Patients with B-Cell Non-Hodgkin Lymphoma (NHL) and Chronic Lymphocytic Leukemia (CLL). Blood 2003; **102**:11: No 4827.
5. **Bakshi NA, Guilbranson R, Garstka D, Bradwell AR, Keren DF.** Serum Free Light Chain (FLC) Measurement Can Aid Capillary Zone Electrophoresis (CZE) In Detecting Subtle FLC M-Proteins. Am J Clin Path 2005; **124**:214-218.

Test questions

1. Are sFLCs abnormal in solitary plasmacytomas of bone?

2. Are sFLC measurements helpful in patients with Waldenström's macroglobulinaemia?

3. Are patients with B-CLL likely to be detected when screening for monoclonal gammopathies using serum FLC assays?

Answers

1. Yes, in about 80% of patients (page 153).

2. This is unknown. In contrast to IgM, however, sFLCs have a short half-life and they are not cryoglobulins (page 156).

3. Yes, quite frequently, because B-CLL is more common than MM (Page 159).

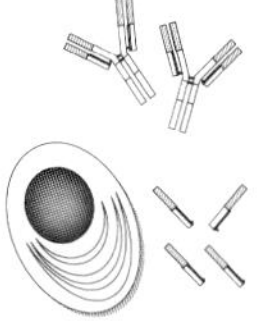

Chapter 19

Monoclonal gammopathies of undetermined significance (MGUS)

19.1. MGUS: Definition and frequency

MGUS denotes the unexpected presence of an intact immunoglobulin monoclonal protein in individuals who have no evidence of MM, AL amyloidosis, Waldenström's macroglobulinaemia, lymphoproliferative disorders, plasmacytoma or related conditions. The term, monoclonal gammopathy, unattributed/unassociated, (MG[u]), is also used.

MGUS is defined as follows:-

1. M-protein in serum <30 g/L
2. Bone marrow clonal plasma cells <10% and low level of plasma cell infiltration in a trephine biopsy (if done)
3. No evidence of other B-cell proliferative disorders
4. No related organ or tissue impairment

MGUS may be found in 1% of the population over 50 years, 3% over 70 years and up to 10% over 80 years of age.[1,2] and is 2-fold higher in African-Americans.[3] Because of the frequency of MGUS, between 50-65% of all monoclonal proteins detected fall into this category and vast numbers go undetected. In a Mayo Clinic study, 73% were IgG, 14% IgM, 11% IgA and 2% biclonal.[1] Rarely, FLC MGUS is found in the urine.[4]

19.2. MGUS and monoclonal free light chains

Although most people with MGUS die from unrelated illnesses, they may transform into malignant monoclonal gammopathies. Patients should, therefore, be followed up on a regular basis to identify early signs of progression. In order to minimise therapeutic harm, treatment is given only when disease develops. During this monitoring phase, symptoms, signs and markers of malignancy are carefully observed, paying particular attention to serum and urine monoclonal proteins.

In a long-term study of outcome in MGUS patients at the Mayo Clinic, 1,384 patients with MGUS have been continually monitored.[5] Since enrolment between the years 1960 and 1994, 115 had progressed, a rate of approximately 1% per year. The most important prognostic factor for progression was the initial size of the serum monoclonal spike. Immunoglobulin class was also important; individuals with IgM and IgA, but not IgG, monoclonal proteins were 5 times more likely to progress. In a recent study by Kyle et al.,[6] looking specifically at 213 patients with IgM MGUS, there was a very high relative risk of progression to Waldenström's macroglobulinaemia (262 fold) or lymphoma (15 fold). Neither study showed any increased relative risk associated with the various immunoglobulin subclasses or urine FLC excretion.

In contrast, other studies have indicated that urine FLC excretion may be an important prognostic marker.[7-8] In an Italian study of 1,231 patients, Bence Jones proteinuria was an independent risk factor for malignant transformation.[9]

Since the amounts of FLC in the urine are restricted by renal catabolism, serum concentrations might be a more reliable predictor of disease progression. Initial studies have indicated that FLC concentrations are raised in the serum of many patients with MGUS.[10-12] Examples from 31 patients are shown in Figure 19.1.[11] 60% of the sera contained monoclonal FLCs as indicated by abnormal κ/λ ratios. Several others had raised concentrations of both FLCs because of renal impairment *(Chapter 20).*

In a study by Tate et al., serum FLC concentrations and/or κ/λ ratios were abnormal in 26 of 32 MGUS patients (*Figure 19.2*).[12] Serum intact immunoglobulin M-protein concentrations ranged from 1.0 to 22g/L. 9 patients had abnormal serum κ/λ ratios but a further 5 with normal serum FLCs had small amounts of urine monoclonal FLCs identified by electrophoretic tests. Presumably, the levels of monoclonal FLCs were insufficient to cause serum abnormalities but accompanying renal leakage allowed detectable amounts to enter the urine. In contrast, when patients with MM have good renal function, urine tests may be normal for monoclonal FLCs, even though plasma cell

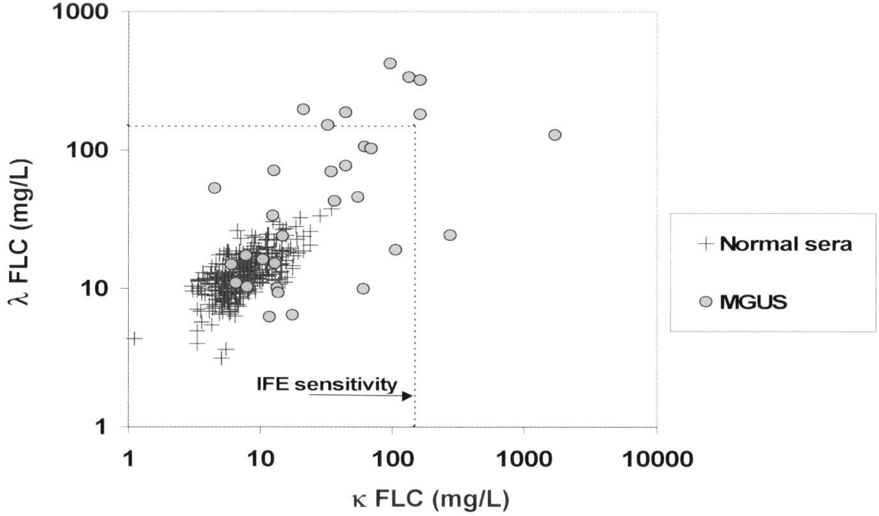

Figure 19.1. Serum FLCs in patients with MGUS. (Courtesy of H Lachmann).

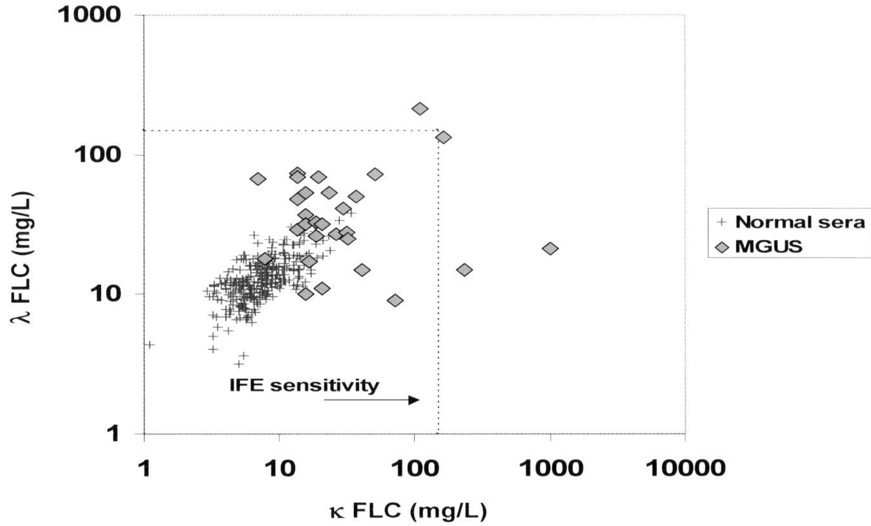

Figure 19.2. Serum FLCs in 32 patients with MGUS.[12]

numbers can be relatively large. Possibly, the same applies to patients with MGUS. It should be born in mind that in patients with LCMM, abnormalities in serum rather than urine FLCs are a more reliable measure of outcome (*Chapters 8 and 12*) and presumably the same applies to FLCs in MGUS. In addition, the urine IFE tests may be falsely identifying intact monoclonal immunoglobulins or ladder banding as monoclonal FLCs *(Chapter 6.6).*

19.3. Risk stratification of MGUS using serum FLC concentrations

The clinical importance of elevated serum FLC concentrations in individuals with MGUS was first noted by J Katzmann in a pilot study at the Mayo Clinic (personal communication). Figures 11.1 and 11.2 *(Chapter 11)* show the κ/λ ratios in MGUS patients who did or did not progress compared with κ/λ ratios in other diseases. Although the κ/λ ratios overlapped, the two groups of MGUS patients had significantly different median values.

Further studies followed,[13-15] and the largest series of patients (1,148) was reported recently.[16-18] Results showed that the risk of progression in patients with abnormal FLC κ/λ ratios was significantly higher (hazard ratio 2.6) than in patients with normal ratios and was independent of the quantity and type of MGUS *(Figure 19.3).* Furthermore, the risk of progression increased as the κ/λ ratio became more extreme *(Figure 19.4).*

The data was used to produce a risk-stratification model based upon immunoglobulin MGUS class, its quantity above or below 15g/L and the presence or absence of an abnormal FLC κ/λ ratio *(Table 19.1).* The risk of progression, with time, after MGUS identification is shown in Figure 19.5.

The explanation for the increased risk from high serum FLC concentrations may

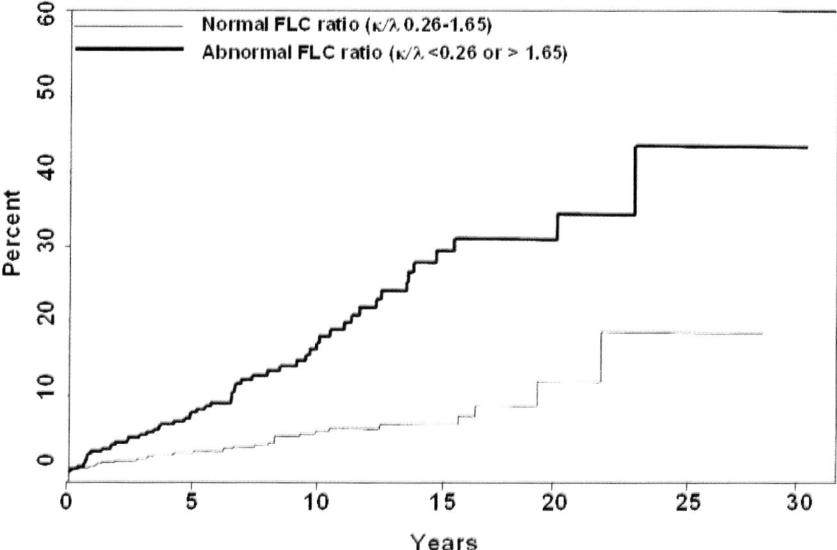

Figure 19.3. Risk of progression based upon MGUS type, its quantity above or below 15g/L and the presence or absence of an abnormal FLC κ/λ ratio.[15] (Copyright American Society of Hematology, used with permission).

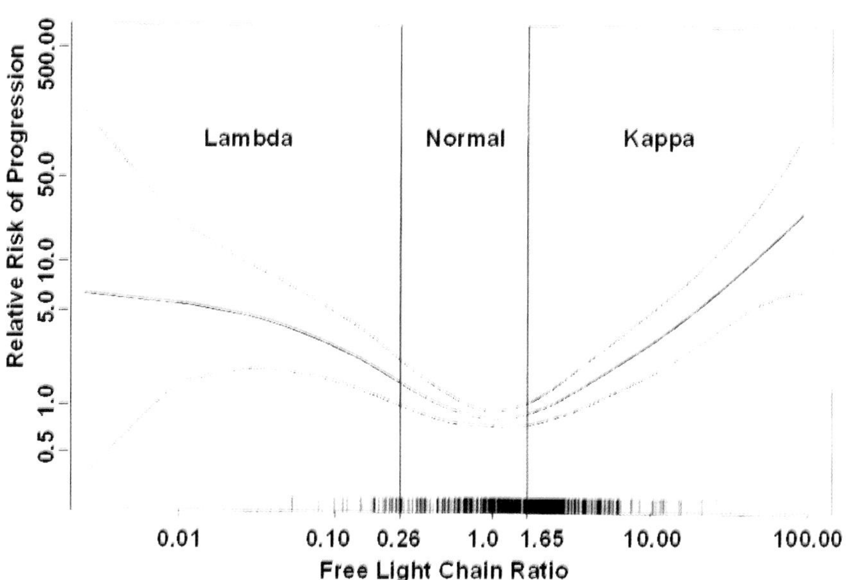

Figure 19.4. Effect of increasingly abnormal FLC κ/λ ratio on the relative risk of progression of MGUS.[15] (Copyright American Society of Hematology, used with permission).

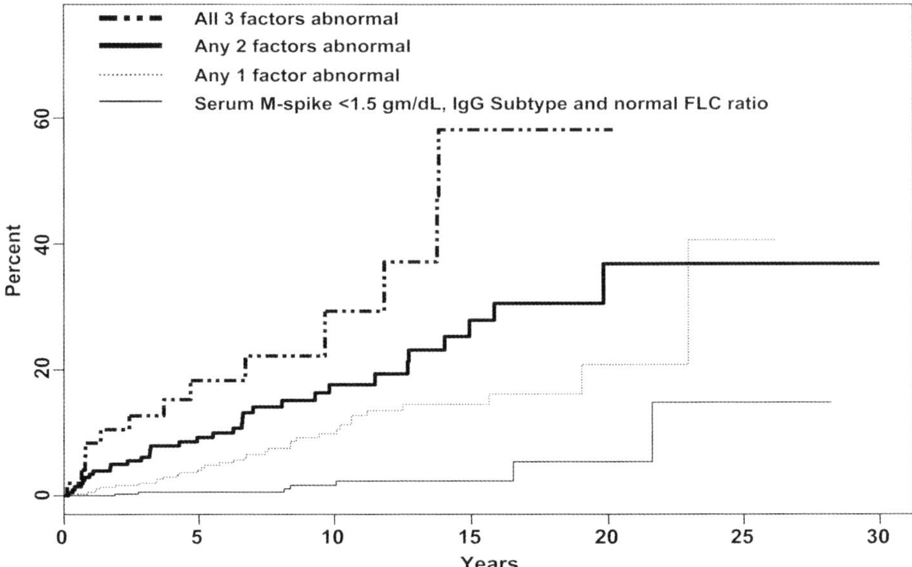

Figure 19.5. Risk of progression to myeloma or related condition in 1148 patients with MGUS.[15] (Copyright American Society of Hematology, used with permission).

Risk Group	No. of patients	Relative risk	Risk of progression at 20 years
Low-risk (Serum M protein <15g/L, IgG subtype, normal FLC ratio (0.26-1.65)	449	1	5%
Low-intermediate-risk (Any 1 factor abnormal)	420	5.4	21%
High-intermediate-risk (Any 2 factors abnormal)	226	10.1	37%
High-risk (All 3 factors abnormal)	53	20.8	58%

Table 19.1. Risk stratification model to predict progression of MGUS.[15]

relate to the clonal evolution of the plasma cells. Genetic and molecular events involved in the transformation of MGUS to MM presumably lead to disordered heavy and light chain immunoglobulin synthesis and abnormal monoclonal FLC production. This is supported by the recent observation that cytogenetic abnomalities were associated with abnormal FLC κ/λ ratios in patients with MM.[19]

These important data have led to considerable debate regarding management guidelines for MGUS. Typical current practice is to monitor all individuals on an annual basis in order to anticipate and prevent debilitating disease progression. Now, it may be preferable to monitor only those individuals at intermediate or high risk. Low risk patients (~ 40%) could be reassured about their test results and not followed up on a long term basis. Their MGUS might be only reassessed when they attend for other illnesses. In contrast, those at high risk might enter drug trials to prevent disease progression.

Possible guidelines were recently discussed in the UK and are shown below *(Table 19.2).* These have yet to be formally adopted.

1. **Low risk** - normal κ/λ ratio, IgG isotype, M-spike <15g/L. Reassurance and discharge. Review MGUS when attending for other illnesses.*
2. **Intermediate risk** - one or two risk factors present. Annual follow-up.+
3. **High risk -** abnormal κ/λ ratio, non-IgG isotype, M-spike >15g/L, 6/12 m follow-up.

* For younger patients - follow-up as for intermediate risk.
\+ No benefit from more frequent early monitoring following diagnosis.
Higher risk associated with higher and/or rising levels of M-spike and more abnormal sFLC ratios.
High sFLC concentrations also associated with risk of renal impairment.

Table 19.2. Possible guidelines for monitoring patients with MGUS.

19.4. Serum free light chain MGUS

Since the monoclonal proteins in MGUS are nearly always intact immunoglobulins and these patients progress to intact immunoglobulin plasma cell dyscrasias, what is the precursor protein for LCMM and AL amyloidosis? There currently appears to be no "FLC MGUS" counterpart for these patients. Occasional reports have described individuals with 'idiopathic' Bence Jones proteinuria who progress to MM.[4] Perhaps there are other individuals who have elevated concentrations of monoclonal serum FLCs that are below the detection limits of electrophoretic tests. Because FLC production is small, such patients might have normal renal function with no urine FLC excretion. The alternative explanation for the origin of LCMM is that they evolve from heavy chain loss in individuals with intact immunoglobulin MGUS. However, this is very rarely seen in clinical practice.

It seems that FLC MGUS may exist as serum FLC κ/λ ratio abnormalities that are undetected by current serum and urine electrophoretic tests. A possible example of such an individual is shown in Figure 19.6. Isolated, minimal urine FLC excretion is usually considered insignificant, but analysis of the corresponding serum indicated an

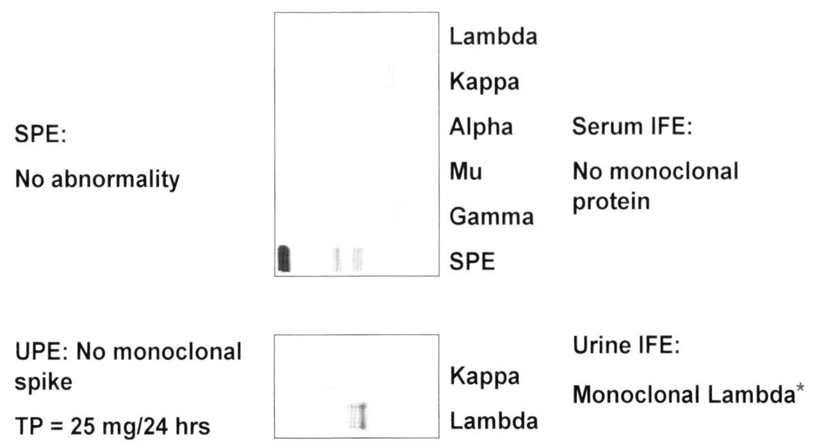

Figure 19.6. Serum and urine IFE on a patient with isolated urine FLC excretion. Serum analysis for FLCs showed an abnormal κ/λ ratio. TP: urine protein excretion. (Courtesy of RA Kyle and JA Katzmann).

abnormality of the κ/λ ratio in this patient.

The existence of FLC MGUS is also apparent from screening studies for monoclonal gammopathies that have incorporated serum FLC measurements. Some individuals have grossly abnormal serum FLC κ/λ ratios but completely normal serum and urine electrophoretic tests *(Chapter 23)*.

The frequency of serum FLC MGUS in a general population has been addressed in a pilot survey at the Mayo Clinic.[20] 901 sera from the Olmsted County MGUS epidemiological study were investigated. All sera selected were negative for serum or urine monoclonal immunoglobulins in the original study (determined from no monoclonal spike by IFE). However, 18 of the samples were abnormal when assessed for serum FLCs. 12 of the sera, with the most abnormal FLC κ/λ ratios (<0.2 or >2.0) were carefully re-assessed by IFE.

One sample had a small IgA band and another a small IgM band hidden in the β region of the gel; 4 had monoclonal λ FLC bands; 3 were equivocal for monoclonal FLCs and 3 were negative. Thus, a total of 7 samples (0.78%) probably had only monoclonal FLCs. These FLC-only MGUS might be the "missing" individuals with preclinical, LCMM or AL amyloidosis. Interestingly, this 0.78% is approximately 20% of the total MGUS incidence in such an age group - a similar percentage to the number of MM patients that are FLC-only (LCMM). This further supports the hypothesis that FLC MGUS are preclinical FLC plasma cell dyscrasias.

Of importance is the observation that the FLC assays identified 2 patients with intact immunoglobulin monoclonal proteins that had been missed in the initial IFE tests. This is an additional reason to use FLC assays in a screening mode.

This study is being expanded to include more individuals in order to answer the following questions:-

1. Are urine FLC concentrations increased in these patients?
2. What is the overall incidence of serum FLC MGUS?
3. Do serum FLC MGUS progress to LCMM or AL amyloidosis?
4. Are they at greater risk of progression than intact immunoglobulin MGUS?

Summary: Elevated monoclonal serum FLCs:-

1. Are found in 0.5-1% of elderly individuals.
2. May identify MGUS patients missed by IFE.
3. Indicate poor outcome in patients with MGUS.
4. May progress to LCMM, AL amyloidosis or other plasma cell dyscrasias.

References

1. **Kyle RA, Rajkumar SV.** Monoclonal gammopathies of undetermined significance. In Hematology/Oncology Clinics of North America: Monoclonal Gammopathies & related disorders. Eds. RA Kyle & M A Gertz; Pub: W B Saunders Co. Philadelphia; 1999; **13**: 1181-1202.

2. **Aguzzi F, Bergami MR, Gasparro C, Bellotti V, Merlini G.** Occurrence of monoclonal components in general practice: Clinical implications. Eur J Haematol 1992; **48**: 192-195.

3. **Langren O, Gridley G, Turesson I, Caporaso NE, Goldin LR, Baris D, Fears TR, Hoover RN, Linet MS.** Risk of monoclonal gammopathy of undetermined significance (MGUS) and subsequent multiple myeloma among African-American and White veterans in the U.S. Blood 2006; 107: 904-906.

4. **Kyle RA, Greipp PR.** "Idiopathic" Bence Jones Proteinuria. New Eng J Med 1982; **306**: 564-567.

5. **Kyle RA, Therneau TM, Rajkumar SV, Offord JR, Larson DR, Plevak MF, Melton LJ.** A long-term Study of Prognosis in Monoclonal Gammopathy of Undetermined Significance. New Eng J Med 2002; **346**: 564-569.

6. **Kyle RA, Therneau TM, Rajkumar SV, Remstein ED, Offord JR, Larson DR, Plevak MF, Melton III LJ.** Long-term follow-up of IgM monoclonal gammopathy of undetermined significance. Blood 2003; **102**: 3759-3764.

7. **Dimopoulos MA, Moulopoulos A, Smith T, Delasalle KB, Alexanian R.** Risk of Disease Progression in Asymptomatic Multiple Myeloma. Amer J Med 1993; **94**: 57-61.

8. **Baldini L, Guffanti A, Cesana BM, Colombi M, Chiorboli O, Damilano I, Maiolo AT.** Role of Different Hematologic Variables in Defining the Risk of Malignant Transformation in Monoclonal Gammopathy. Blood 1996; **87**: 912-918.

9. **Cesana C, Klersy C, Barbarano L, Nosari AM, Crugnola M, Pungolino E, Gargantini L, Granata S, Valentini M, Morra E.** Prognostic factors for Malignant Transformation in Monoclonal Gammopathy of Undetermined Significance and Smouldering Multiple Myeloma. J Clin Oncol 2002; **20**: 1625-1634.

10. **Marien G, Oris E, Bradwell AR, Blanckaert N, Bossuyt X.** Detection of Monoclonal Proteins in Sera by Capillary Zone Electrophoresis and Free Light Chain Measurements. Clin Chem 2002; **48**: 1600-1601.

11. **Lachmann HJ, Gallimore R, Gillmore JD, Smith L, Bradwell AR, Hawkins PN.** Detection of monoclonal free light chains by nephelometry in systemic AL amyloidosis. Clin Chem 2002; **48**: A164: pE45.

12. **Tate RJ, Gill D, Cobcroft R, Hickman PE.** Practical considerations for the Measurement of Free Light Chains in Serum. Clin Chem 2003; **49**: 1252-1257

13. **Rajkumar SV, Kyle RA, Therneau TM, Bradwell AR, Melton III LJ, Katzmann JA.** Presence of Monoclonal Free Light Chains in Serum Predicts Risk of Progression in Monoclonal Gammopathy of Undetermined Significance. Blood 2003;**102** (11): 3481

14. **Rajkumar SV, Kyle RA, Therneau TM, Clark RJ, Bradwell AR, Melton LJ III, Larson DR,**

Plevak MF, Katzmann JA. Presence of monoclonal free light chains in the serum predicts risk of progression in monoclonal gammopathy of undetermined significance. Br J Haem 2004; **127**: 308-310.

15. Rajkumar SV, Kyle RA, Therneau TM, Melton LJ III, Bradwell AR, Clark RJ, Larson DR, Plevak MF, Dispenzieri A, Katzmann JA. Presence of an Abnormal Serum Free Light Chain Ratio is an Independent Risk Factor for Progression in Monoclonal Gammopathy of Undetermined Significance (MGUS). Blood 2005: **104** (11): 3647.

16. Rajkumar SV, Kyle RA, Therneau TM, Melton LJ III, Bradwell AR, Clark RJ, Larson DR, Plevak MF, Dispenzieri A, Katzmann JA. Serum free light chain ratio is an independent risk factor for progression in monoclonal gammopathy of undetermined significance. Blood 2004: **106**: 812-817.

17. Munshi NC. Determining the undetermined. Editorial, Blood 2004: **106**: 767-768.

18. Rajkumar VS. MGUS and Smoldering Multiple Myemloma: Update on Pathogenesis, Natural History, and Management. Hematology (Am Soc Hematol Educ Program). 2005; p340-345.

19. Cavallo F, Rasmussen E, Zangari M, Tricot G, Fender B, Fox M, Burns M, Barlogie B. Serum Free-Lite Chain (sFLC) Assay in Multiple Myeloma (MM): Clinical Correlates and Prognostic Implications in Newly Diagnosed MM Patients Treated with Total Therapy 2 or 3 (TT2/3). Blood 2005; **106** (11): 3490: p974a.

20. Katzmann JA, Clark RJ, Rajkumar VS, Kyle RA. Monoclonal free light chains in sera from healthy individuals: FLC MGUS. Clin Chem 2003; **49**: A-74: pA24.

Test Questions

1. How should patients with a serum FLC MGUS be managed?
2. What clinical decisions should be made about MGUS patients who have associated monoclonal serum FLCs?
3. Why are FLC MGUS rarely seen?
4. What are the clinical benefits of MGUS risk stratification?

Answers

1. Unknown at present, but annual follow-up is prudent (page 169).
2. The risk of progression should be assessed and long-term monitoring discussed with the patient (page 169).
3. Because the amounts of FLCs produced are below the sensitivity of electrophoretic tests and are insufficient to exceed the proximal tubular reabsorption mechanisms and overflow into urine (page 169).
4. Patients at high risk of progression can be more closely monitored while low-risk patients can be discharged from follow-up clinics (Page 169).

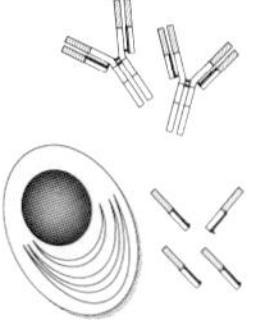

Section 3

Diseases with increased polyclonal free light chains

Chapter 20

Renal diseases and free light chains

20.1. Introduction

Elevated polyclonal FLCs in serum (associated with normal κ/λ ratios) result from increased polyclonal production, reduced renal clearance or a combination of both mechanisms. Increased production is due to proliferation of plasma cells and/or their progenitors and is frequently associated with polyclonal hypergammaglobulinaemia. This is a common finding in patients with liver diseases, connective tissue disorders, chronic infections, etc. A complete list of the relevant diseases is given in Chapter 29.

Reduced clearance of sFLCs results from impaired renal glomerular filtration and is a frequent finding. This can be seen even in apparently healthy, elderly individuals who may have normal serum creatinine concentrations but elevated polyclonal sFLCs from slight renal damage.

Frequently, acute and chronic inflammatory diseases are associated with some degree of renal impairment. The combination of increased production and reduced renal clearance leads to particularly high sFLC concentrations, classically observed in patients with SLE. Although not documented, it is likely that many patients with chronic inflammatory diseases and associated renal impairment will be found to have very high concentrations of polyclonal sFLCs, but with substantially normal κ/λ ratios.

20.2. Effect of renal impairment on serum free light chain concentrations

The normally rapid renal clearance of sFLCs of 2-6 hours is increased to 2-3 days in complete renal failure (*Chapter 3*).[1] Removal from the circulation then occurs through pinocytosis by cells of the reticulo-endothelial system in the liver and elsewhere *(Chapter 13)*. As the glomerular filtration rate (GFR) falls, sFLC concentrations rise and may be 20-30 times normal in end-stage renal failure.

The relationship between sFLC concentrations and GFR is shown in a series of correlation coefficients in Table 20.1 and Figures 20.1 and 20.2. The MDRD index (Modification of Diet in Renal Disease) of GFR produces a poorer correlation with FLC levels than serum creatinine levels but better that the Cockroft-Gault formula.[2,3] Cystatin C concentrations have the highest correlation with FLC levels and arguably are the most accurate simple measure of GFR *(Figure 20.2)*.[4]

20.3. Effect of renal impairment on serum κ/λ ratios

As both serum κ and λ FLC levels increase with deteriorating renal function their relative amounts change slightly. While glomeruli clear monomeric κ molecules approximately 3 times faster than dimeric λ molecules *(Chapter 3)*, pinocytosis removes both proteins at the same rate. With deteriorating renal function κ/λ ratios gradually increase *(Chapters 3.4, 5.1 and Table 5.3)* and eventually equal the κ:λ production rates

	Kappa	Lambda
Serum creatinine	0.697	0.701
Cockroft-Gault formula	0.521	0.490
MDRD	0.631	0.613
Cystatin C	0.778	0.727

Table 20.1. Relationship (correlation coefficient - R^2) between serum FLC concentrations and different markers of glomerular filtration rate in 107 patients with chronic renal failure. MDRD: Modification of Diet in Renal Disease.

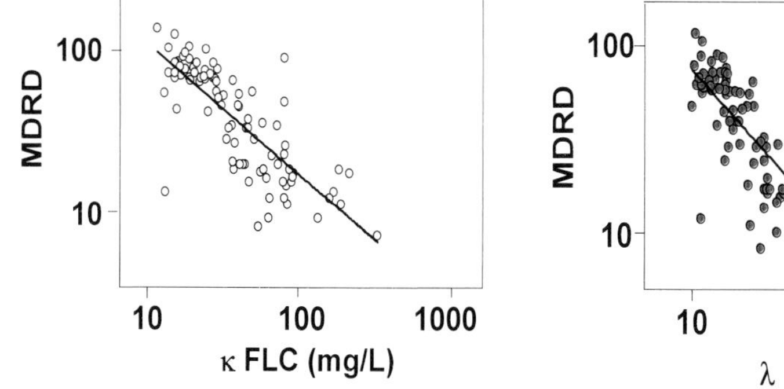

Figure 20.1. Correlation between serum κ and λ concentrations and the MDRD index of glomerular filtration in 107 patients with chronic renal failure *(from Table 20.1)*. MDRD: Modification of Diet in Renal Disease.

of approximately 1.8:1 in end-stage renal failure.

The effect of renal impairment on κ/λ ratios is seen in several patient groups:-

1. κ and λ concentrations increase with age in apparently normal individuals because of minor degrees of renal impairment *(Figure 5.1)*. This is associated with an increase in the median κ/λ ratio from 0.49 to 0.70 in older people *(Table 20.2)*. This is shown as a change in the κ/λ ratios from 0.6 on a κ/λ plot *(Figure 20.3)*.

2. Patients in chronic renal failure, but without FLC monoclonal gammopathies, have slightly higher κ/λ ratios than normal individuals. As renal function deteriorates the amounts of κ FLC cleared by the kidneys progressively fall relative to λ FLCs. This is manifest as an increase in median κ/λ ratios as FLC concentrations rise *(Figure 20.4)*.

3. Patients with AL amyloidosis caused by λ FLC monoclonal gammopathies tend to have κ/λ ratios closer to the normal range population than κ-producing patients *(Figure 20.5)*. There is also asymmetry of κ compared with λ FLC concentrations in patients with LCMM *(Figure 8.2)* and MGUS *(Figure 19.4)*. The patients with these diseases frequently have some degree of renal failure so that κ concentrations are relatively high. Individuals with normal renal function clear κ molecules more quickly.

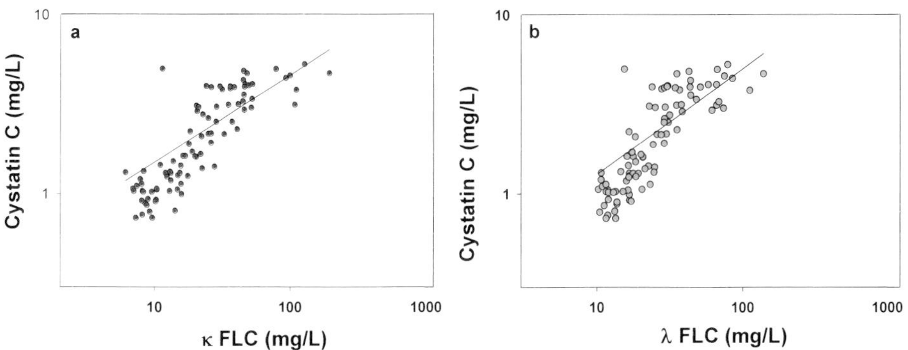

Figure 20.2. Correlation between (a) κ and (b) λ concentrations and cystatin C concentrations in 107 patients with chronic renal failure *(from Table 20.1)*.

Age (years)	κ FLC (mg/L)	λ FLC (mg/L)	FLC κ/λ
20-29	6.3	12.4	0.49
30-39	7.2	13.6	0.55
40-49	7.5	12.8	0.58
50-59	6.4	11.3	0.59
60-69	6.9	11.8	0.70
70-79	8.0	11.9	0.65
80-90	9.1	15.1	0.64

Table 20.2. Changes in median serum FLC κ/λ ratios with increasing age in apparently normal individuals. Data from Figure 5.1.

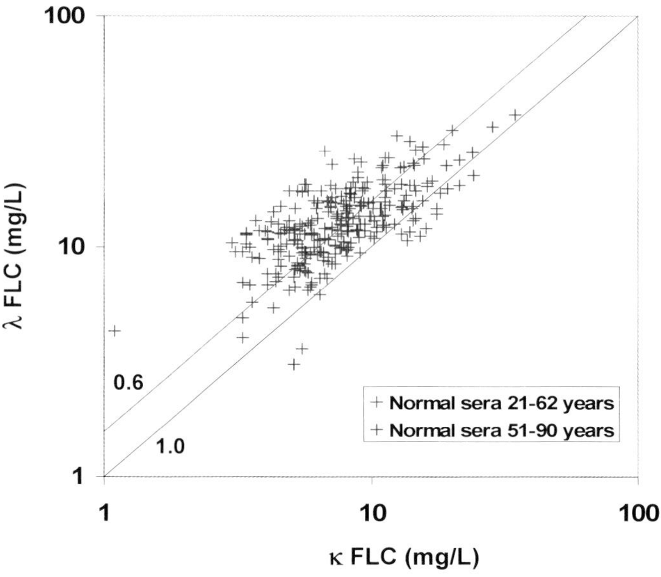

Figure 20.3. Serum FLCs in 282 normal sera. Normal range data from Figure 5.1. The diagonal axes labelled 1.0 and 0.6 are set at the κ/λ ratios of 1.00 and 0.6 respectively. The latter is the approximate median value for normal individuals.

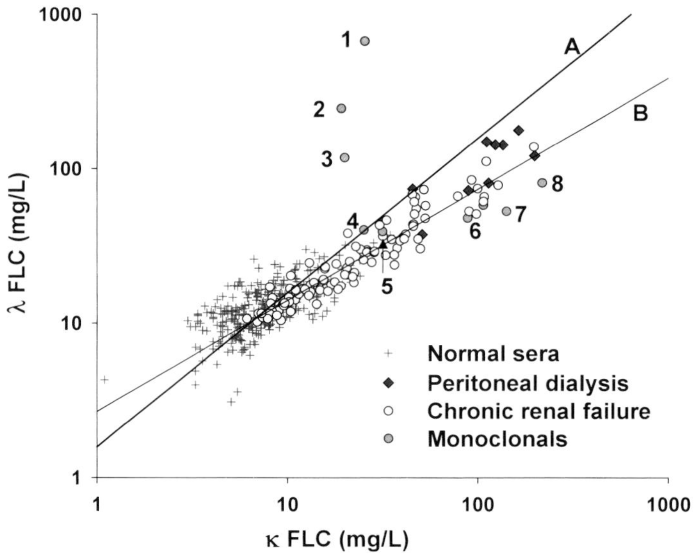

Figure 20.4. Elevated serum free light chain concentrations in 107 patients with varying degrees of chronic renal failure. Numbers 1-8 refer to patients with monoclonal gammopathies shown in Table 20.4. Line A is at a κ/λ ratio of 0.6 and line B is the κ/λ ratio in patients with renal failure.

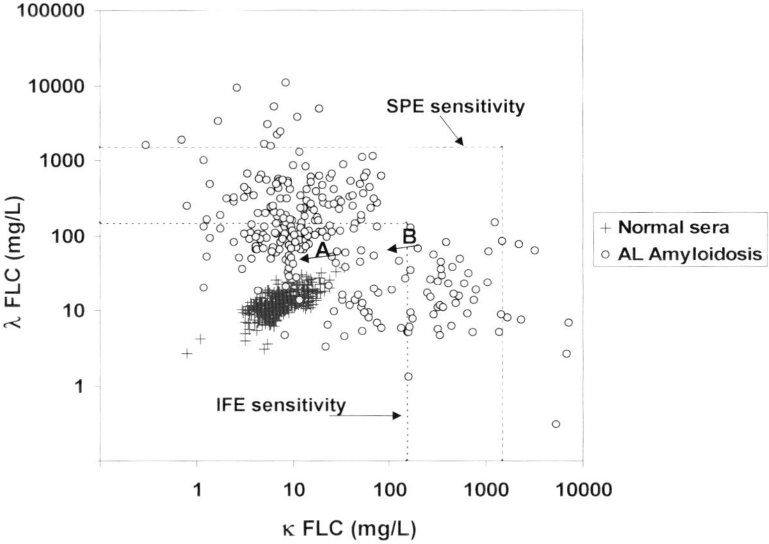

Figure 20.5. Serum FLCs in patients with AL amyloidosis, many of whom have renal impairment. The λ–producing patients tend to cluster against the normal samples because of increased κ levels due to reduced renal clearances. A and B show potential changes in FLC concentrations with recovery of normal renal function.

The change in κ/λ ratios with increasing renal impairment is of clinical relevance when interpreting borderline results. Patients might be misclassified as having minor κ monoclonal gammopathies because of slightly increased κ/λ ratios when, in fact, they have renal impairment. Equally, patients with minor λ monoclonal gammopathies could have normal κ/λ ratios because of the relative increase in κ concentrations *(Figure 20.5: A and B)*.

The relationship between cystatin C concentrations and κ/λ ratios is shown in Figure 20.6 and Table 20.3. A correction factor for the κ/λ ratios based on cystatin C assessments of the glomerular filtration rate may be of help in patients with borderline κ/λ ratios who have renal impairment. The formula for this correction factor is:-

$$\text{Corrected } \kappa/\lambda \text{ ratio} = \text{uncorrected } \kappa/\lambda - \{(\text{cystatin C} - 0.6) \times 0.16\}$$

It should be noted that this correction factor has not been validated clinically and is not relevant to the vast majority of patients. Its use will probably only apply to patients with borderline results who have changing renal function. In screening studies, a wide range for the κ/λ ratio might be used so that patients with renal impairment are not misdiagnosed as having monoclonal gammopathies *(Chapter 23)*.

20.4. Removal of serum free light chains by dialysis

The pore size of haemodialysis membranes (dialysers) allows removal of small to medium-sized protein molecules from the blood. Membranes typically have a molecular

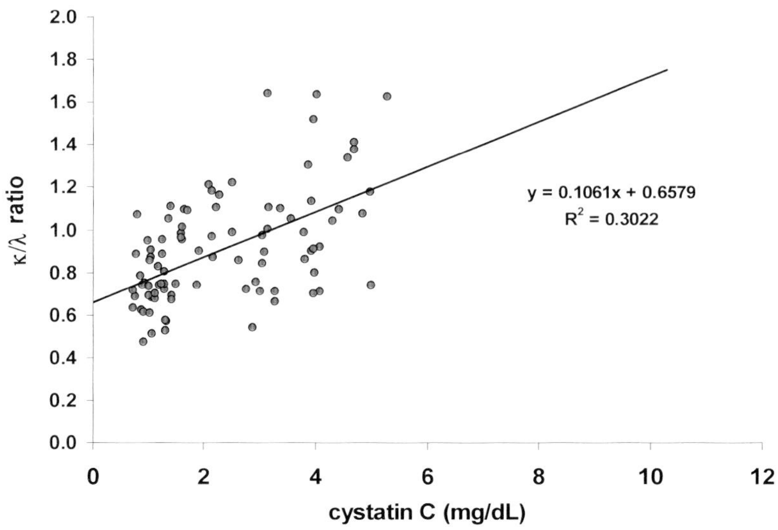

Figure 20.6. Relationship between κ/λ ratios and cystatin C in patients with chronic renal failure.

cystatin C (mg/L)	Correction factor	95% confidence limits
1.5mg/L	-0.14	(0.12-0.17)
2.0mg/L	-0.22	(0.19-0.26)
3.0mg/L	-0.38	(0.32-0.45)
4.0mg/L	-0.54	(0.45-0.63)
5.0mg/L	-0.70	(0.58-0.82)

Table 20.3. Suggested subtracted correction factors for κ/λ ratios based upon the use of cystatin C concentrations as a measure of renal impairment.

weight cut-off of 15-20kDa so the filtration efficiency for FLCs is relatively modest. However, some dialysers are more permeable and others adsorb FLCs on to the membranes. Figure 20.7 shows the reduction in serum FLC concentrations in 40 patients with chronic renal failure over a 4-hour dialysis period using a high-flux polysulphonate membrane. 60% of κ and 37% of dimeric λ molecules were removed and median κ/λ ratios changed from 1.23 to 0.7.[5]

The quantities of FLCs in the filtrate fluid accounted for approximately 60% of the observed reductions in serum concentrations while the remainder was adsorbed onto the filtration membranes.[6] Multiple sampling of the dialysate fluid during the 4-hour haemodialysis period showed slowly reducing FLC concentrations as serum levels fell *(Figure 20.8)*. Dialysate fluid κ/λ ratios changed from 1.6 to 1.4 during the dialysis period as greater amounts of the smaller monomeric κ molecules were preferentially cleared. Some dialysers are more efficient at FLC removal because of larger pore sizes

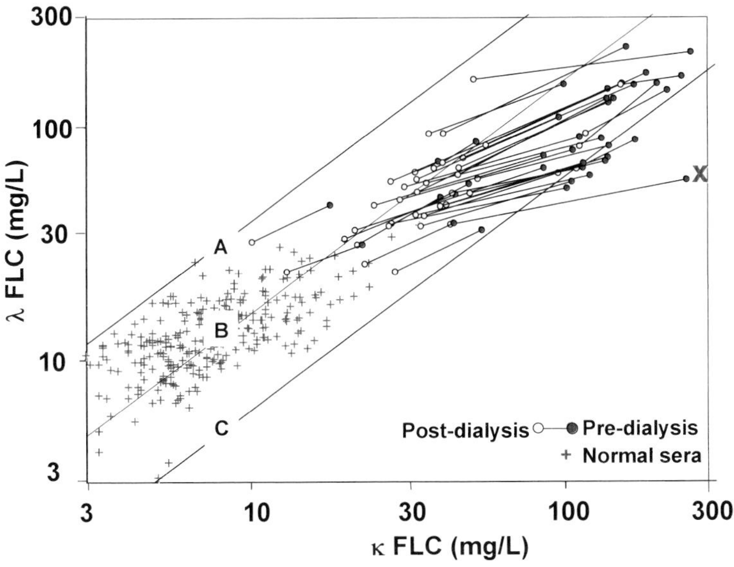

Figure 20.7. Reduction of sFLCs in 40 patients with chronic renal failure undergoing four hours of haemodialysis. Patient X had an IgAκ monoclonal gammopathy with monoclonal κ FLCs. A, B and C show axes for κ/λ ratios of 0.2, 0.6 and 2.0 respectively.

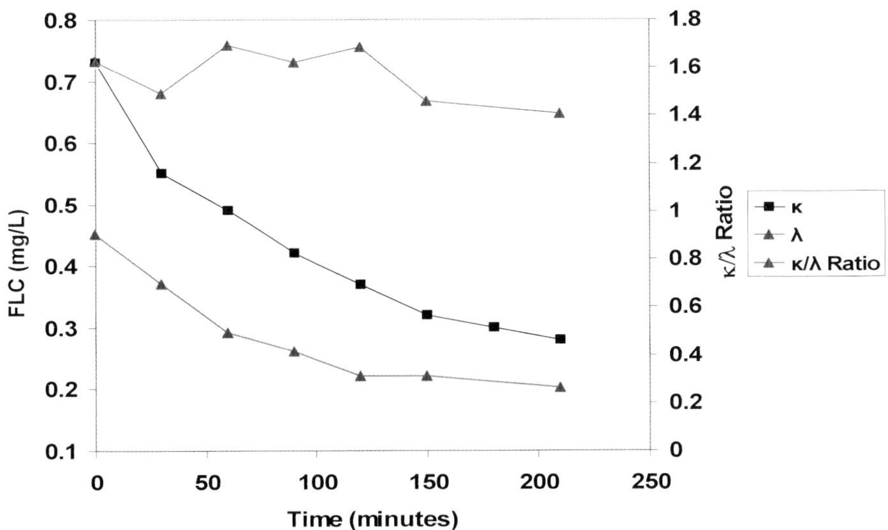

Figure 20.8. Concentrations of FLCs in the dialysate fluid of a patient, sampled every 30 minutes, during 4 hours of haemodialysis.

and different suface charges and may be useful for patients with LCMM who are in acute renal failure *(Chapter 14).*

Peritoneal dialysis is less efficient at removing FLCs *(Figure 20.4).* The fluid volumes exchanged during this process are much less than in haemodialysis, which presumably accounts for the poor removal.

The clinical consequences of elevated sFLCs in renal impairment are unclear. Reports have suggested that the elevated FLCs lead to reductions in immune function and should therefore be classified as uraemic toxins.[7] Indeed, studies have shown that FLCs are inflammatory proteins.[8] It is thought that their toxicity may partly account for the relatively poor survival of many patients undergoing chronic haemodialysis.

There is an additional concern about the toxicity of the high FLC load on the kidneys in patients during the progression to end-stage renal failure. As the nephron mass declines with increasing renal impairment the remaining nephrons, which are hyperfiltrating, are exposed to increasing levels of FLCs. This may contribute to an accelerating decline in renal function.[9]

20.5. Monoclonal free light chains in chronic renal failure

It is of interest that 8 of 107 (7%) patients in chronic renal failure in Figure and Table 20.4 had monoclonal gammopathies. None were associated with clinically apparent plasma cell dyscrasias and, indeed, only one had been identified prior to the study. 3 of the patients had FLC-only MGUS. 5 other patients had intact immunoglobulin monoclonal proteins identified by serum IFE of which 2 had associated FLC MGUS.

From this study, it appears that many patients in chronic renal failure have FLC MGUS.[10] It is possible that these patients have monoclonal FLCs contributing to their renal disease. Dingli et al., (2005) showed that there was a relationship between focal and segmental glomerulosclerosis and plasma cell disorders in a study of 13 patients.[11] It was considered likely that some of the pathological damage was due to monoclonal FLCs. Studies of renal biopsies in patients with chronic renal disease have shown that AL-amloidosis is under-recognised and approximately 3% of biopsies have monoclonal light chains deposited in renal tissues without systemic features.[12,13] Such patients require chemotherapy, but monitoring treatment from repeated biopsies is impractical.

Patient	Kappa	Lambda	κ/λ ratio	IFE
1	25.42	671.77	0.04	Normal
2	19.1	246.77	0.08	Normal
3	19.88	118.13	0.17	IgGλ
4	25.15	40.31	0.62	IgGκ
5	33.06	46.58	0.71	IgGλ
6	31.52	39.41	0.80	IgGκ
7	141.32	53.15	2.66	IgGκ
8	216.91	81.31	2.67	Normal

Table 20.4. Analysis of 8 samples with monoclonal gammopathies (5 with monoclonal light chains only) in 107 patients with chronic renal failure *(from Figure 20.4).*

Serum FLC analysis should allow these patients to be identifed early and monitored for the appropriate chemotherapy in order to eliminate their clonal disease.[14] It may be that these patients should not be transplanted until their clonal plasma cell disorder is properly treated as the donated kidney may not survive long.[15,16]

Case-matched studies are required to determine whether the prevalence is higher than in a normal population *(Chapter 19).* It may be that individuals with serum FLC MGUS accumulate in the chronic renal disease population. While their renal impairment is readily identified, the underlying cause(s) is not necessarily established.

Clinical case history No 10. Influence of renal function on sFLC concentrations.[17]

A 55-year-old woman presented with uncomplicated IgGκ MM and was given three courses of VAD followed by high dose melphalan and a PBSCT. She was well immediately following the transplant but then developed a degree of renal impairment. Careful attendance to fluid and electrolyte balance restored normal renal function.

While in hospital, she was monitored daily with sFLCs in an on-going investigation into their role as markers of treatment responsiveness (*Figure 20.9 and Chapter 13*). The effect of high dose melphalan was to reduce both κ and λ FLCs to below normal concentrations with a favourable relative reduction in the tumour FLC levels. Subsequently, from day 15, as bone marrow engraftment took place, both FLCs increased and the κ/λ ratio normalised. Then, the FLCs increased above normal with a rising κ/λ ratio indicating some renal impairment. This observation was supported by an increase in serum creatinine concentrations. After day 22, FLC concentrations normalised and the κ/λ ratio fell, alongside serum creatinine levels.

In this patient, the combination of serial sFLC concentrations and serum creatinine

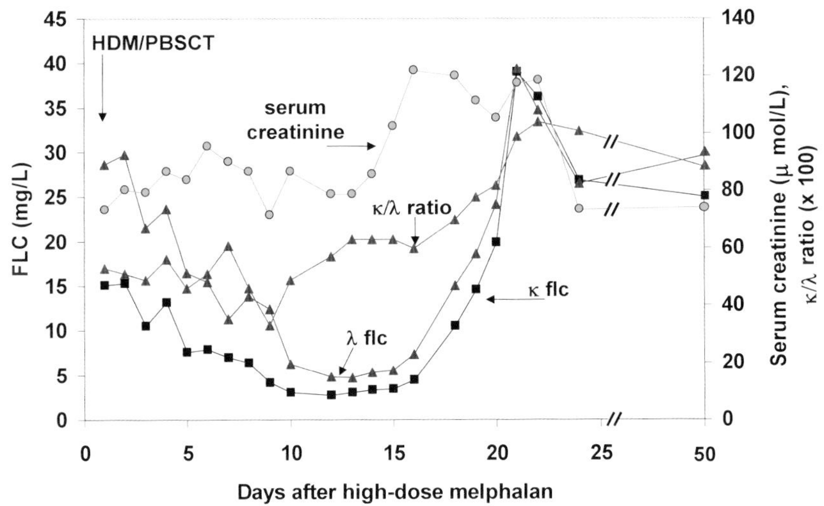

Figure 20.9. Changes in FLCs and creatinine while monitoring a patient with MM after high-dose melphalan and PBSCT (Courtesy of G Pratt, Heartlands Hospital, Birmingham).[17]

measurements allowed assessment of renal dysfunction and bone marrow recovery. Changes in the κ/λ ratio may need to be corrected for renal impairment if there is confusion about interpreting the results. In addition, since patients with plasma cell dyscrasias are frequently elderly and are treated with nephrotoxic drugs, repeated measurements of sFLCs might assist in assessing renal function.

Summary: In patients with renal impairment:

1. Polyclonal sFLC levels rise as glomerular filtration rate falls.
2. Concentrations may increase 30-40 fold.
3. κ/λ ratios increase slightly with decreasing renal function.
4. Monoclonal FLCs are frequently found in patients with chronic renal failure.
5. Serum FLCs can be effectively removed by haemodialysis.

References

1. **Abraham GN, Waterhouse C.** Evidence for defective immunoglobulin metabolism in severe renal insufficiency. Amer J Med Sci 1974; **268**: 227-233.

2. **Levey AS, Bosch JP, Lewis JB, Green T, Rogers N, Roth D.** A More Accurate Method To Estimate Glomerular Filtration Rate from Serum Creatinine: A New Prediction Equation. Ann Intern Med 1999; **130**: 461-470.

3. **Cockroft DW, Gault MH.** Prediction of creatinine clearance from serum creatinine. Nephron 1976; **16**: 31-41.

4. **Katzmann JA, Clark RJ, Abraham RS, Bryant S, Lymp JF, Bradwell AR, Kyle RA.** Serum Reference Intervals and Diagnostic Ranges for Free κ and Free λ Immunoglobulin Light Chains: Relative Sensitivity for Detection of Monoclonal Light Chains. Clin Chem 2002; **48**: 1437-1444.

5. **Reid SD, Cockwell P, Hewins P, Millard JL, Mead GP, Bradwell AR**. Haemodialysis removes free light chains from serum. Clin Chem 2005; **51** (6): suppl: D-12.

6. **Cohen G, Rudnicki M, Schmaldienst S, Horl WH**. Effect of dialysis on serum/plasma levels of free immunoglobulin light chains in end-stage renal disease patients. Nephrol Dial Transplant 2002; **17**: 879-883.

7. **Cohen G, Rudnicki M Horl WH.** Uraemic toxins modulate the spontaneous apoptotic cell death and essential functions of neutrophils. Kidney Int 2001; **59** (Suppl 78): S48-S52.

8. **Van Der Heijden M, Kraneveld A, Redegeld F.** Free immunoglobulin light chains as target in the treatment of chronic inflammatory diseases. Eur J Pharmacol 2006. *In Press.*

9. **Kritz W, LeHir M.** Pathways to nephron loss starting from glomerular diseases - Insights from animal models. Kid International 2005; **67**: 404-419.

10. **Reid SD, Cockwell P, Millard J, Chandler K, Hutchison CA, Mead GP, Bradwell AR.** MGUS incidence in a chronic kidney disease population. 2006; *Submitted.*

11. **Dingli D, Larson DR, Plevak MF, Grande JP, Kyle RA.** Focal and segmental glomerulosclerosis and plasma cell proliferative disorders. Am J Kidney Dis 2005; **46** (2): 278-282.

12. **Sanders PW, Herrera GA, Kirk KA, Old CW, Galla JH.** Spectrum of Glomerular and Tubulointerstitial Renal Lesions Associated with Monotypical Immunoglobulin Light Chain Deposition. Lab Invest 1991; **64** (4): 527-537.

13 **Novak L, Cook WJ, Herrera GA, Sanders PW.** AL-amyloidosis is underdiagnosed in renal biopsies. Nephrol Dial Transplant 2004; **19**: 3050-3053.

14. **Montseny J-J, Kleinknecht D, Meyrier A, Vanhille P, Simon P, Pruna A, Eladari D.** Long-term outcome according to renal histological lesions in 118 patients with monoclonal gammopathies. Nephrol Dial Transplant 1998; **13**: 1438-1445.

15. **Leung N, Lager DJ, Gertz MA, Wilson K, Kanakiriya S, Fervenza FC.** Long-term outcome of renal transplantation in light-chain deposition disease. Am J Kidney Dis 2004; **43** (1): 147-153.

16. Tanenbaum ND, Howell DN, Middleton JP, Spurney RF. Lambda light chain deposition in a renal allograft. Transplant Proc 2005; **37** (10): 4289-4292.

17. Pratt G, Mead GP, Godfrey KR, Hu Y, Evans ND, Chappell MJ, Lovell R, Bradwell AR. The tumor kinetics of multiple myeloma following autologous stem cell transplantation as assessed by measuring serum-free light chains. Leukemia & Lymphoma 2006; **47** (1): 21-28.

Test Questions

1. What is the mechanism of increase in serum FLC levels in renal impairment?
2. How are increases in polyclonal and monoclonal FLCs differentiated?
3. Why are κ/λ ratios slightly increased in patients with renal failure compared with patients having normal renal function?
4. Which is more efficient for FLC removal: plasma exchange or haemodialysis?
5. Why may patients with chronic kidney disease have unexpected monoclonal FLCs?

Answers.
1. Increase in serum half-life from reduced glomerular filtration (Page 174).
2. By use of a κ/λ log plot and κ/λ ratios (Page 174).
3. Faster removal of κ molecules reduces with increasing renal failure (Page 175).
4. Haemodialysis (Page 177).
5. Light chain deposition is not easily identified in renal biopsies so the clone of plasma cells remains unrecognised, and IFE fails to identify low concentration serum FLCs (Page 180).

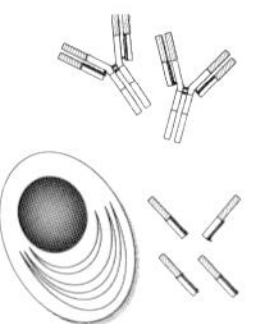

Chapter 21

Immune stimulation and elevated polyclonal free light chains

21.1. Introduction

Diseases associated with generalised increased B-cell activation frequently have high concentrations of polyclonal immunoglobulins and coexisting high polyclonal sFLCs. The different conditions are listed in Chapter 29.[1]

The relationship between polyclonal hypergammaglobulinaemia and elevated polyclonal serum FLCs was demonstrated in 25 patients studied at the Mayo Clinic.[2] In some patients, concentrations of both FLCs were highly elevated, although, κ/λ ratios were always within the normal range (*Figure 21.1*). Total immunoglobulin concentrations were as high as 54g/L while maximum FLC concentrations were 273mg/L for κ and 307mg/L for λ. The correlation between immunoglobulin and sFLC levels was modest. This may have been due to impaired renal function elevating the FLC concentrations in some patients. However, data on glomerular filtration rates was not available.

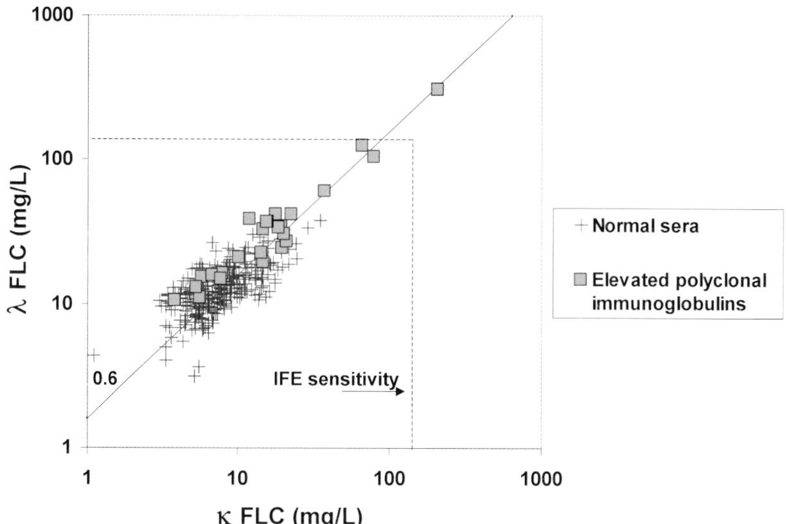

Figure 21.1. Serum FLCs in 25 patients with polyclonal hypergammaglobulinaemia, compared with normal individuals. (Courtesy of RA Kyle and JA Katzmann).[2]

One interesting aspect of polyclonal FLCs is whether they are bioactive molecules in inflammatory disease processes. This has been mooted for some time but the availablity of a simple serum assay has re-awakened this area of research.

21.2. Rheumatic diseases

Many rheumatic diseases feature polyclonal B-cell activation, high concentrations of autoimmune antibodies and polyclonal elevations of serum immunoglobulins. Excess polyclonal FLCs have been detected in the urine of these patients and indeed, their measurement may be useful for assessing disease activity. Presumably, serum analysis of FLCs in such patients would be more reliable. This may be particularly applicable to patients with SLE, many of whom have high concentrations of urine polyclonal FLCs.[3-5] Since these patients frequently have renal impairment, sFLC concentrations may be highly elevated.

Hoffman et al. investigated the relationship between sFLCs and other markers of disease activity in patients with rheumatic diseases.[7] Figure 21.2 shows the concentrations of sFLCs in the different disease groups. Patients with intercurrent illnesses were excluded from analysis to ensure that the changes were due exclusively to the disease under study.

High FLC concentrations were found in rheumatoid arthritis, SLE, Sjögren's

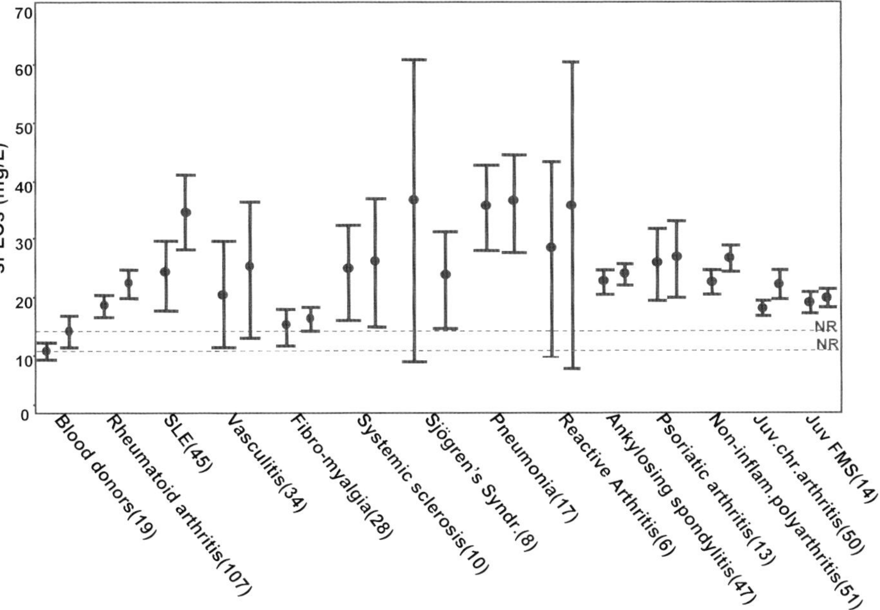

Figure 21.2. Serum FLCs in different diseases compared with blood donors Bars show range and mean concentrations of κ (red) and λ (blue). Juv chr arthritis: juvenile chronic arthritis. Juv FMS: juvenile fibromyalgia syndrome. Numbers of individuals studied are shown in brackets. (Courtesy of U Hoffmann).[7]

syndrome, vasculitis and systemic sclerosis compared with control groups of 28 patients with fibromyalgia and 19 blood donors ($p<0.05$). Furthermore, sFLC concentrations were more frequently elevated than intact immunoglobulins. In all individuals, κ/λ ratios were normal, indicating polyclonal synthesis. It was also found that sFLCs were more frequently elevated than C-reactive protein in patients with SLE, Sjögren's syndrome and systemic sclerosis. However, the numbers of patients in some groups were insufficient for statistical analysis.

As might be expected, there was a positive correlation between concentrations of sFLCs and creatinine in all patient groups. Predictably, FLC concentrations were higher in SLE patients who had renal involvement compared with those having normal renal function (*Figure 21.3*).

Clinical scores of SLE correlated with sFLC levels, particularly when the disease was active. In a subsequent prospective study, the clinical scores (ECLAM) in 8 patients were compared with a variety of laboratory parameters.[8] sFLC concentrations showed a strong correlation with disease activity *(Figure 21.4)* which was not observed for C-reactive protein or ESR. Further studies are ongoing.

Gottenberg J-E et al.,[9] studied 139 patients with Sjögren's Syndrome *(Figure 21.5)* compared with the 8 patients studied by Hoffmann *(Figure 21.2)*. 20% of the patients had raised sFLC levels and concentrations were highest in association with SSB autoantibodies. Also, patients with systemic disease had higher levels than those with only glandular involvement. Interestingly, a further 15 patients with Sjögren's syndrome had monoclonal FLCs, a higher proportion than might be expected by chance. Since some of these patients progress to maltomas, abnormal κ/λ FLC ratios might be a

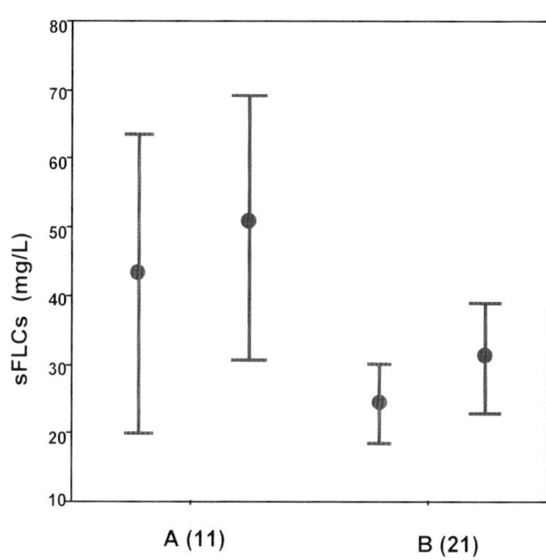

Figure 21.3. Serum FLC in SLE (A) with and (B) without renal involvement . The numbers of individuals studied are shown in brackets. Bars show range and mean concentrations of κ (red) and λ (blue). (Courtesy of U Hoffmann).[8]

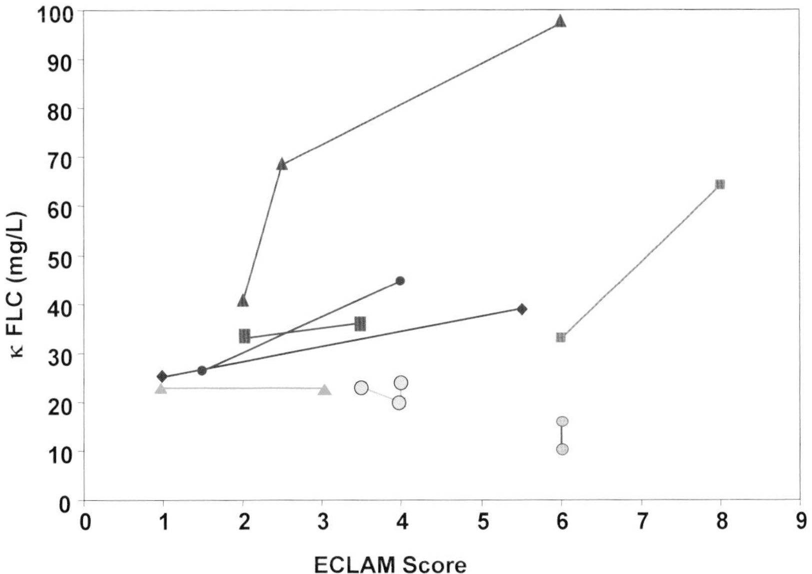

Figure 21.4. Follow up of 8 patients with SLE showing a strong correlation between disease acitivity measured by ECLAM scores and serum FLC κ concentrations. (Courtesy of U Hoffmann).[8]

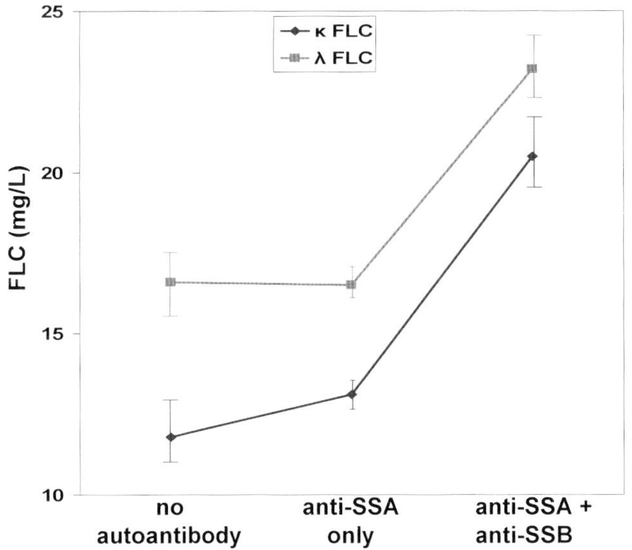

Figure 21.5. Serum FLCs in relation to the presence of SSA and SSB antibodies in patients with Sjögren's syndrome. (Courtesy of X Mariette).[9]

useful marker for tumour development *(Table 18.2)*. Longitudinal studies are underway.

21.3. Diabetes Mellitus.

Two studies have identified a relationship between urine FLC concentrations and rapidly progressive diabetes mellitus. Thus, 20 years ago, it was noted that patients with proliferative retinopathy had both higher urine κ FLC excretion (λ FLC assays were not available) than those without retinopathy and more than patients with proteinuria from other causes.[10] There was an associated elevated κ FLC/albumin excretion ratio. Subsequently, the same authors suggested that elevated FLC/albumin excretion ratios were an early indication of diabetic nephropathy and they directly implicated a renal cause.[11] This was supported by the finding of normal serum FLC concentrations. However, in the absence of sensitive serum assays this interpretation was perhaps premature and increased FLC production could be a contributory factor.

A recent study by our group analysed FLC levels in both serum and urine of diabetic patients attending an early diabetes clinic.[12] Of 88 patients studied, mean FLC levels were higher in serum compared with a normal population (κ 19.9mg/L vs. 8.4mg/L, λ 17.4mg/L vs. 14.5mg/L: $p<0.0001$) (*Figure 21.6*) and were also higher in urine (κ 49.3mg/L vs. 5.5mg/L, λ 7.7mg/L vs. 3.17mg/L: $p<0.002$) *(Figure 21.7)*. Both κ and λ urinary FLC concentrations showed a positive correlation with albumin/creatinine excretion ratios ($r = 0.69$, and 0.58 respectively). 49% of the patients had abnormal urine FLC concentrations compared with 24% having abnormal albumin/creatinine ratios. This supports the previous observation that increased urine FLCs may be a marker of early diabetic nephropathy.

The finding of increased serum FLCs indicates either increased production and/or reduced renal clearance. There is some evidence for reduced clearance because many of the patients had reduced glomerular filtration rate as evidenced by a reduced MDRD

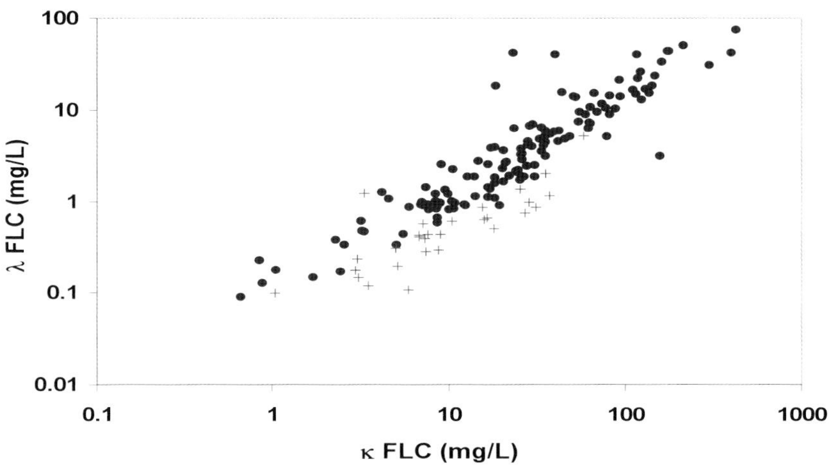

Figure 21.6. Serum FLC concentrations in patients with diabetes mellitus (blue) compared with the normal population (red). (Courtesy of C Hutchison).[12]

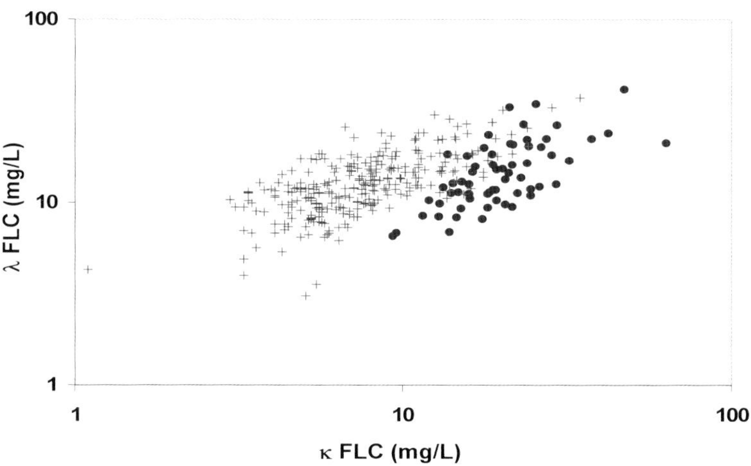

Figure 21.7. Urine κ and λ FLCs in patients with diabetes mellitus (blue) compared with normal urine FLC concentrations (red). (Courtesy of C Hutchison).[12]

index *(Chapter 20)*. Further evidence supporting renal impairment was the elevated κ/λ ratios in some patients *(Figure 21.6)*. However, some patients had normal MDRD indices with high concentrations of sFLCs indicating increased production. This is suggestive of generalised inflammation/vasculopathy. Perhaps retinopathy and nephropathy are the most readily observed clinical signs of a generalised inflammatory process that is apparent from raised FLC production.

Since polyclonal FLCs are potentially nephrotoxic, increased concentrations may contribute to rapidly progressive nephropathy. It has also been suggested that monoclonal FLCs may play a role in some patients' renal disease.[13] Indeed, mesangial monoclonal FLC deposits observed in the renal biopsies of patients with renal impairment may be similar in appearance to those found in diabetic glomerulosclerosis.[14] Furthermore, FLC MGUS is frequently observed in patients with renal impairment *(Chapter 20)*, so it may be an additional risk factor for progressive nephropathy in diabetes mellitus.

In conclusion, diabetic patients have significant FLC abnormalities in serum and urine that may be involved in the pathogenesis of diabetic nephropathy.

21.4. Other diseases with elevated polyclonal free light chains

There was one early study of sFLCs in other acute or chronic inflammatory diseases,[6] and a recent study of a few patients with acute pneumonia *(Figure 21.8)*.[8] As expected, polyclonal sFLCs were elevated. In the latter study, the median κ/λ ratio was higher than in other disease groups suggesting modest impairment of renal function *(Chapter 20)*.

21.5. Free light chains as bioactive molecules in inflammatory diseases

Since FLCs are part of the binding site of intact immunoglobulin molecules they have bioactivity. This has been observed for both polyclonal and monoclonal FLCs and has

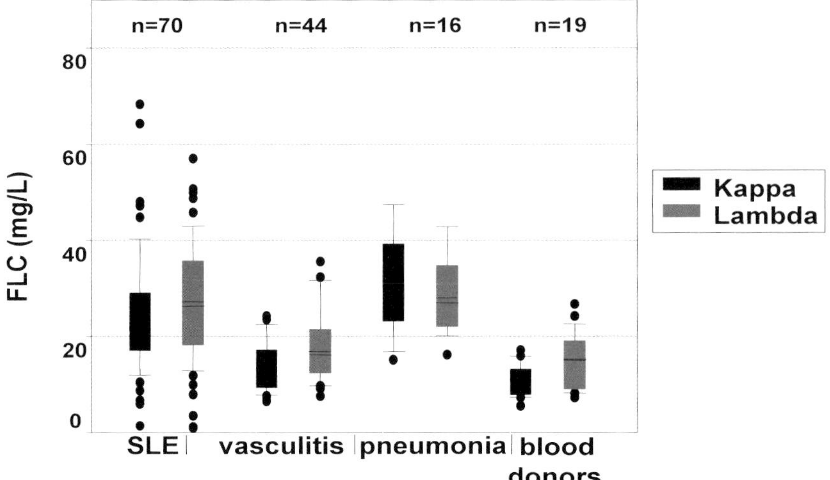

Figure 21.8. Serum FLCs in patients with pneumonia compared with other diseases. The slight increase in κ compared with λ concentrations may be related to renal impairment. (Courtesy of U Hoffman)[8]

recently been reviewed.[15]

For instance, the biological activities of FLCs have been shown in immediate hypersensitivity-like responses and contact sensitivity dermatitis. Since FLCs can activate mast cells (which contain a range of biologically active molecules), their potential for causing inflammatory and other diseases such as asthma is high. Possibly, FLCs are one of the components in the active inflammatory processes that are apparent in chronic renal failure. Removal of FLCs in these patients using 'protein-losing' dialysers may be important.

Finally, different monoclonal FLCs have been shown to bind individual target molecules. They can stimulate anti-angiogenic activity, have proteolytic potential and can be used to target proteins in lung cancer and other diseases. The complementarity determining regions of FLCs have sufficient variability and flexibility to bind any biological molecule.

References

1. **Dispenzieri A, Gertz MA, Therneau TM, Kyle RA.** Retrospective Cohort Study of 148 Patients with Polyclonal Hypergammaglobulinaemia. Mayo Clin Proc 2001; **76**: 476-487.

2. **Katzmann JA, Clark RJ, Abraham RS, Bryant S, Lymp JF, Bradwell AR, Kyle RA.** Serum Reference Intervals and Diagnostic Ranges for Free k and Free l Immunoglobulin Light Chains: Relative Sensitivity for Detection of Monoclonal Light Chains. Clin Chem 2002; **48**: 1437-1444.

3. **Epstein, WV, Tan M.** Increase of L-chain proteins in the sera of patients with systemic lupus erythematosus and the synovial fluids of patients with peripheral rheumatoid arthritis. Arthritis Rheum 1966; **9**: 713-719.

4. **Hopper JE, Sequeira W, Martellotto J, Papagiannes E, Perna L, Skosey JL.** Clinical Relapse in Systemic Lupus Erythematosus: Correlation with Antecedent Elevation of Urinary Free Light-Chain

Immunoglobulin. J Clin Immunol 1989; **9**: 338-50.

5. **Hopper JE, Golbus J, Meyer C, Ferrer GA.** Urine free light chain in SLE: Clonal markers of B-cell activity and potential link to in vivo secreted IG. J Clin Immunol 2000; **20**: 123-137.

6. **Sölling K, Sölling J, Romer FK.** Free Light Chains of Immunoglobulins in Serum from Patients with Rheumatoid Arthritis, Sarcoidosis, Chronic Infections and Pulmonary Cancer. Acta Medica Scand 1981; **209**: 473-477.

7. **Hoffman U, Opperman M, Küchler S, Ventur Y, Teuber W, Michels H, Welcker, Landenberg PV, Helmke K.** Free immunoglobulin light chains in patients with rheumatic diseases. Z Rheumatol 2003; **62**, Suppl.1: PFr-40, p1051.

8. **Urban S, Oppermann M, Reucher SW, Schmolke M, Hoffmann U, Hiefinger-Schindlbeck R, Helmke K.** Free light chains (FLC) of immunoglobulins as parameter resembling disease activity in autoimmune rheumatic diseases. Proc. of EULAR, June 2004 (www.EULAR.ORG).

9. **Gottenberg J-E, Aucouturier F, Busson M, Cohen-Solal J, Goetz J, Sibilia J, Mariette X**. Serum Immunoglobulin Free Light-Chain Assessment in Patients with Primary Sjogren's Syndrome. Personal communication.

10. **Teppo AM and Groop L.** Urine excretion of plasm proteins in diabetic subjects. Increased excretion of kappa light chains in diabetic patients with and without proliferative retinopathy. Diabetes 1985; **34** (6): 589-594.

11. **Groop L, Mäkipernaa A, Stenman S, DeFronzo RA, Teppo A-M.** Urinary excretion of kappa light chains in patients with diabetes mellitus. Kid Int 1990; **37**: 1120-1125.

12. **Hutchison CA, Bradwell AR, Reid SD, Cockwell P, Mead GP, Barnett AH.** Free light chain abnormalities in diabetic patients with and without microalbuminuria. *In Press*

13. **Dillon JJ, Sedmak DD, Cosio FG.** Rapid-onset diabetic nephropathy in type II diabetes mellitus. Ren Fail 1997; **19** (6): 819-822.

14. **Sanders PW, Herrera GA, Kirk KA, Old CW, Galla JH.** Spectrum of Glomerular and Tubulointerstitial Renal Lesions Associated with Monotypical Immunoglobulin Light Chain Deposition. Lab Invest 1991; **64** (4): 527-537.

15. **van der Heijden M, Kraneveld A, Redegeld F.** Free immunoglobulin light chains as targets in the treatment of chronic inflammatory diseases. Eur J Pharm 2006; *In Press: published on line.*

Test questions

1. Do conditions causing hypergammaglobulinaemia produce increases in serum free light chain measurements?

2. How are unexpected increases in polyclonal free light chains evaluated?

3. Why are sFLCs highly elevated in patients with SLE?

4. Why might urine FLCs be an early marker of renal disease in diabetes mellitus?

Answers

1. Free light chain production normally increases alongside increased production of the intact immunoglobulin molecules (page 184).

2. Assess renal status first and if the high light chain levels remain unexplained, there may be an occult inflammatory disease process (page 185).

3. Because of increased production and reduced renal clearance (page 186).

4. Because hyperfiltering glomeruli leak albumin. This competes with normal FLC removal in the proximal tubules thereby displacing it into the urine (page 188).

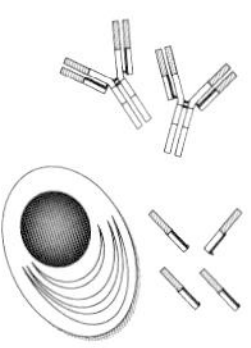

Chapter 22

Cerebrospinal fluid and free light chains

During inflammation of the central nervous system there is usually synthesis of intrathecal immunoglobulins. Since the blood-brain barrier acts as a molecular size filter, they gradually accumulate in the cerebrospinal fluid (CSF) where they can be detected as oligoclonal bands on electrophoretic gels or can be quantitated by protein assays.

When determining clinical relevance, the abnormal immunoglobulins need to be assessed in the context of any serum immunoglobulins which may have diffused into the CSF from the blood. For example, if the patient's serum contains monoclonal immunoglobulins produced in the bone marrow, small amounts will cross the blood-brain barrier making interpretation of CSF oligoclonal bands difficult. Similarly, if there is inflammation of the meninges, serum proteins will enter the CSF more readily and CSF proteins will not only be of intrathecal origin. Hence, CSF measurements are always made in relation to serum protein levels. In the case of immunoglobulin quantification, CSF/blood immunoglobulin ratios are compared with CSF/blood albumin ratios because albumin is never synthesised in the brain.

While these techniques are generally reliable there are clinical discrepancies and interpreting CSF oligoclonal bands on electrophoretic gels is time consuming and may be difficult.[1] Consequently, there has been interest in alternative markers of intrathecal inflammation, particularly CSF FLCs.[2-6] They are produced alongside intact immunoglobulins and accumulate in the CSF but they do not leak into the CSF from the blood, in significant amounts, because of their low serum concentrations.

The detection methods for CSF FLCs have included iso-electric focusing, quantitation by enzyme immunoassays and nephelometry, but results have not been of additional clinical benefit. With the development of sensitive and specific FLC nephelometric assays, there has been renewed interest in their measurement in CSF.

Fischer et al.,[7,8] studied CSF/serum pairs from 95 patients who had been investigated for intrathecal immunoglobulin synthesis. Of these, 24 were negative for oligoclonal immunoglobulin synthesis and 71 were positive, comprising 49 with multiple sclerosis and 22 with other neurological diseases *(Figure 22.1)*. The median κ concentrations in the patients with neurological diseases were higher. When samples with increased albumin leakage were excluded, there was no overlap between normal and disease groups (cut-off level of κ concentrations: 0.5mg/L). This indicated that determination of κ FLC concentrations in CSF provided information similar to that of oligoclonal band measurements, providing samples with raised albumin levels were excluded. The combination of κ CSF/serum ratios and albumin CSF/serum ratios for each sample was assessed *(Figure 22.2)*. Only two normal samples were misclassified. They concluded that CSF κ FLCs measurements may be a useful diagnostic procedure for detecting and potentially monitoring intrathecal immunoglobulin synthesis.

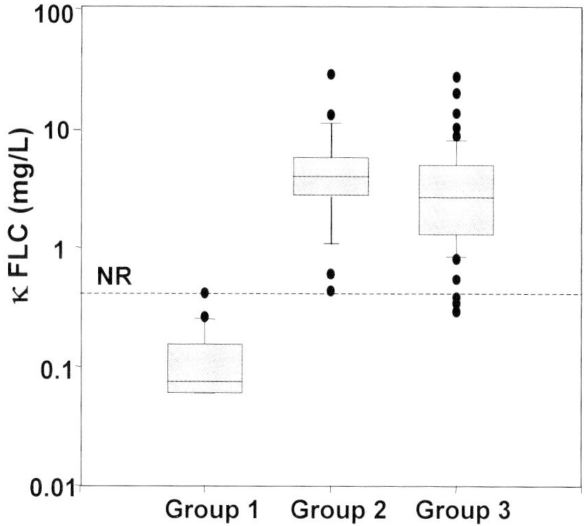

Figure 22.1. Box plot of κ FLC concentration (mg/L) in CSF from (1) normal individuals, (2) patients with multiple sclerosis and (3) other neurological diseases.[7] NR: upper limit of normal range for κ in the CSF was 0.5mg/L. (Courtesy of KJ Lackner).

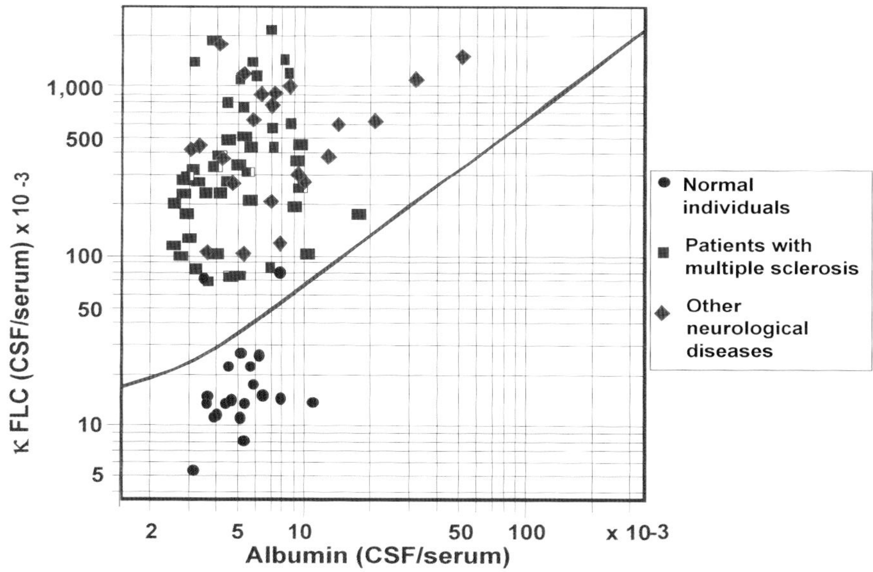

Figure 22.2. Quotients of κ FLC concentrations in CSF and serum plotted against the respective albumin quotients.[7] Samples are from patients in Figure 22.1. (Courtesy of KJ Lackner).

An editorial accompanying the article by Fischer et al.,[8] discussed the use of CSF FLC measurements in relation to existing tests for oligoclonal immunoglobulin bands.[9] Some scepticism was voiced by the author, but *"not with a closed mind"*.

More recently, Desplat-Jego et al., have published similar findings.[10] In 89 patients studied, the FLC κ index (CSF/serum ratios compared with albumin CSF/serum ratios) was more sensitive but less specific than the comparable IgG CSF index or CSF oligoclonal bands. 2 patients were only positive by the FLC κ index so it was a useful complementary test for the diagnosis of multiple sclerosis. It was considered that because the CSF FLC assay was easy, rapid and automated, it could be included in CSF studies in patients with suspected intrathecal inflammation.

References

1. **Luxton RW, McLean BN, Thompson EJ.** Isoelectric focusing versus quantitative measurements in the detection of intrathecal local synthesis of IgG. Clin Chim Acta 1990; **187**: 297-308.
2. **DeCarli C, Menegus MA, Rudick A.** Free light chains in multiple sclerosis and infections of the CNS. Neurology 1987; **37**: 1334-1338.
3. **Vladutiu AO.** κ Light Chains in Spinal Fluid for Diagnosing Multiple Sclerosis. JAMA 1994; **272**: 242-243.
4. **Lamers KJ, de Jong JG, Jongen PJ, Kock-Jansen MJ, Tuenesen MA, Prudon-Rosmulder EM.** Cerebrospinal fluid free kappa light chains versus IgG findings in neurological disorders: qualitative and quantitative measurements. J Neuroimmunol 1995; **62**: 19-25.
5. **Krakauer M, Schaldemose H, Jensen NJ, Sellebjerg F.** Intrathecal synthesis of free immunoglobulin light chains in multiple sclerosis. Acta Neurol Scand 1998; **98**: 161-165.
6. **Jenkins MA, Cheng L, Ratnaike S.** Multiple sclerosis: use of light-chain typing to assist diagnosis. Ann Clin Biochem 2001; **38**: 235-241.
7. **Arneth B, Fischer C, Koehler J, Birklein F, Lackner KJ.** Kappa Free Light Chains in Cerebrospinal Fluid as Markers of Intrathecal Immunoglobulin Synthesis. Clin Chem and Lab Med 2003; **41**: A107: p7.85.
8. **Fischer C, Arneth B, Koehler J, Lotz J, Lackner K.** Kappa Free Light-chains in Cerebrospinal Fluid as Markers of Intrathecal Immunoglobulin Synthesis. Clin Chem 2004; **50** (10): 1809-1813.
9. **Thompson EJ.** Quality versus Quantity: Which Is Better for Cerebrospinal Fluid IgG?. Editorial. Clin Chem 2004; **50** (10): 1721-1722.
10. **Desplat-Jego S, Feuillet L, Pelletier J, Bernard D, Cherif AA, Boucrout J.** Quantification of Immunoglobulin Free Light Chains in CerebroSpinal Fluid by Nephelometry. J Clin Imm 2005; **25** (4): 338-345.

Test question

1. Are raised free light chains in the cerebrospinal fluid of clinical relevance?

Answer

1. Yes, they are indicative of intrathecal immunoglobulin synthesis and are clinically useful (page 192).

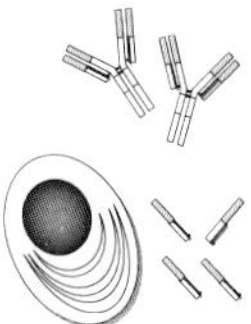

Section 4

General applications of free light chain assays

Chapter 23

Screening studies using serum free light chain assays

23.1. Introduction

Whether or not to measure serum FLCs at the time of the initial diagnostic request for, *'possible myeloma - please investigate'*, is an important issue. By tradition, SPE and/or IFE tests have been performed first, sometimes alongside IgG, IgA and IgM measurements. SPE can detect intact immunoglobulin monoclonal proteins in the 2-5g/L range which is more than adequate to identify all IIMM patients. Some centres screen with IFE because it is ten times more sensitive. However, it is non-quantitative and many low-level MGUS proteins are detected that are unlikely to progress to malignancy, provided their sFLC levels are also normal *(Chapter 19)*.[1] Some laboratories measure total serum κ and λ in the initial screen but this is inadequate *(Chapter 6)*.

The SPE tests are preferably performed alongside UPE but in the majority of patients urine is not available. Nevertheless, even with this ideal strategy many patients with NSMM, AL amyloidosis and other FLC-associated disorders are still missed. It is, therefore, logical to test for sFLCs on receipt of the first blood sample. The results will also provide baseline values for subsequent disease monitoring.

Hence, a strategy of using SPE combined with sFLC analysis, *"up-front"*, allows identification of all clinically significant monoclonal gammopathies apart from occasional patients with AL amyloidosis. It also reduces the detection rate of clinically unimportant MGUS samples (identified by IFE), with the attendant problems of informing and managing anxious patients.

This chapter discusses the current and potential screening options for identifying monoclonal proteins. As a general rule, intact immunoglobulin monoclonal proteins can be identified using SPE (or CZE) while monoclonal light chain diseases should be identified using sFLC assays. The combination of these two tests produces good diagnostic accuracy and urine tests are rarely needed at initial clinical presentation *(Chapter 24)*.

23.2. Diagnostic protocols for monoclonal gammopathies

The accuracy of different diagnostic protocols used for identifying monoclonal gammopathies are shown in Table 23.1. The basis of the numerical analysis is as follows:-

1. SPE identifies all patients with IIMM. By definition, they have at least 10g/L of monoclonal protein which is much greater than the sensitivity of the assays (2-5g/L). The test fails to identify approximately 30% of LCMM patients (the other 70% have sFLC bands or hypogammaglobulinaemia) and all NSMM *(Chapter 9)*. Approximately 50% of AL amyloidosis patients are abnormal by SPE *(Chapter 15)*. Many intact immunoglobulin MGUS individuals are also identified.

2. The combination of SPE and IFE is more sensitive but fails to identify a few patients with LCMM and all patients with NSMM. 70% of patients with AL amyloidosis are identified but those producing FLC only are frequently missed. Many MGUS individuals are identified but monoclonal proteins of less than 2-5g/L are of little clinical consequence if sFLCs are normal *(Chapter 19)*.[1]

3+4. The addition of UPE to either of the above protocols identifies ~30% more patients with LCMM and many patients with AL amyloidosis. No additional MGUS patients are identified because they rarely produce sufficient monoclonal FLCs to exceed the renal threshold and enter the urine *(Chapter 19)*. Also, since serum tests for FLCs are clinically more useful than UPE tests, these protocols are illogical *(Chapter 24)*.

5. sFLC analysis identifies FLC monoclonal gammopathies but cannot be used alone. It is, by definition, a test for FLCs and not for intact monoclonal immunoglobulins.

Accuracy of diagnostic tests at clinical presentation				
	Protocols	**Myeloma**	**AL amyloidosis**	**MGUS**
1	**SPE alone**	**90**	**50**	**45**
2	**SPE, serum IFE**	**95**	**70**	**80**
3	**SPE and UPE**	**95**	**75**	**70**
4	**SPE, UPE, serum and urine IFE**	**97**	**90**	**80**
5	**FLC alone**	**96**	**95**	**65**
6	**SPE and FLC**	**99**	**98**	**85**
7	**SPE, FLC, serum IFE**	**99**	**99**	**100**

Table 23.1. Approximate diagnostic sensitivity of tests for monoclonal gammopathies (see relevant chapters for details).

Approximately 35% of patients with MGUS and about 5% of patients with IIMM do not have excess FLC production *(Figures 10.1 to 10.3)*.

6. Arguably, the optimum protocol is to use SPE to identify all the intact monoclonal immunoglobulins and sFLC immunoassays to identify all the monoclonal FLCs. Approximately 20% of NSMM patients will be missed with this strategy *(Chapter 9)*. Such patients are non-producers or non-excretors and may have frame-shifts in the light chain DNA causing protein shape distortion.[2] Nearly all patients with AL amyloidosis and LCDD are identified *(Chapters 15 and 17)*. Some additional MGUS individuals are identified who produce only monoclonal FLC. Their clinical importance is not yet known but FLC MGUS is probably the precursor of LCMM and AL amyloidosis and may have a relatively poor outcome *(Chapter 15)*. Patients with renal impairment are also identified *(Chapter 20)*.
7. The addition of serum IFE to protocol 6 is not likely to identify any more patients with MM. It identifies approximately 10% additional AL amyloidosis patients *(Chapter 15)*. It also identifies some MGUS individuals with minor monoclonal intact immunoglobulins who are unlikely to progress to overt disease if there is no accompanying abnormal FLC κ/λ ratio *(Chapter 19)*. The extra cost, the inconvenience of performing the test and problems interpreting the clinical relevance of minor MGUS bands may not be justified in most clinical laboratories.

In the unlikely event that SPE and serum FLC tests are normal but the clinical picture still suggests a monoclonal gammopathy, urinalysis for FLCs is required. However, caution should be exercised when considering the clinical importance of minor urine FLC bands when serum FLC tests are normal *(see below and Chapter 24)*. After a monoclonal protein has been identified, IFE is required to characterise the heavy chain type. The light chain type can be identified by the serum κ/λ ratio or from the IFE gels.

Summary:-

A useful screening test protocol for monoclonal gammopathies comprises a combination of SPE and serum FLC assays. This identifies nearly all patients with clinically significant intact monoclonal immunoglobulins including the 20-30% of patients who only produce monoclonal FLCs, and removes the need for urine tests.

23.3. Screening studies using serum free light chain analysis

Several studies have evaluated the use of sFLC assays, alongside other tests, as part of the initial diagnostic screen for monoclonal gammopathies. These are described below.

Bakshi and colleagues used a combination of CZE and sFLC analysis.[3] 1,003 consecutive unknown samples were studied. 39 contained monoclonal proteins by CZE and 33 had abnormal κ/λ ratios to give a total of 55 abnormal sera.

16 samples (11 κ and 5 λ) were abnormal for monoclonal proteins only by sFLC analysis *(Figure 23.1 and Table 23.2)*. Subsequent IFE showed that 5 of the 16 samples were abnormal, although some had barely visible bands, but 11 samples were clearly only abnormal by FLC assays. Of the 39 samples that were positive by CZE, 17 were

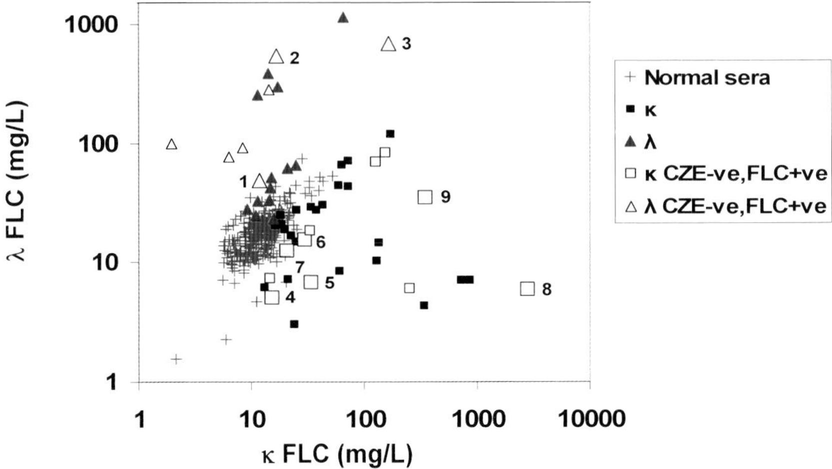

Figure 23.1 κ/λ ratios in 55 abnormal sera from a CZE and FLC screening study of 1,003 patients. Sera with monoclonal intact immunoglobulins are shown as dark symbols and samples containing only abnormal FLC κ/λ ratios are shown as yellow symbols. Numbers against large symbols refer to additional tumour patients identified using FLC tests *(Table 23.2).*

associated with abnormal FLC κ/λ ratios. In every case, the FLC test results concurred with the light chain type of the intact monoclonal immunoglobulin.

9 of the extra monoclonal gammopathy patients identified from abnormal κ/λ ratios were eventually shown to have plasma cell dyscrasias: 3 with MM, 4 with B-CLL/small cell CLL, 1 aplastic anaemia and 1 lymphoma. 7 samples were not associated with significant diseases and were classified as FLC MGUS only *(Chapter 19)*.

Addition of the FLC analysis to the CZE test in this screening trial increased the yield of lymphocyte and plasma cell proliferative diseases by 56%. The authors noted that the study emphasised the utility of FLC testing for patients with monoclonal proteins where CZE was essentially non-diagnostic.

Forsyth et al.[4] studied 925 consecutive serum samples referred to a UK District General Hospital. 79 sera were "suspect" by SPE and of these, IFE was positive in 57. FLC ratios were abnormal in an additional 52 sera. Six of these had monoclonal bands confirmed by IFE. In 2 others, with κ/λ ratios of 50 and 193, subsequent urine tests and bone marrow biopsies confirmed the presence of κ LCMM. At the time of analysis, 9% additional monoclonal proteins had been identified with sFLC assays and other results were being followed up (*Figure 23.2*). Other patients had borderline elevations of the κ/λ ratio due to renal impairment *(Chapter 20)*. Such minor abnormalities need to be considered in the context of reference ranges for hospitalised patients *(Chapter 5)*.

In this study, comparison was made between the utility of serum and urine tests for monoclonal FLCs. 370 (40%) of the serum samples were accompanied by urine samples. Of these, 141 (38%) had suspicious UPE tests and were further analysed by

nº	κ	λ	κ/λ Ratio	CZE	IFE	Diagnosis
5 sera : Capillary zone electrophoresis (CZE) negative but lambda FLC positive						
1	11.8	48.5	0.24	Hypoalbuminaemia	Normal	B-CLL/SLL
2	163.0	681.0	0.24	Polyclonal with β–γ bridging	Tiny IgM lambda	Aplastic anaemia
3	16.9	537.0	0.03	Normal pattern	λ light chain	λ Light chain myeloma
	8.5	91.5	0.09	Normal pattern	IgAλ (too small to measure)	MGUS
	14.3	279.0	0.05	Normal pattern	Normal	MGUS
11 sera : Capillary zone electrophoresis (CZE) negative but kappa FLC positive						
4	15.3	5.1	3.04	Normal pattern	Normal	B-CLL/SLL
5	33.8	6.8	4.94	Hypogammaglobulinaemia	Normal	B-CLL/SLL
6	29.7	15.6	1.90	Normal pattern	Normal	Possible early B-CLL/SLL
7	21.0	12.4	1.69	Mild protein loss pattern	NI	B-NHL, possible MZL or PCL
8	2830.0	5.9	482.94	Mild protein loss pattern/reactive	Free κ in serum & urine	κ Light chain myeloma
9	350.0	35.0	10.00	Oligoclonal bands	Normal	Nonsecretory myeloma
	155.0	83.1	1.87	Polyclonal-chronic inflammation	Normal	Borderline ?MGUS
	127.0	68.9	1.84	Polyclonal-chronic inflammation	Broad IgG κ (tiny)	Borderline ?MGUS
	33.4	18.5	1.81	Normal	Normal pattern	Borderline ?MGUS
	14.6	7.3	1.99	Normal	Normal	Borderline ?MGUS
	255.0	6.1	42.08	Hypogammaglobulinemia	Normal	FLC MGUS

Table 23.2. Clinical and laboratory data in 16 patients (confirmed monoclonal lymphoproliferative diseases) that were normal by CZE but abnormal by serum FLCs [3]. NI: Not indicated, B-CLL: B-cell chronic lymphocytic leukaemia, SLL: B-cell small lymphocytic leukaemia, LPL: lymphoplasmacytic lymphoma, MZL: marginal zone lymphoma. Case numbers refer to the patients also shown in Figure 23.1.

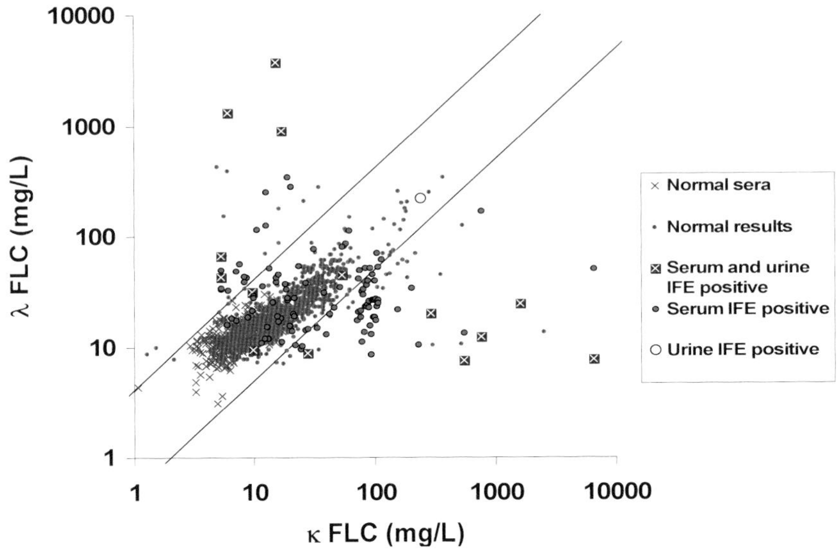

Figure 23.2. FLCs in 925 sera screened at Derby, UK.[4] Normal results are the FLC levels in samples with normal SPE. (Courtesy of P Hill).

urine IFE. Only 15 of these urine samples (4% of the total tested) had confirmed monoclonal FLC indicating that 126 tests were performed unnecessarily (*Figure 23.3)*. In 11 of the samples there was a corresponding serum FLC abnormality but 4 were normal. One of the 4 samples was associated with a serum IgGλ of 7g/L that was identified by IFE but had been missed on the initial SPE. The remaining 3 samples had urine FLC concentrations of approximately 50mg/L. Two normalised as the patients recovered from their illnesses and the 4th patient has persisting FLC proteinuria but is asymptomatic and has no evidence of a B-cell disorder. Hence, none of the 'urine only' monoclonal FLCs were of clinical importance.

On the basis of these results the hospital practice has changed to a policy of no urine tests for monoclonal gammopathies. This has allowed all patients to have proper assessments for monoclonal FLCs, has improved operational efficiencies and increased costs by £4 on a patient-by-patient basis.

Augustson et al.[5] studied 217 consecutive samples referred to a district general hospital. They found an extra 8 monoclonal gammopathies by abnormal sFLC κ/λ ratios. Three of these patients had LCMM which were missed by the routine SPE tests and resulted in serious diagnostic delays. Subsequently, the study was increased to 996 patients and results were similar to other screeing studies *(Figure 23.4*). 50 samples had raised FLCs with normal κ/λ ratios and 30 samples had abnormal κ/λ ratios that are currently under investigation.

Smith et al., reported results on 312 consecutive samples from Seattle hospitals in the USA.[6] Serum FLC tests identified a higher percentage of true positive and true negative samples and a lower percentage of false positive and false negative samples than SPE.

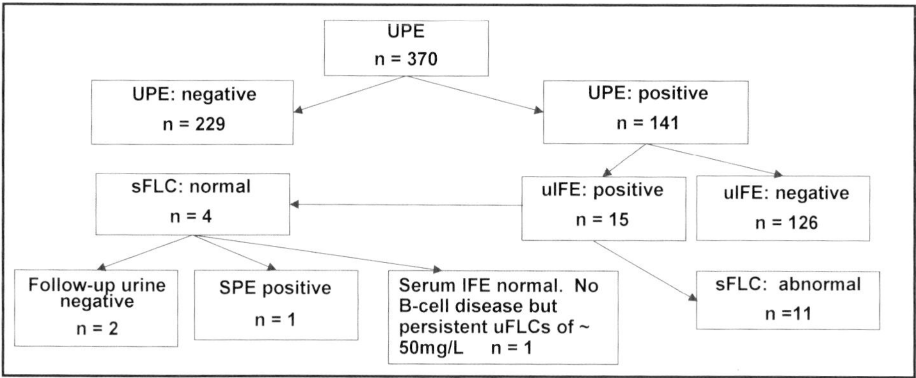

Figure 23.3. Test results on 370 urines screened for monoclonal proteins at a UK Hospital.[4] Of 925 sera sent for screening, 370 (40%) had accompanying urine samples of which 126 were suspicious by UPE but were negative by urine IFE. (Courtesy of P Hill).

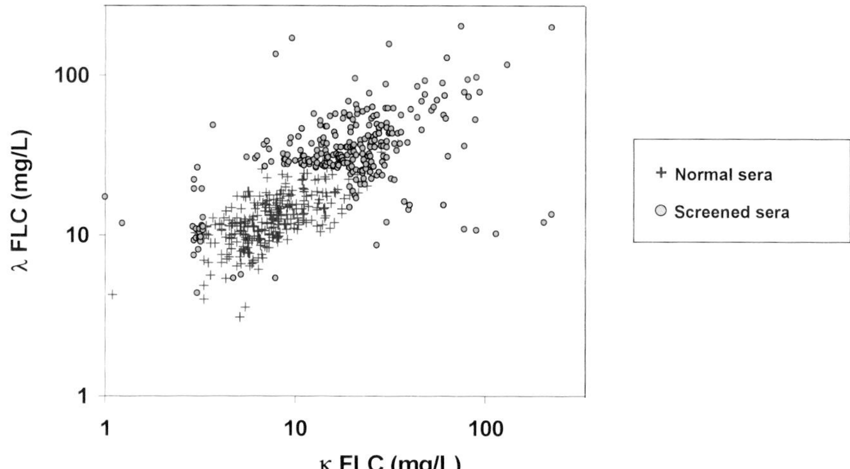

Figure 23.4. Test results on 996 sera screened for monoclonal proteins at Nuneaton, UK.[5] Patient samples in the normal range have been excluded.

The two assays in combination offered the most reliable results *(Figure 23.5)*.

Foray and Chapuis-Cellier studied 75 patients with FLC monoclonal gammopathies.[7] They observed 6 patients who were normal by urine tests but had abnormal sFLC results. They concluded that the assays should be used whenever FLC diseases were suspected.

The results from the 5 studies described above are consistent. Adding sFLC assays to the SPE tests, in routine screening, increased the tumour pick-up rate by approximately one patient per 100 samples tested. Some of the additional patients identified had significant changes to therapy on the basis of the earlier diagnosis.

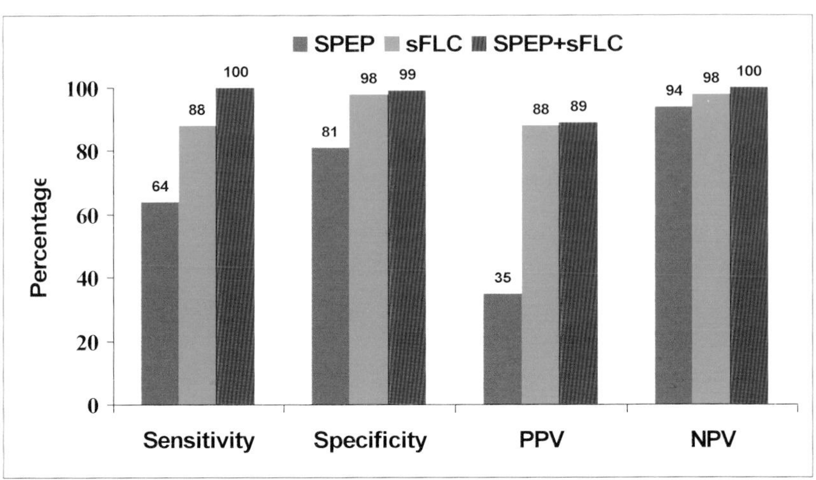

Figure 23.5. Combined assay performance of SPE and sFLC assays for identifying monoclonal gammopathies in a screening study. PPV: Positive predictive value, NPV: Negative predictive value. (Courtesy of DE Smith).[6]

23.4. Audit of serum free light chain usage

Katzmann et al.[8] performed an audit of sFLC analysis for the year 2003, on patients attending The Mayo Clinic *(Table 23.3)*. Of the 1,020 tests, 88% had plasma cell disorders. All 121 patients who had no plasma cell disorder had normal κ/λ ratios, in spite of a complex variety of different diseases tested. Thus, there were no false positive results in this study. At diagnosis, the sensitivity for AL amyloidosis by serum κ/λ ratios was 91% compared with 69% for serum IFE and 83% for urine IFE. Serum κ/λ ratios plus serum IFE produced a sensitivity of 99% which was not improved by adding urine IFE *(see Table 15.1)*. For 5 NSMM patients at clinical presentation, all had abnormal

1020 sample requests	
121	normal individuals had normal κ/λ ratios
899	**with plasma cell disorders comprising:-**
330	multiple myeloma
269	AL amyloidosis (91% sensitivity at diagnosis)
114	MGUS (44% sensitivity)
72	Smouldering myeloma (88% sensitivity)
22	Plasmacytoma
20	Nonsecretory myeloma (all of 5 at diagnosis were abnormal)
9	Waldenström's macroglobulinaemia
7	Light chain deposition disease (100% sensitivity)
56	Miscellaneous

Table 23.3. Audit of serum FLC requests at the Mayo Clinic for the year 2003.[7]

κ/λ ratios (100%). 5 of the 6 NSMM patients who had normal serum FLCs had achieved complete clinical remission after PBSCT and had normal bone marrow plasma cell content. The conclusion was that the performance of the FLC assays, in a prospective analysis, matched the results from published retrospective validation studies.

Summary:

1. Screening symptomatic patients using SPE and sFLC immunoassays is a clinically sensitive strategy for identifying patients with monoclonal gammopathies.
2. Extra patients with monoclonal FLCs are identified and require further investigation.
3. Adding sIFE or urine tests to the initial screen is of little extra clinical consequence.
4. The combination of CZE and FLC immunoassays allows automated screening of symptomatic patients for monoclonal gammopathies.

References

1. **Rajkumar SV, Kyle RA, Therneau TM, Melton LJ III, Bradwell AR Clark RJ, Larson DR, Plevak MF, Dispenzieri A, Katzmann JA.** Serum free light chain ratio is an independent risk factor for progression in monoclonal gammopathy of undetermined significance. Blood 2005: **106**: 812-817.
2. **Coriu D, Weaver K, Schell M, Eulitz M, Murphy CL,Weiss DT, Solomon A.** A molecular basis for nonsecretory myeloma. Blood 2003; **104** (3): 829-831.
3. **Bakshi NA, Guilbranson R, Garstka D, Bradwell AR, Keren DF.** Serum Free Light Chain (FLC) Measurement Can Aid Capillary Zone Electrophoresis (CZE) In Detecting Subtle FLC M-Proteins. Am J Clin Path 2005; **124**: 214-218.
4. **Forsyth JM, G. Hill PG, Rai BS, Mayne S, Mead GP.** Serum Free Light Chain Measurement Can Replace Urine Electrophoresis in the Detection of B Cell Proliferative Disorders. Blood 2005; **106** (11): 5081: p352b.
5. **Augustson BM, Katsavara H, Reid SD, Mead GP, Shirfield M, Bradwell AR.** Monoclonal gammopathy screening: Improved sensitivity using the serum free light chain assay. Haematologica 2005; **90** (s1): PO1302: p195.
6. **Smith DE, Abadie J, Bankson D, Mead GP.** Assessment of Serum Free Light Chain Assay for Screening for Plasma Cell Disorders. Blood 2005; **106** (11): 2563: 720a.
7. **Foray V, Chapuis-Cellier C.** Contribution of serum free light chain immunoassays in diagnosis and monitoring of free light chain monoclonal gammopathies. Immuno-analyse et Biologie Specialisee 2005; **20**: 385-393.
8. **Katzmann J, Abraham RS, Dispenzieri A, Lust JA, Kyle RA.** Diagnostic performance of Quantitative Kappa and Lambda Free Light Chain Assays in Clinical Practice. Clin Chem 2005; **51** (5): 878-881.

Test Questions

1. How many extra patients with monoclonal immunoglobulins are detected when screening symptomatic patients with sFLC assays?
2. How do serum FLC assays fit into routine testing for monoclonal protein?

Answers
1. About 50% more than by SPE and 1% extra in the population (Page 197).
2. FLC tests should be added to SPE tests (page 202).

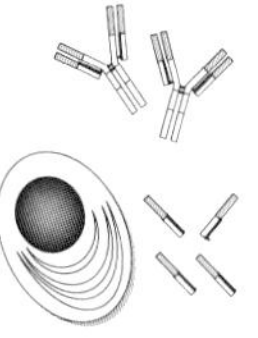

Chapter 24

Serum versus urine tests for free light chains

24.1. Introduction

The purpose of this chapter is to bring together all the arguments for the use of serum rather than urine for FLC measurements. The preceding chapters have covered many of the issues, and in some detail, but they are scattered throughout the book rather than being focussed into a single coherent discussion. Since there is a residue of informed opinion that continues to favour urine over serum measurements, it is time to persuade them otherwise. An analogy with diabetes mellitus is helpful. 30 years ago, all patients were monitored using urine glucose tests. Now they are monitored using blood glucose because of its overwhelming clinical advantages. Similar arguments apply to serum FLC measurements.

"If free light chains are in the urine they are always in the serum first".

24.2. Renal threshold for free light chain excretion

As described in Chapter 3, sFLCs are primarily cleared through the renal glomeruli and then metabolised in the proximal tubules of the nephrons. Only when the tubular absorptive capacity is exceeded are significant amounts of FLCs seen in the urine as "overflow proteinuria". Since the normal production is about 500mg/day and the renal absorptive capacity is 10-30g/day, production must increase many times before urine contains significant amounts of FLCs.[1]

The effect of renal tubular absorption on urine FLC concentrations is shown in Figure 24.1. Serum and urine FLC concentrations were compared in 4 patients undergoing treatment.[2] Patients 1 and 2 had large amounts of serum and urine FLCs with good correlations between changes in concentrations. In patients 3 and 4, urine excretion was minimal and unchanging over many months while serum levels could be used to monitor the changing tumour burden. Urine results in these latter patients were normal because there was no renal impairment and, therefore, no overflow proteinuria.

The concentrations of monoclonal serum FLCs necessary to cause overflow proteinuria was studied by Nowrousian et al., in patients attending a MM clinic.[3] In 131 samples from patients with elevated serum κ concentrations, 82 had urine FLCs by IFE

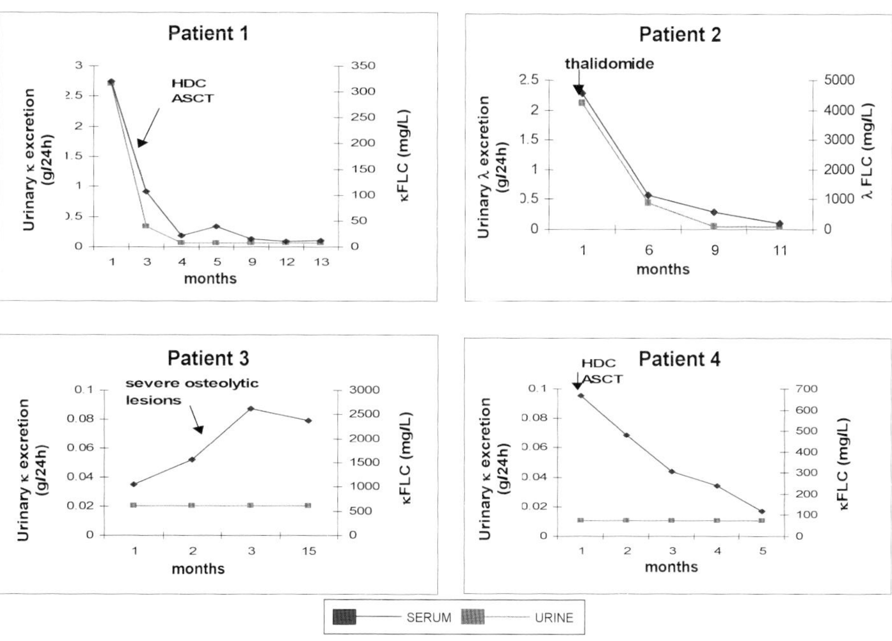

Figure 24.1. Serum and urine FLCs in 4 patients with LCMM. Serum tests were useful even when urine FLC excretion was minimal in patients 3 and 4.[2]

while 49 were normal *(Figure 24.2)*. The median serum κ concentrations associated with monoclonal FLCs in urine was 113mg/L (range 7-39,500) and 40mg/L (range 6-710) for normal urines. Monoclonal λ FLC producing patients had median serum values of 278mg/L (range 5-7,060) for positive urines and 44mg/L (range 3-561) for negative urines. The wide range of renal thresholds observed presumably reflected different degrees of renal damage.

Thus, for κ-producing patients, serum levels associated with abnormal urine FLCs were 5-fold above normal (upper limit of normal range: 19.4mg/L). For λ patients serum levels were elevated 10-fold above normal (upper limit of normal range: 26.3mg/L) when the urine was abnormal. The higher serum threshold levels for λ producing patients can be explained by the dimerisation of λ molecules limiting their filtration through the glomerular membranes *(Chapter 3.4)*. This study also showed the extra sensitivity of the serum tests when evaluating disease stage *(Figure 10.3)*.

Thus, when FLC production is below the renal clearance threshold, serum tests are more reliable than urinalysis. This may be particularly relevant for identifying patients with residual disease when urine assessments indicate complete remission *(Chapter 12)*.[1]

24.3. Problems collecting satisfactory urine samples

Even if there is significant urine excretion of FLCs, accurate quantification requires

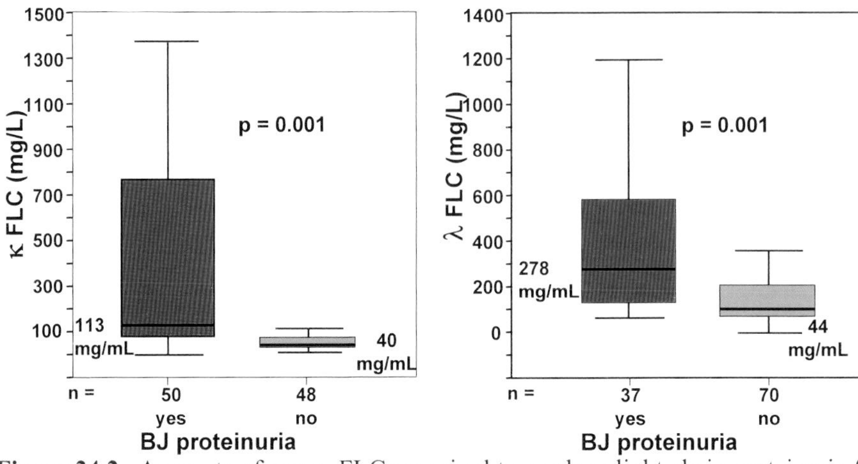

Figure 24.2. Amounts of serum FLCs required to produce light chain proteinuria for κ and λ myelomas. Median, 95% and ranges are shown. (Courtesy of MR Nowrousian)[3] .

a proper 24-hour urine collection. This may be particularly difficult because:-

- Accurate timing of the collection is hard for ill patients.
- Large volumes are produced in polyuric patients - perhaps larger than the bottle volume.
- Night-time collections are difficult for patients with painful or fractured bones.
- Problems occur sending voluminous urines to the laboratory by post.
- Collections may be awkward in front of friends or work colleagues.

Hence, even if there is significant renal leakage of FLCs, urine measurements may not be as reliable as those in serum. Figure 24.3 compares serum and urine results in a patient with LCMM who is relapsing. The concentrations of the FLCs in both fluids are considerably elevated indicating that the renal threshold is exceeded (compared with patients 3 and 4 in Figure 24.1). However, the urine measurements are highly variable and do not show a definitive rise until day 160. In contrast, the steady rise in serum FLC concentrations from day 40 indicates relapse of the tumour 3-4 months earlier. Presumably, the 24-hour urine collections were inaccurate, but there may have been additional inaccuracies in the UPE measurements (*see below*).

24.4. Problems measuring urine samples

Urine FLC measurements are normally based upon electrophoretic tests (*Table 4.1 and Chapter 6*). These may require samples to be concentrated prior to analysis by up to 100-fold. They are then analysed by UPE and scanning densitometry or by IFE. The methods are manual and relatively time-consuming or semi-automated.

Additional problems with urine samples include (*Chapter 6.6*):-

- High background staining in the presence of heavy proteinuria.
- Ladder banding - false bands that may hide monoclonal FLCs.

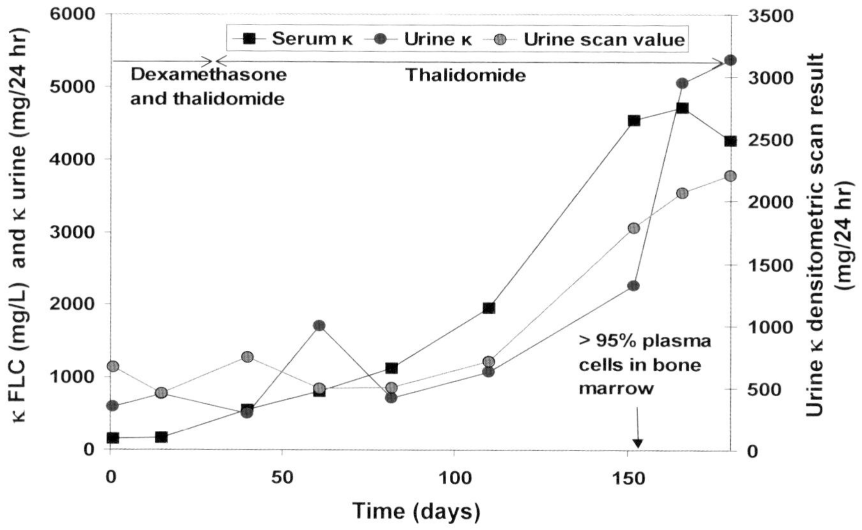

Figure 24.3. Serum and urine FLCs in a patient with LCMM. Disease relapse can be identified 3 months earlier using serum rather than urine samples. (Courtesy of G Wieringa, Christie Hospital, Manchester, UK).

- Difficulties identifying the correct band amongst other protein bands.
- Poor precision compared with immunoassays.
- Non-specificity of antibodies used on IFE.

As an alternative to urine electrophoretic tests, FLC immunoassays can be used for urine samples. Nowrousian et al., compared the sensitivity of urine FLC analysis with urine IFE.[3] 98 κ and 107 λ samples that had abnormal serum κ/λ ratios were studied. Urines negative by IFE contained a median of 23 mg/L of κ (range 0-251) and 9mg/L of λ (range 1-196) by FLC immunoassays. Urines positive by IFE contained a median of 448 mg/L of κ (range: 5-70,800) and 313 mg/L of λ (range: 17-11,100) by FLC immunoassays *(Figure 24.4)*.

These results indicate that urinalysis by FLC immunoassays and IFE may be complementary. However, the ranges of FLC concentrations and κ/λ ratios in normal urines are far wider than in serum so serum tests are more reliable (*Chapter 5.3*). Furthermore, urine FLC immunoassays do not solve any of the renal threshold and urine collection problems indicated above. Similar findings have been reported elsewhere and it was concluded that urine IFE was more reliable for detecting monoclonal diseases than urine FLC analysis.[4]

There are, of course, many other problems with urinalysis. Urine is less easily handled than serum; samples may be unpleasant; they need to be stored in large volumes if further analysis is required, and FLCs are more prone to precipitation in urine than in serum.

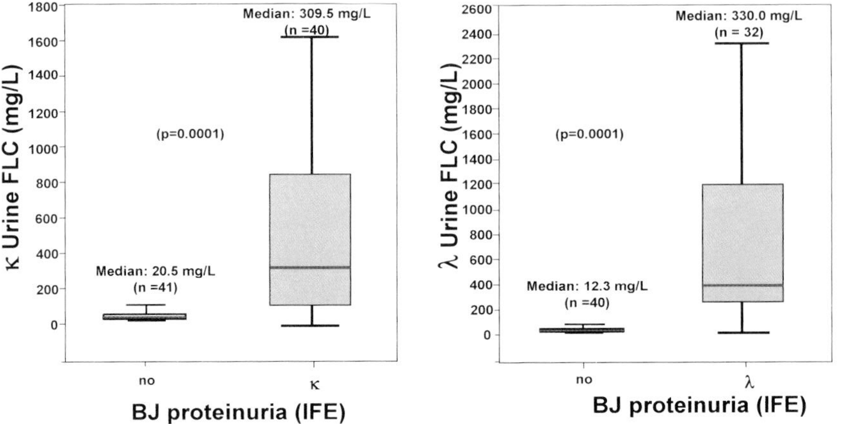

Figure 24.4. Comparison of FLC immunoassays and IFE for detecting urine FLCs.[3] Median, 95% and ranges of FLCs are shown. (Courtesy of MR Nowrousian).

24.5. Clinical benefits of serum free light chain analysis

The improved sensitivity of serum over urine FLC measurements has had a major impact on the ease of diagnosis and/or monitoring of the following diseases:-

1. Light chain multiple myeloma (*Chapter 8*).
2. Nonsecretory multiple myeloma (*Chapter 9*).
3. AL amyloidosis (*Chapter 15*).
4. Light chain deposition disease (*Chapter 17*).
5. Monoclonal gammopathy of undetermined significance (*Chapter 19*).

Figure 24.5 shows serum FLC concentrations in a variety of diseases at the time of clinical diagnosis. Patients with NSMM are in white. By definition, there are no detectable monoclonal proteins by both SPE and UPE tests in these patients. Hence, patients with monoclonal FLCs at or below these concentrations but with other types of plasma cell dyscrasias are not likely to be detected by conventional methods. Figure 24.5 also includes samples from many patients with AL amyloidosis and IIMM who were in remission by IFE.

Table 24.1 analyses the diagnositic sensitivity of serum tests (IFE plus sFLCs) for the different monoclonal gammopathies. There are no additional clinically significant diseases identified with urine tests. This shows that sFLC analysis can replace urinalysis when these diseases are being considered.

Serum FLC analysis offers additional clinical benefits:-

1. Rapid assessment of treatment responses in MM (*Chapter 13*) and AL amyloidosis (*Chapter 15*).
2. Identification of complete remission/residual disease in MM (*Chapters 8 and 12*).
3. Monitoring LCMM patients who are in renal failure (*Chapter 14*).
4. Risk stratification of patients with MGUS (Chapter 19).

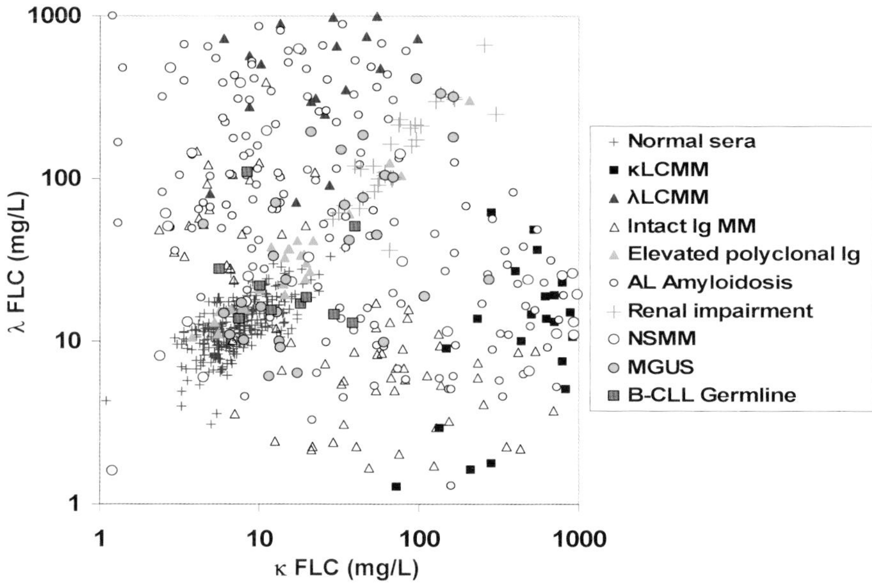

Figure 24.5. Serum FLCs in patients with low production rates. By electrophoretic tests, serum FLCs are usually undetectable or unquantifiable in most of these patients. (See relevant chapters for details of the patient data).

Disease	Serum tests positive	Additional diagnoses using urine tests
LCMM	100%	none (Chapter 8.1)
NSMM	70%	none (Chapter 9.2)
IIMM	100%	none (Chapter 10.2)
AL	99%	none (Chapter 15.2)
LCDD	~90%	none (Chapter 17.2)
MGUS	100%	none (Chapter 19)

Table 24.1. The sensitivity of serum electrophoretic tests combined with sFLC analysis ensures that urinalysis offers no additional benefits for disease diagnosis.

24.6. Organisational and cost benefits of serum free light chain analysis

As well as improved clinical outcomes, there are organisational and cost benefits of introducing serum FLC assays. The laboratory issues were analysed at the Christie Hospital in Manchester, UK. Superior analytical performance of the serum assays, faster reporting times and reduced laboratory costs were found *(Table 24.2)*.[5] Cost benefits in relation to clinical outcomes were not analysed in this study but may accrue from earlier diagnosis and treatments that reduce morbidity.

	Serum free light chains	Urine densitometry
Sensitivity	1.5mg/L	50mg/L
Precision	5%	>15%
Analysis time	15 minutes	1 hour
Reporting turnaround	1 hour	1 week
Cost per year (700 requests)	£6,500	£4,500
Extra staff costs per year	£0	£1,000
24hr urine bottle usage	Not relevant	£1,000
Storage needs	30cm^3	10m^3

Table 24.2. Analytical and cost/benefit study of serum and urine FLC tests.[5]

Hill et al.,[6] evaluated the costs of changing from urine electrophoretic tests to serum FLC immunoassays in routine screening of patients for monoclonal gammopathies *(Chapter 23).* They considered that on a patient-by-patient basis the costs were increased by £4. But, in their study only 40% of serum samples were accompanied by urines so the overall costs increased more. However, better clinical governance was achieved and more clinical diagnoses were made.

One relatively simple clinical situation that may be improved by measuring serum FLCs is in determining the underlying pathology of patients presenting with acute renal failure *(Chapter 14).* When MM is suspected, the normal procedure is to perform SPE and UPE. If results are positive for a monoconal gammopathy then a renal biopsy may be necessary. As an alternative, it might be appropriate to request an urgent serum FLC analysis. This would identify all patients with a FLC cause for their renal impairment. If MM were suspected, a bone marrow biopsy could be performed rather than a renal biopsy. This is a less risky procedure and may be preferable in some patients. Serum FLC analysis alone is also cheaper than the combined serum and urine IFE tests that are currently requested.

24.7. Is there any remaining role for urine tests?

Serum tests for FLCs are occasionally normal when urine tests are abnormal. Some of the discrepancies may be explained on technical grounds or on sampling errors *(Chapter 6.6).* For instance, when monitoring patients, 24-hour urine collections may be taken earlier than the corresponding serum samples. Since FLC concentrations can fall rapidly following treatment *(Chapter 13)*, urine samples collected a few days before attending the clinic for serum FLC analysis could produce quite different results. The sensitivity of the urine measurements is also highly dependent upon technique. Obviously, highly sensitive IFE gels identify more samples than UPE used in routine hospital practice.

The frequency of discordant results has been analysed in patients with AL amyloidosis.[7] 260 sera and corresponding urine samples from patients with AL amyloidosis were studied. 5 samples had normal serum κ/λ FLC ratios but more than 200mg/day of urine FLCs *(Table 24.3).* The serum samples were taken during the period

Sample	Urine IFE	Urine FLC g/day	Urine κ (mg/L)	Urine λ (mg/L)	Serum κ/λ ratio
1	Lambda	0.53	70.2	53.5	0.31
2	Lambda	0.7	211	152	0.45
3	Lambda	0.21	96.5	69.8	0.62
4	Lambda	0.38	130	98	0.70
5	Lambda	0.41	117	42.6	0.72

Table 24.3 Results in 5 patients with AL amyloidosis who had abnormal urine FLCs by IFE but normal serum FLC κ/λ ratios.

of the 24-hour urine collection to avoid errors of timing and all gels were carefully analysed retropectively.

Some of the serum FLC results in the 5 patients were borderline abnormal and concentrations of the urine FLCs were minimal in all other patients. Since the normal serum reference range for FLCs was based on a screening study that included all samples tested, it may be that when monitoring patients, narrower normal range criteria can be used *(Chapter 5)*. Moreover, low concentration urine monoclonal proteins in patients with normal serum FLC concentrations and κ/λ ratios are of doubtful clinical importance. International guidelines indicate that urine FLC concentrations below 1g/L are of little relevance *(Chaper 25)*.

In a routine screening study comparing serum with urine analysis, approximately 1% of patients had normal serum κ/λ ratios but minor monoclonal FLCs in the urine by IFE *(Chapter 23, Figure 23.3)*[6] Follow-up of these 4 patients showed that the urine monoclonal proteins were inconsequential. It may be unwise to treat patients with chemotherapy based only upon a minor urine monoclonal band detected by IFE when serum FLC tests are normal.

The effect of renal failure on serum κ/λ ratios needs to be considered in patients with borderline results. This is discussed in detail in Chapter 20. Slower clearance of κ molecules occurs when glomerular filtration is impaired so that κ/λ ratios increase slightly. It may be appropriate to use measurements of cystatin C to correct the κ/λ ratios in some of these patients.

If a choice has to be made between serum or urine tests then serum is clearly preferable for the reasons given above.[8] When both serum and urine tests are available, it is always clinically reassuring to have two separate tests giving the same results. Clearly, samples do occasionally get incorrectly analysed, mislabelled or misplaced, so supporting evidence for making a diagnosis or changing treatment is always helpful. In the context of a stem cell transplant in MM patients,for example, the additional cost of performing both serum and urine tests is inconsequential.

The impact of serum FLC analysis is important and all new national and international guidelines include recommendations on its use *(Chapter 25)*.

Summary: Table 24.4

Serum versus urine measurements	
Serum	**Urine**
Easy to collect	Difficult to collect
κ/λ ratio little affected by renal function	Renal function affects levels
Easily analysed	Samples need concentrating
Easily stored	More difficult to store
More frequently abnormal in NSMM and AL amyloidosis	Less frequently abnormal
More sensitive for monitoring patients	Less sensitive for monitoring patients
Of prognostic importance in MGUS	Of uncertain importance in MGUS

References

1. **Bradwell AR, Carr-Smith HD, Mead GP, Harvey TC, Drayson MT.** Serum test for assessment of patients with Bence Jones myeloma. Lancet 2003; **361**: 489-491.

2. **Alyanakian M-A, Abbas A, Delarue R, Arnulf B, Aucouturier P.** Free Immunoglobulin Light-chain Serum Levels in the Follow-up of Patients With Monoclonal Gammopathies: Correlation With 24-hr Urinary Light-chain Excretion. Am J of Haem 2004; **75**: 246-248

3. **Nowrousian MR, Brandhorst D, Sammet C, Kellert M, Daniels R, Schuett P, Poser M, Mueller S, Ebeling P, Welt A, Bradwell AR, Buttkereit U, Opalka B, Flasshove M, Moritz T, Seeber S.** Serum Free Light Chain Analysis and Urine Immunofixation Electrophoresis in Patients with Multiple Myeloma. Clin Cancer Res 2005; **11** (24): 8706-8714.

4. **Viedma JA, Garrigos N, Morales S.** Comparison of the sensitivity of 2 automated immunoassays with immunofixation electrophoresis for detecting urine Bence Jones proteins. Clin Chem. 2005; **51** (8): 1505-1507.

5. **Carr-Smith HD, Harland B, Anderson J, Overton J, Wieringa G, Bradwell AR.** The effect on laboratory organisation of introducing serum free light chain assays. Clin Chem 2004; **50** (6): C-22: pA76

6. **Hill PG, Forsyth JM, Rai BS, Mayne S, Mead GP**. Serum free light chain measurement can replace urine electrophoresis for detecting B cell proliferative disorders. Clin Chem 2005; **51** (6): B-6.

7. **Stubbs P.** The Binding Site Ltd., *Personal communication.*

8. **Carr-Smith HD, Mead GP, Bradwell AR.** Serum free light chain assays as a replacement for urine electrophoresis. Haematologica 2005; **90** (1): 107: PO404.

Test Questions

1. Is there any remaining role for urine tests?

2. Why are patients with excess monoclonal serum κ FLCs more likely to have positive urine results?

3. How do the costs of serum FLC immunoassays compare with urine tests?

Answers

1. Yes, but probably only as supporting evidence for minimal tumour burden in patients with MM (page 210).

2. Monomeric κ molecules filter through the glomeruli more readily than dimeric λ molecules (page 205).

3. Two studies indicated similar costs on a patient-by-patient basis (page 209).

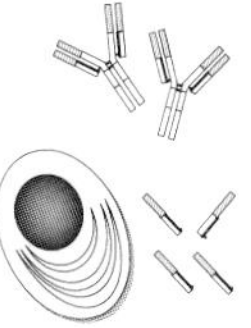

Chapter 25

Guidelines for use of serum free light chain assays

There are several new International and National guidelines for identifying and managing patients with plasma cell dyscrasias. These are being widely adopted for assessing new patients and for patient entry into clinical trials. This chapter provides an overview with an emphasis on the serum FLC component. Classification criteria for the less common plasma cell dyscrasias (some of which do not yet include the use of serum FLCs) are described in Chapter 18.

25.1. International Guidelines for the classification of MM and MGUS[1]

The most recent guidelines were published in 2003 and comprise the following:-

Symptomatic multiple myeloma

- M-protein in serum and/or urine.
- Bone marrow (clonal) plasma cells or plasmacytoma.
- Related organ or tissue impairment (end organ damage, including bone lesions*).

Nonsecretory multiple myeloma

- No M-protein in serum and/or urine with immunofixation.
- Bone marrow clonal plasmacytosis >10% or plasmacytoma.
- Related organ or tissue impairment (end organ damage, including bone lesions*).

Asymptomatic myeloma (smouldering myeloma)

- M-protein in serum >30g/L: and/or
- Bone marrow clonal plasma cells >10%.
- No symptoms, related organ or tissue impairment (no end organ damage, including bone lesions*).

Monoclonal gammopathy of undetermined significance (MGUS)

- M-protein in serum <30g/L
- Bone marrow clonal plasma cells <10% and low level of plasma cell infiltration in a trephine biopsy (if done)

- No evidence of other B-cell proliferative disorders.
- No related organ or tissue impairment (no end organ damage, including bone lesions).

***Criteria for end organ damage in MM - CRAB** (**C**alcium increased, **R**enal insufficiency, **A**naemia or **B**one lesions).

- **C**alcium levels increased: serum calcium >0.25mmol/L above the upper limit of normal or >2.75mmol/L.
- **R**enal insufficiency: creatinine >173mmol/L.
- **A**naemia: haemoglobin 2g/dL below the lower limit of normal or haemoglobin <10g/dL.
- **B**one lesions: lytic lesions or osteoporosis with compression fractures.
- **Others**: symptomatic hyperviscosity, AL amyloidosis, recurrent bacterial infections (>2 episodes in 12 months).

25.2. UK Myeloma Forum, Nordic Myeloma Study Group and the British Committee for Standards in Haematology[2]

The guidelines include the following use of serum FLC measurements:-

Investigation and diagnosis.

Quantification of serum FLCs and κ/λ ratio can be used as an alternative to measuring urine FLCs. Serum FLCs are particularly useful for the diagnosis of LCMM and patients in whom the serum and urine is negative on IFE (NSMM).[3,4]

Measuring responses to therapy.

Serum FLCs are useful for monitoring LCMM and NSMM.[3,4] Serum FLCs may also be helpful in monitoring responses in the many patients with IIMM.[5] Because of the short half-life of sFLCs this can give an earlier indication of response to therapy than changes in intact monoclonal immunoglobulins.

25.3. International Staging System for Multiple Myeloma[6]

In May 2005, the International Staging System for Multiple Myeloma was published. This is based upon serum albumin and serum β2 microglobulin alone *(Table 25.1)*.[6] Because of detailed analysis, wide international agreement and simplicity, it is likely to be adoped quickly.

Earlier staging systems included concentrations of monoclonal immunoglobulins. It has now been realised that they have little relevance to MM outcome. The same is true for monoclonal serum FLC concentrations but abnormal κ/λ ratios do statistically relate to the extent of the disease *(Chapter 10; Fig 10.13)*. Nowrousian et al., compared the presence or absence of abnormal serum FLC κ/λ ratios with urine monoclonal FLCs in 364 paired serum and urine samples alongside SWOG staging.[7] They showed that serum FLC κ/λ ratios were more frequently abnormal than urine monoclonal FLCs but both parameters correlated with the assessment of the disease stage. Interestingly, κ patients were more likely to present in Stage I. This may be because urine tests become positive at lower serum κ concentrations than λ because of their faster glomerular clearance *(Chapter 24.2)*. Such patients would, therefore, be identified earlier. It may also be that

Stag	Criteria	Median survival
I	Serum β_2M < 3.5mg/L. Serum albumin >35g/L	62 months
II*	Not stage I or III	44 months
III	Serum β_2M >5.5mg/L	16 months

Table 25.1. New International Staging System.[6] *There are 2 categories for stage II: serum β_2M <3.5mg/L but serum albumin <35g/L; or serum β_2M 3.5 to 5.5mg/L, irrespective of the serum albumin level.

the pre-renal load of FLCs is an additional predictor of disease outcome in MM patients because it relates to development of myeloma kidney in a significantly high proportion.[8-11] Whether κ/λ ratios provide an independent marker of outcome that is clinically useful remains to be determined.

25.4. New "Uniform Response Criteria for MM" incorporating FLCs[12-14]

There have been extensive international discussions on guidelines that utilise the high sensitivity of serum FLC measurements. One important new recommendation is to change the way that the κ/λ ratios are reported. Subtraction of the tumour FLC from the non-tumour FLC provides a single value that is easy to report and understand. It also provides an interpretable result when the non-tumour FLC is either below the detection limit or is fluctuating widely. It is similarly helpful when interpreting high concentrations of the alternate FLC that are seen in patients with impaired renal function (*Chapter 20.2*). Limited clinical studies indicate no loss of clinical utility.[13] The response criteria will be published in full soon[14], while below is their current status:-

Table 1. Rationale for the development of uniform response criteria

1. Facilitate precise comparisons of efficacy between new treatment and strategies in trials
2. *Incorporation of the serum free light chain assay*
3. *Stricter definitions of complete response*
4. Incorporate standard definition of near compete response
5. Stricter definition of disease progression
6. *Enable greater inclusion of patients with oligo-secretory and nonsecretory disease*
7. Provide clarifications, improve detail, and correct inconsistencies in prior response criteria

Table 2. Diagnostic criteria for multiple myeloma requiring systemic therapy

1. Presence of an M-component* in serum and/or urine plus clonal plasma cells in the bone marrow and/or a documented clonal plasmacytoma

   Plus one or more of the following:**
2. **C**alcium elevation (>11.5 gms/dl)
3. **R**enal insufficiency (creatinine>2mg /dl)
4. **A**nemia (Hemoglobin <10gms /dl or 2gms <normal)
5. **B**one disease (lytic or osteopenic)

* *In patients with no detectable M-component, serum FREELITE chain (FLC) assays can substitute and satisfy this criterion. For patients with no serum or urine M-component, the baseline bone marrow must have >30% plasma cells. These patients are referred to as "nonsecretory myeloma".*

** Must be attributable to the underlying plasma cell disorder

Table 3. Practical Details of Response Evaluation

Laboratory tests for measurement of M proteins.

Serum M-protein level is quantitated using densitometry on SPE except in cases where the SPE is felt to be unreliable such as in patients with IgA monoclonal proteins migrating in the beta region. If SPE is not available for routine M-protein quantitation during therapy, then nephelometry or turbidimetry can be accepted. However, this must be explicitly reported; nephelometry can be used only for individual patients to access response; SPE and nephelometric values cannot be used interchangeably.

Urine M protein measurement is estimated using 24-hour UPE only. *Random or 24 hour urine tests measuring κ and λ FLC measurements are not reliable and are not recommended.*

Definitions of measurable disease

Response criteria for all categories and subcategories of response except CR are applicable only to patients who have "measurable" disease defined by at least one of the following 3 measurements:-

Serum M protein =/>1 gm/dL (> 10 gm/L)

Urine M protein =/>200 mg/24 hours

Serum FLC assay: Involved FLC =/> 10 mg/dL (>100 mg/L)

Response criteria for complete response (CR)

These are applicable to patients who have abnormalities on one of the three measurements. Note that patients who do not meet any of the criteria for measurable disease as listed above can only be assessed for CR and cannot be assessed for any of the other response categories

Serum M protein detectable on IFE

Urine M protein detectable on IFE

Abnormal serum FLC κ/λ ratio (<0.26 or >1.65)

Follow-up to meet criteria for partial response or stable disease

It is recommended that patients undergoing therapy be tracked monthly for the first year of new therapy and every alternate month thereafter

Patients with "measurable disease" as defined above by SPE and UPE need to be followed by both SPE and UPE for response assessment and categorization

Except for assessment of complete response, patients with measurable disease restricted to the SPEP will need to be followed only by SPE; correspondingly patients with measurable disease restricted to UPE will need to be followed only by UPE

Patients with measurable disease in either SPEP or UPE, or both, will be assessed for response only based on these two tests and not by FLC assays. FLC response criteria are only applicable to patients without measurable disease in the serum or urine, and to fulfil the requirements in the category of stringent CR.

To be considered CR, both serum and urine IFE must be done and be negative regardless of the size of baseline M protein in the serum or urine; patients with negative UPE values pre-treatment still require UPE testing to confirm CR and exclude light chain (or Bence-Jones) escape.

Skeletal survey is required only if clinically indicated; Bone marrow is required only for categorization of CR, and for patients with nonsecretory disease

Table 4. International Myeloma Working Group Uniform Response Criteria: Complete Response and Other Response Categories

Note that all response categories require two consecutive assessments done at anytime before the institution of any new therapy.

* Refer to Table 3 for definitions of measurable disease.

Response Subcategory	Response Criteria
Complete Response (CR)	· Negative IFE in the serum and urine *and:-* · Disappearance of any soft tissue plasmacytomas *and:-* · < 5% plasma cells in bone marrow
Stringent CR (sCR)	CR as defined above plus:- · *Normal FLC ratio and:-* · Absence of clonal cells in BM by immunohistochemistry or immunofluorescence
Very Good Partial Response (VGPR)	Serum and urine M-component detectable by IFE but SPE-ve or:- · 90 or greater reduction in serum M-component and urine M-component <100 mg per 24 hours
Partial Response	50% reduction of serum M protein *and:-* · Reduction in 24-hour urinary M protein by =/>90% or to =/<200 mg per 24 hours and · If present at baseline, a =/>50% reduction in size of soft tissue plasmacytomas · *If the serum and urine M-protein are unmeasurable*, a >50% decrease in the difference between involved and uninvolved FLC levels is required in place of the M-protein criteria* · *If serum and urine M-protein are unmeasurable, and sFLCs are also normal, =/>50% reduction in plasma cells is required in place of M-protein, provided baseline BM plasma cell percentage is =/>30%*
Stable Disease	Not meeting criteria for complete response, near complete response, partial response, or progressive disease

Table 5. Response Evaluation for Patients proceeding to Stem Cell Harvesting and Transplantation

Timing	Recommended testing of M-component, serum FLCs and CRAB features.
Post-Induction	At least one assessment pre-harvest. If harvest occurs during induction then assessment should be immediately pre-transplant.
Post-Harvest	At least one assessment post-harvest if cytoreductive therapy used for harvest and/or if patient proceeding directly to maintenance only
Post-Transplant	One measurement required at =/<100 days. This re-staging requires bone marrow biopsy

Table 6. International Myeloma Working Group Uniform Response Criteria: Disease Progression and Relapse from Complete response*

* All relapse categories require two consecutive assessments done at anytime before the institution of any new therapy.

** Patients developing two or more of the CRAB features without increases in monoclonal protein or free light chain levels are also considered to progressive disease.

Relapse Subcategory	Relapse Criteria
Progressive disease.* (Includes primary progressive disease and disease progression on or off therapy; To be used for calculation of time to progression and progression-free survival endpoints.	**Any one or more of the following:** · Increase of =/>25% from baseline in - Serum M-component and/or (the absolute increase must be =/> 0.5 g/dL) - Urine M-component and/or (the absolute increase must be =/>200 mg/24 hours - *Difference between involved and uninvolved FLC levels. The absolute increase must be >10 mg/L.* - Bone marrow plasma cell %. The absolute % must be =/> 10%. **PLUS any one or more of:** **Direct indicators of increasing disease and/or end organ dysfunction (CRAB features)**** 1. Development of new soft tissue plasmacytomas or bone lesions 2. Definite increase in size of existing plasmacytomas or bone lesions. A definite increase is defined as a 50% (and at least 1 cm) increase as measured serially by the sum of the products of the cross diameters of the measurable lesion. 3. Hypercalcemia (>11mg/dL) 4. Decrease in haemoglobin of 20gm/L or more. 5. Rise in serum creatinine by 2mg/dL or more.
Relapse from CR.* (To be used only if the endpoint studied is "Disease free survival"; otherwise CR patients should also be evaluated using criteria for progressive disease).	**Any one or more of the following:** · Reappearance of serum and urine M protein by IFE, SPE or UPE · Development of =/>5% plasma cells in the bone marrow · Appearance of any other sign of progression (i.e. new plasmacytoma, lytic bone lesion, or hypercalcemia see below)

25.5. USA National Academy of Clinical Biochemistry guidelines for the use of tumor markers in monoclonal gammopathies[15]

Serum FLC measurements are useful for the diagnosis and follow up of NSMM, MGUS and AL amyloidosis. They are more sensitive than urine tests in patients with LCMM and in other patients with MM who may have coexistent SLE or renal impairment.

25.6. Guidelines for AL amyloidosis

A Consensus Opinion from the 10th International Symposium on Amyloid and Amyloidosis.[16] Definition of Organ Involvement and Treatment Response in Immunoglobulin Light Chain Amyloidosis (AL):

Complete response (CR)

Serum and urine negative for a monoclonal protein by IFE

Serum FLC κ/λ ratio normal.
Marrow contains < 5% plasma cells.

Partial response (PR)

If serum M component > 0.5g/dL, a 50% reduction.
If FLCs in the urine with a visible peak and =>100 mg/day, a 50% reduction.
If serum FLC >10 mg/dL* (100mg/L): reduction by =>50 %.

Progression

From CR, any detectable monoclonal protein or abnormal FLC κ/λ ratio (light chain must double).
From PR or stable response, 50% increase in serum M protein to > 0.5g/dL or 50% increase in urine M protein to > 200mg/day; a visible peak must be present.
Serum FLC increase of 50% to >10mg/dL.

Stable disease

No CR, no PR, no progression

UK Guidelines[17] (Similar guidelines have been adopted in France).[18]

The report includes comments on serum FLC measurements as follows:-

1. Serum FLCs are abnormal in 98% of patients with systemic AL amyloidosis including those that cannot be identified by conventional methods. Patients should be assessed for serum FLCs during the diagnostic procedure.
2. Serum FLC measurements appear to be the most effective current method of monitoring patients.
3. Changes in amyloid load correlate with changes in FLC concentrations and with survival.
4. Treatment should be continued, when feasible, until serum FLC concentrations have fallen by at least 50-75%.
5. Treatment strategies are best guided by their early effect on concentrations of serum FLCs.

25.7. Guidelines for assessing outcome in MGUS.[19]

Until recently there have been no useful markers for predicting outcome in MGUS because they lacked statistical power. Recently, Rajkumar et al. have shown that the combination of immunoglobulin MGUS class, its quantity above or below 15g/L and the presence or absence of an abnormal FLC κ/λ ratio can be used for risk stratification *(Chapter 19)*. Data from this study is likely to be used in future guidelines for MGUS management.

References

1. **Kyle RA, Child JA, Durie BGM, Blade J, Boccadoro M, Ludwig H et al.** Criteria for the classification of monoclonal gammopathies, multiple myeloma, and related disorders: a report of the International Myeloma Working Group. Br J Haem 2003; **121**: 749-757.

2. **Smith A, Wisloff F, Samson D on behalf of the UK Myeloma Forum, Nordic Myeloma Study Group and the British Committee for Standards in Haematology.** Guidelines on the diagnosis and management of Multiple Myeloma 2005. Br J Haem 2006; **132**: 410-451.

3. **Bradwell AR, Carr-Smith HD, Mead GP, Harvey TC, Drayson MT.** Serum test for assessment of patients with Bence Jones myeloma. Lancet 2003; **361**: 489-491.

4. **Drayson MT, Tang LX, Drew R, Mead GP, Carr-Smith HD, Bradwell AR.** Serum free light-chain measurements for identifying and monitoring patients with nonsecretory multiple myeloma. Blood 2001; **97** (9) 2900-2902.

5. **Mead GP, Carr-Smith HD, Drayson MT, Morgan GT, Child JA, Bradwell AR.** Serum free light chains for monitoring multiple myeloma. Br J Haem 2004; **126**: 348-354.

6. **Greipp PR et al.** International Staging System for Multiple Myeloma. J Clin Oncology 2005; **23**: 3412-3420.

7. **Nowrousian MR, Brandhorst D, Sammet C, Kellert M, Daniels R, Schuett P, Poser M, Mueller S, Ebeling P, Welt A, Bradwell AR, Buttkereit U, Opalka B, Flasshove M, Moritz T, Seeber S.** Serum Free Light Chain Analysis and Urine Immunofixation Electrophoresis in Patients with Multiple Myeloma. Clin Cancer Res 2005; **11** (24): 8706-8714.

8. **Engelhardt M, Rapple D, Weis A, Bisse E, Thorst G.** Serum Free Light Chain (FLC) Measurement in Multiple Myeloma (MM) Patients (pts) Correlate with Known Monoclonal Paraprotein, Disease Stage and Therapy Response. Blood 2004; **104** (11): 4907.

9. **Cavallo F, Rasmussen E, Zangari M, Tricot G, Fender B, Fox M, Burns M, Barlogie B.** Serum Free-Lite Chain (sFLC) Assay in Multiple Myeloma (MM): Clinical Correlates and Prognostic Implications in Newly Diagnosed MM Patients Treated with Total Therapy 2 or 3 (TT2/3). Blood 2005; **106** (11): 3490: 974a.

10. **Hassoun H, Reich L, Klimek VM, Dhodapkar M, Cohen A, Kewalramani T, Riedel ER, Hedvat CV, Teruya-Feldstein J, Filippa DA, Fleisher M, Nimer SD, Comenzo RL.** The Serum Free Light Chain Ratio after One or Two Cycles of Treatment Is Highly Predictive of the Magnitude of Final Response in Patients Undergoing Initial Treatment for Multiple Myeloma. Blood 2005; **106** (11): 3481: 972a.

11. **Hassoun H, Reich L, Klimek VM, Dhodapkar M, Cohen A, Kewalramani T, Zimman R, Drake L, Riedel ER, Hedvat CV, Teruya-Feldstein J, Filippa DA, Fleisher M, Nimer SD, Comenzo RL.** Doxorubicin and dexamethosone followed by thalidomide and dexamethasone is an effective well tolerated initial therapy for multiple myeloma. Br J Haem 2006; **132**: 155-161.

12. **Rajkumar SV, Kyle RA.** Conventional therapy and approach to management. Best Pract Res Clin Haematol. 2005; **18**: 585-601.

13. **Kumar S, Gertz MA, Hayman SR, Lacy MQ, Dispenzieri A, Zeldenrust SR, Lust JA, Greipp PR, Kyle RA, Fonseca RS. Rajkumar VS.** Use of the Serum Free Light Chain Assay in Assessment of Response to Therapy in Multiple Myeloma: Validation of Recently Proposed Response Criteria in a Prospective Clinical Trial of Lenalidomide Plus Dexamethasone for Newly Diagnosed Multiple Myeloma. Blood 2005; **106** (11): 3479: 971a.

14. **Durie BGM, Harousseau J-L, San Miguel J, Blade J, Barlogie B, Anderson K, Greipp PR, Westin J, Sonneveld P, Ludwig H, Garton G, Powles R, Sirohi B, Boccadaro M, Pilarski L, Merlini G, Joshua D, Vesole D, Kyle RA, Alexanian R, Tricot G, Attal M, and Rajkumar SV on behalf of the International Myeloma Working Group.** Uniform Response Criteria for Multiple Myeloma. Leukaemia *In Press.*

15. **Gupta S, Comenzo RL, Hoffman BR, Fleisher M.** National Academy of Clinical Biochemistry Guidelines for the use of Tumor Markers in Monoclonal Gammopathies. 2005 nacb.org.

16. **Gertz MA, Comenzo R, Falk RH, Fermand JP, Hazenberg BP, Hawkins PN, Merlini G, Moreau P, Ronco P, Sanchorawala V, Sezer O, Solomon Al, Grateau G.** Definition of Organ Involvement and Treatment Response in Immunoglobulin Light Chain Amyloidosis (AL): A Consensus Opinion From the 10th International Symposium on Amyloid and Amyloidosis. Am J Hematology 2005; **79**: 319-328.

17. **Bird JM, Cavenagh J, Samson D, Mehta A, Hawkins P, Lachmann H**. Guidelines on the diagnosis and management of AL amyloidosis. Br J Haem 2004; **125**: 681-700.

18. **Jaccard A, Moreau P, Aucouturier P, Ronco P, Fermand J-P, Hermine O.** Amylose immunoglobulinique. Hematologie. 2003; **9** (6): 485-495.

19. **Rajkumar SV, Kyle RA, Therneau TM, Melton LJ III, Bradwell AR Clark RJ, Larson DR, Plevak MF, Dispenzieri A, Katzmann JA.** Serum free light chain ratio is an independent risk factor for progression in monoclonal gammopathy of undetermined significance. Blood 2005; **106**: 812-817.

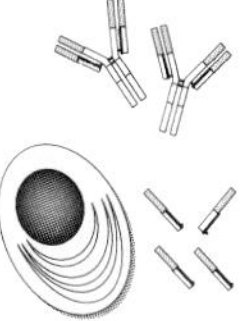

Section 5

Practical aspects of serum free light chain testing

Chapter 26

Implementation and interpretation of free light chain assays

26.1. Why measure free light chains in serum?

It is logical to measure serum FLCs in the situations listed below. Justification can be found in the relevant chapters. Some of the indications are well established while others are still under evaluation.

- Diagnostic test when suspecting a monoclonal gammopathy *(Chapters 6 and 23).*
- Replacement of urine tests for Bence Jones protein *(Chapters 8 and 24).*
- Monitoring of patients that cannot be assessed by electrophoretic tests *(Section 2).*
- Rapid assessment of treatment responses *(Chapter 13).*
- Assessment of residual disease and complete responses *(Chapter 12).*
- Risk stratification for progression in MGUS *(Chapter 19).*
- Monitoring MM patients in renal failure undergoing haemodialysis *(Chapter 14).*

FLCs are preferably measured in serum rather than urine. Urine samples have a wider normal range, are more difficult to collect and process and are less sensitive when FLC production is low *(Chapter 24).* Both FLCs should be measured and κ/λ ratios calculated. Results should be reported on log/log graphs that include normal range data and results from a variety of clinical conditions *(Figure 26.1).*

26.2. Getting started

There are many implementation issues to be considered: clinical, technical, educational, political, etc. Laboratories are familiar with the introduction of new tests

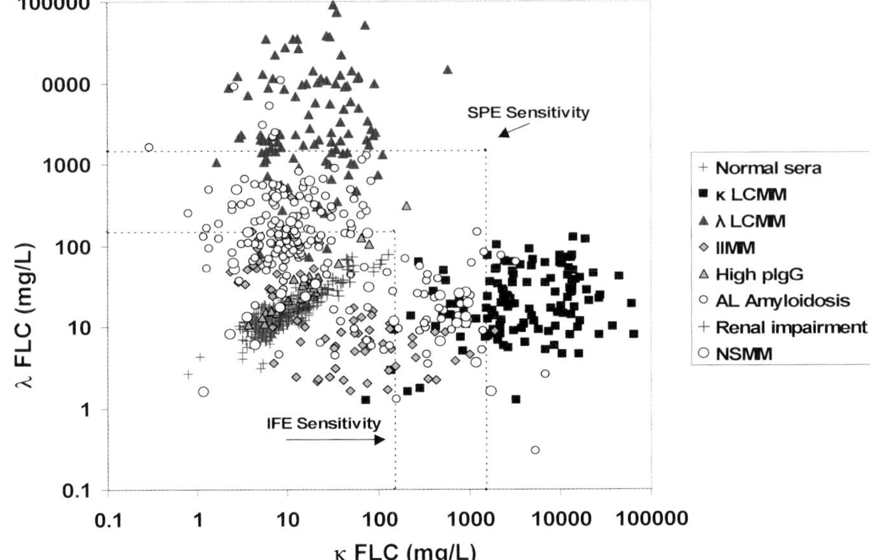

Figure 26.1. Serum FLCs in a selection of clinical conditions.

so it is not appropriate for these issues to be discussed here. Implementation of FLC tests normally come under the category of '*service development*'. Because FLCs are widely measured in urine they can usually be introduced without seeking new test approval.

In analytical terms, FLC molecules are stable in serum, kits are available for many routine laboratory instruments and clinical interpretation of the results is well established. Practical issues directly related to FLC analysis are discussed below and in Chapters 27 and 28.

Pre-analytical

Serum or plasma samples can be used and FLCs are stable for many weeks when stored at 4°C. Longer-term storage should be at -20°C with preservatives *(Chapter 4)*. There is minimal variation in FLC concentrations in samples taken from patients at different times of the day.

Analytical

FLC kits are available for use on many instruments. Results are generally more precise on the large clinical chemistry analysers. Details can be found in Chapter 27. External quality control schemes are available and should be used (*Chapter 28*).

Post-analytical

Reporting of results for diagnosis should be on κ/λ log plots that include normal range data and results from a variety of clinical situations *(Figure 26.1)*. Serial monitoring should include both FLCs and κ/λ ratios. It may be useful to include a renal function marker such as serum creatinine or cystatin C.

26.3. Use and interpretation of serum free light chain results

A. Screening symptomatic patients for monoclonal gammopathies

Serum FLC analysis should be used alongside SPE and sIFE tests and then >99% of patients with monoclonal gammopathies are identified. Results are considered abnormal when they are outside the following normal ranges:-

Serum κ concentrations: 3.3-19.4mg/L
Serum λ concentrations: 5.7-26.3mg/L
Serum κ/λ ratio: 0.26-1.65

Patients' results separate into different categories depending upon several factors: whether the clone is κ or λ, the presence of renal failure or polyclonal hypergammaglobulinaemia and the degree of bone marrow impairment from the growing tumour or from drug therapy (*Figure 26.2*). An accompanying table for this figure provides a simplistic guide to interpretation of results (*Table 26.1*).

1. **Normal samples.** Serum κ, λ and κ/λ ratio are all within the normal ranges. If accompanying serum electrophoretic tests are normal it is most unlikely that the patient has a monoclonal gammopathy.
2. **Abnormal κ/λ ratios.** Support the diagnosis of a monoclonal gammopathy and require an appropriate tissue biopsy. Borderline elevated κ/λ ratios occur with renal impairment and may require appropriate renal function tests.

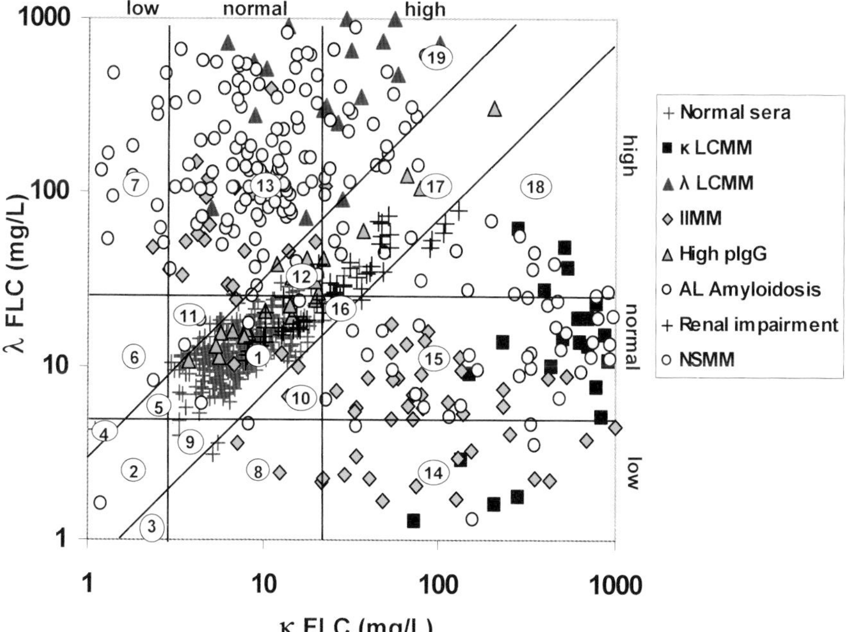

Figure 26.2. Serum κ and λ concentrations in a selection of clinical conditions. Patients are categorised according to FLC concentrations and κ/λ ratios. *See Table 26.1 for interpretation.* The axes are truncated for clarity compared with Figure 26.1.

	Kappa	Lambda	κ/λ Ratio	Interpretation
1	Normal	Normal	Normal	Normal serum
2	Low	Low	Normal	BM suppression without MG
3			High	MG with BM suppression
4			Low	
5		Normal	Normal	Normal serum or BM suppression
6			Low	MG with BM suppression
7		High	Low	
8	Normal	Low	High	
9			Normal	Normal serum or BM suppression
10		Normal	High	MG with BM suppression
11			Low	
12		High	Normal	pIg or renal impairment
13			Low	MG without BM suppression
14	High	Low	High	MG with BM suppression
15		Normal	High	MG without BM suppression
16			Normal	pIg or renal impairment
17		High	Normal	
18			High	MG with renal impairment
19			Low	

Table 26.1. Classification of monoclonal gammopathies according to serum FLC concentrations (*also see Figure 26.2*). BM: bone marrow. MG: monoclonal gammopathy.

3. **Low concentrations of κ, λ or both.** Indicate bone marrow function impairment.
4. **Elevated concentrations of both κ and λ with a normal κ/λ ratio.** May be due to the following:-
    - renal impairment (common).
    - over-production of polyclonal FLCs from inflammatory conditions (common).
    - biclonal gammopathies of different FLC types (rare).
5. **Elevated concentrations of both κ and λ with an abnormal κ/λ ratio.** Suggest a combination of monoclonal gammopathy and renal impairment.

B. Replacement of urine electrophoretic tests for FLCs

Many clinical studies have shown that urine FLC tests offer no additional benefit over serum FLC tests in assessing patients with NSMM, LCMM, IIMM, AL amyloidosis and MGUS. Laboratory comparison of the sensitivity of serum FLC tests with urine tests indicates greater sensitivity for serum tests. Occasional patients have normal serum FLC results but minor monoclonal FLCs in the urine. However, their clinical relevance is doubtful.

C. Monitoring patients using serum FLC assays

Patients with monoclonal gammopathies can be monitored serially using the tumour FLC and the κ/λ ratio. As an alternative, the numerical value of the concentration of the tumour (involved) FLC, minus the non-tumour (uninvolved) FLC appears satisfactory

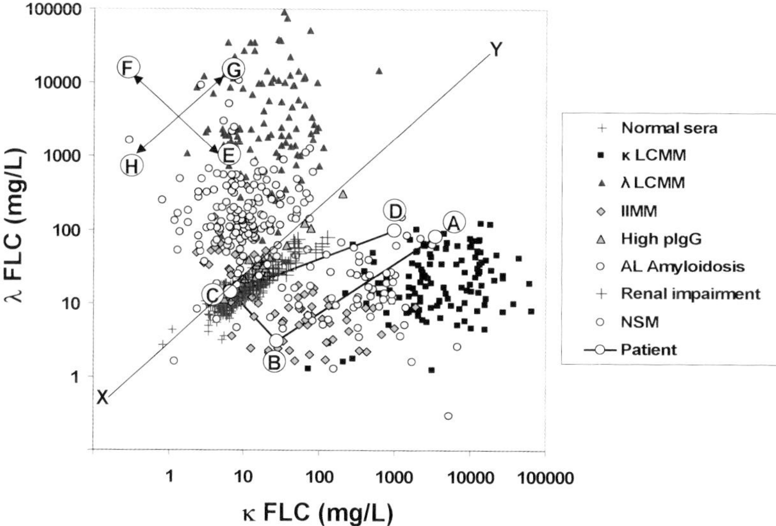

Figure 26.3. Changes in sFLCs during treatment of a patient with MM. Results at presentation (A), after high-dose melphalan showing treatment response and bone marrow suppression (B), in complete remission (C) and in relapse with renal impairment from FLC (D). For explanations of E-F: G-H see text. X---Y = normal κ/λ ratio.

This subtracts the polyclonal FLC component. This technique of FLC assessment is recommended in the new response criteria for monitoring MM.

Results from serum FLC measurements can be presented in different ways. Figure 26.3 shows changes in serum FLC concentrations in a patient with MM from the time of presentation to disease relapse. At presentation (A), κ concentrations were highly elevated at 3,500mg/L and the non-tumour FLC was mildly elevated because of FLC deposition in the kidneys. While under treatment (B), both sFLC concentrations fell because of bone marrow suppression but there was selective tumour cell killing reflected in a reduction of the κ/λ ratio. Successful treatment is shown by return of the FLC concentrations and κ/λ ratio to normal (C). At subsequent relapse (D), the tumour FLC and the κ/λ ratio increased, as might be expected, but the alternate FLC also increased as a result of renal impairment from chemotherapy and FLC deposition in the nephrons.

The normal κ/λ ratio is marked as **X---Y**. Changes away from this axis indicate decreasing (E) or increasing λ tumour FLCs (F). Changes parallel to the κ/λ ratio axis and both FLC concentrations increasing (G), indicate renal impairment. Similarly, decreasing concentrations indicate renal function recovery, with the addition of bone marrow suppression if below the normal range (H).

Another way to present the results is against time. Data should include κ, λ and κ/λ ratios (*Figure 26.4)*, perhaps with the addition of other markers such as intact immunoglobulins. Examples of patients being monitored using serum FLCs can be found in the relevant chapters. An Excel spreadsheet addition is available from The

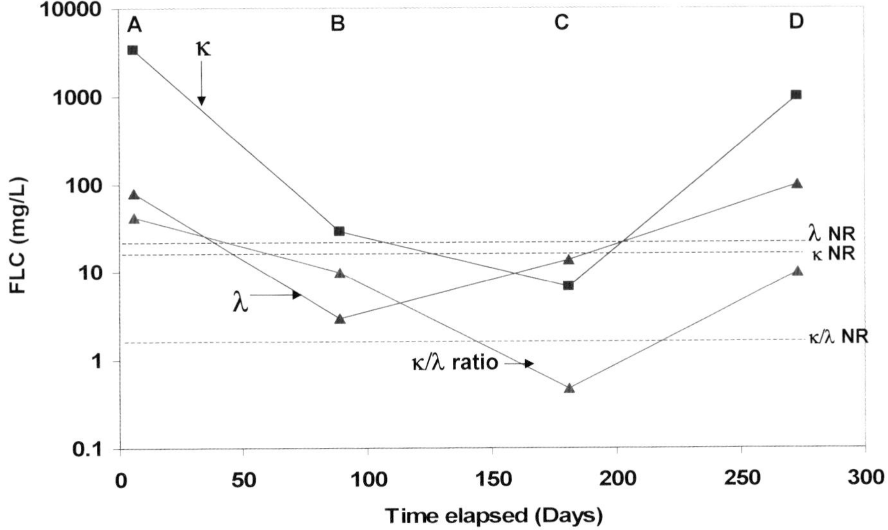

Figure 26.4. Data from the patient shown in Figure 26.3. Results at clinical presentation (A), after high-dose melphalan showing treatment response and bone marrow suppression (B), in complete remission (C) and in relapse with renal impairment from FLC damage (D).

Binding Site for longitudinal plotting of patients' results over time.

26.4. Limitations of serum free light chain analysis

While serum FLC immunoassays have many advantages over electrophoretic tests, there are limitations. When results give doubt, monoclonal FLCs should be assessed by SPE and IFE. Difficulties that may occur are described below. Details can be found in the relevant chapters of the book.

1. Clonality assessment

Using FLC immunoassays, monoclonal FLCs are determined by abnormal κ/λ ratios. This is clearly different from the assessment of bands on electrophoretic gels. Arguably, κ/λ ratios are preferable because numerical limits are easily established while visual impressions of bands on gels are more difficult to assess and quantitate.

In some situations analysis of κ/λ ratios is preferable. For example, patients with NSMM have highly abnormal κ/λ ratios yet electrophoretic tests are normal. In AL amyloidosis *(Chapter 15)* and LCDD *(Chapter 17)*, serum FLCs are the actual molecules causing the disease.

Rare patients have monoclonal FLC bands when tested by urine IFE which are not abnormal by serum FLC immunoassays *(Chapter 24)*. These monoclonal bands are of little clinical relevance and can probably be safely ignored.

2. Inaccuracy of free light chain measurements

Each monoclonal protein is structurally unique, so results depend upon how well the antibodies recognise molecular variants and polymeric conformations. Some of these variants may give rise to inaccuracies in measurement. Historically, this line of argument has been used to discredit the measurement of intact monoclonal immunoglobulins by nephelometry. However, experience has shown that this has not invalidated their utility and widespread acceptance in a clinical setting. The same can now be said for serum FLC immunoassays. Nevertheless, in some patients huge discrepancies are seen between monoclonal FLCs measured by immunoassays and other techniques, particularly in urine samples. In the latter fluid, FLC immunoassays may give higher concentration values than other methods of FLC measurement (*Chapter 5*).

3. Standardisation

While current standards may well be accurate, there are no international standards or traceable international materials. Although every effort might be made by the manufacturers to ensure good quality, the assays may drift with time and in an unpredictable manner. Local standards and reference materials should be used with the assays, when possible.

4. Non-linearity of monoclonal free light chain proteins

This refers to variations in quantification that occur when a sample is diluted and the result is different from the starting value. A number of factors may be involved. Details can be found in Chapter 4 and include the following:-

- Monoclonal FLCs of unusual shape, partially missed by the antisera (see below).
- Antibody bias to one form of the FLC proteins.
- Antisera cross-reactivity with intact immunoglobulins.
- Non-specific assay interference (lipids, haemoglobin etc).
- Use of unsuitable materials for assay calibrators.

5. Different batches of antisera

Consideration should be given to apparent changes in serum FLC concentrations that might occur when changing to a different batch of antisera. Batches are made to react in a characterised manner with a variety of standards and control sera. These are manufactured to defined limits that are achieved during kit production. Within these limits there is some small but quantifiable variation.

In addition, each monoclonal FLC is unique and will react in its own particular manner in the assays. While great effort is made during manufacture to maintain lot-to-lot consistency, antisera cannot be made to recognise every individual monoclonal FLC equally. Some structurally abnormal molecules may not, therefore, be reproducibly measured. In such circumstances, the previous sample should be re-run alongside the new sample, using the new batch of antiserum, and the results compared.

6. Presence of polyclonal free light chains

Raised polyclonal FLCs lead to an overestimation of monoclonal FLCs. This is particularly apparent in patients with renal failure in whom the polyclonal, non-tumour FLC is greatly elevated (*Chapter 20*). However, κ/λ ratios are likely to remain abnormal if monoclonal FLCs are present. Borderline results may need to be corrected against serum creatinine (or a better marker of impaired glomerular filtration such as cystatin C) in patients with renal failure.

7. Biclonal gammopathies of different light chain types

Approximately 1-2% of patients with MM have bi-clonal gammopathies. When the FLC types differ (~50%), so that the patient has both types of FLC, κ/λ ratios can be normal. It is likely that both FLC concentrations would be elevated so the clinician would be alerted to an abnormality. The issue can be resolved by testing the sample by IFE and identifying two monoclonal bands of different light chain types. Renal function should also be determined to assess the degree of polyclonal elevation of FLCs from reduced glomerular clearance.

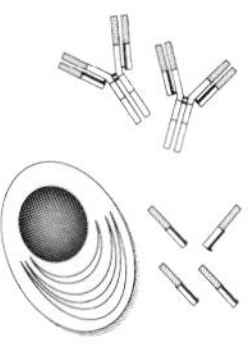

Chapter 27

Instrumentation for free light chain immunoassays

Introduction

Serum FLC concentrations can be measured on many different laboratory analysers. All use latex-enhanced assays to allow detection of FLCs at low but clinically important concentrations. Details of the applications are given in this chapter and an outline can be found in Chapter 4.

Nephelometers and turbidimeters have similar levels of sensitivity and precision for serum proteins but vary in their ability to handle samples, clean reaction cuvettes, identify antigen excess, etc. Immunology and smaller clinical chemistry laboratories tend to use nephelometers that are dedicated to protein measurements but sample handling is relatively slow. Such instruments may not have 'open' channels, so technical assistance is frequently required to implement the FLC tests.

Large clinical laboratories tend to use multifunctional chemistry instruments that analyse proteins turbidimetrically. These instruments are usually more precise and stable than dedicated protein analysers and may be more 'user-friendly' for new assay implementation. However, some external assistance is usually required to ensure proper running of the assays and interpretation of results.

Inevitably, there are occasional assay related 'issues' that lead to customer questions or complaints. Analysis of The Binding Site database has showed that approximately 50% of problems were related to inadequate maintenance of the analysers or incorrect parameter programming. About 20% were due to problems with calibrators and 15% were related to samples behaving in a non-linear manner. The precision values shown in the tables below for each instrument are those found in experienced laboratories. If attained precision figures are significantly worse, then the instrument or the programming may be at fault. It should be noted that the majority of complaints have been restricted to two instruments. This is largely because they have been more widely used.

Exact information on the performance of the assays and their implementation is contained in the package inserts. Parameters may change slightly with different batches.

27.1. Bayer Advia 1650™

This is an open instrument but some assistance may be required to input the FLC assay protocols. Assay performance is good *(Table 27.1)*. It is linear across the measuring range, has good sensitivity and curve stability and shows good intra-run and inter-run precision. Results compare well with those from other instruments.

	Kappa	**Lambda**
Range: 1/5 (κ); 1/8 (λ)	3.5 - 56mg/L	7.0 - 93.4mg/L
Sensitivity neat	0.75mg/L	0.88mg/L
Assay time	13.5 min	13.5 min
Precision: within-run	5.1% at 5.82mg/L	1.7% at 4.66mg/L
	2.8% at 18.0mg/L	4.3% at 12.3mg/L
	3.9% at 22.5mg/L	2.6% at 34.4mg/L
	3.2% at 34.9mg/L	1.6% at 65.7mg/L
Precision: between-run	5.0% at 13.9mg/L	3.8% at 26.3mg/L
	4.4% at 30.5mg/L	2.7% at 50.4mg/L

Table 27.1. Assay performance on the Bayer Advia 1650.

References

1. **Wands C, Powell M, Jupp R.** The Development of Serum Free Light Chain Immunoassay on Bayer Advia 1650. Proceedings of ACB National Meeting, 2003; **No.2**: p47.

2. **Carr-Smith HD, Harland B, Anderson J, Overton J, Wieringa G, Bradwell AR.** Evaluation of latex-enhanced turbidimetric reagents for measuring free immunoglobulin light chains on the Bayer Advia 1650. Clin Chem 2004; **50** (6): Suppl, A82: C-44.

27.2. Beckman Coulter IMMAGE® and IMMAGE® 800

The IMMAGE is a rate nephelometer that measures plasma proteins by homogeneous immunoassay. The instrument has two basic modes of operation; a fully automated 'Beckman' mode, controlled by the manufacturer and a ‘user-defined’ reagent mode. The latter allows assays to be developed by individual laboratories.

The Binding Site provides FLC kits for use in ‘user-defined’ mode. Each contains a pre-prepared, six level calibrator set, κ or λ latex reagents and product information. Support is usually required for setting up the assays and some disposable components and buffers are required from Beckman Coulter.

The assays use serum samples diluted to 1/10 and the instrument can be programmed to analyse samples at 1/5 or 1/50 if the initial dilution is unsatisfactory. Higher sample dilutions must be prepared off-line. The 1/10 dilutions cover the FLC concentrations found in most samples and antigen excess capacity is good (*Table 27.2).*

Assay trouble shooting

1. **Cuvette fogging.** Latex particles accumulate on the cuvettes so they must be changed regularly (every 1,200 Freelite tests).

2. **Washer probe.** This needs particular attention. It must be clean, free from corrosion and correctly aligned.
3. **Syringes and buffer lines:** Check there is no leakage or air bubbles.
4. **Buffers:** The No 1 system diluent must be used.

	Kappa	Lambda
Range at 1/10	6-180mg/L	8-270mg/L
Sensitivity at 1/5	3mg/L	4mg/L
Assay time	10 min	10 min
Precision:within-run	2.5% at 18mg/L	6.4% at 32mg/L
	3.4% at 27mg/L	4.1% at 47mg/L
	2% at 57mg/L	2.4% at 99mg/L
Precision:between-run	12.5% at 20mg/L	6.7% at 34mg/L
	7.2% at 27mg/L	9.4% at 65mg/L
	6.4% at 58mg/L	2.9% at 101mg/L

Table 27.2. Assay performance on the Beckman Coulter IMMAGE.

References

1. **Tate JR, Gill D, Cobcroft R, Hickman PE**. Practical Considerations for the Measurement of Free Light Chains in Serum. Clin Chem 2003; **49**: 1252-1257.

2. **Harris J, Tang LX, Showell PJ, Carr-Smith HD, Drew R, Bradwell AR.** Assays for immunoglobulin free light chains in serum on the Beckman IMMAGE™. Clin Chem 2000; **46**: 701: pA180.

3. **Ong S, Sethi S.** Assessment of free light chains in serum on the Beckman IMMAGE™. Clin Chem 2003; **49** (6): D59: pA106.

27.3. The Binding Site Minineph™ (Mark 2)

This is a small, manual nephelometer that has been modified for serum FLC analysis. The calibration curves are stored on magnetic swipe-cards. Once loaded into the instrument's memory, curve validity is confirmed by assaying control samples. Patient samples are analysed individually by semi-automated addition of reagents into cuvettes within the instrument. The assays show good linearity, readily identify antigen excess situations and have good agreement with the BNII. The instrument may find use in laboratories with low work loads (<10 samples per day) or when the cost of a larger instrument cannot be justified.

Reference

1. **Showell PJ, Matters DJ, Long JM, Carr-Smith HD, Bradwell AR.** Evaluation of latex-enhanced nephelometric reagents for measuring free immunoglobulin light chains on a modified Minineph™. Clin Chem 2002; **48**: Suppl. A-67: pA17.

27.4. Dade Behring BNII™

The BNII is a nephelometer designed for measuring plasma proteins by homogeneous immunoassays. The instrument can be programmed for non-Dade Behring assays using

	Kappa	Lambda
Range at 1/20	5.5-88mg/L	7.6-120mg/L
Sensitivity at 1/5	1.4mg/L	1.9mg/L
Assay time	6 min	6 min
Precision:within-run	7.3% at 11mg/L	9.1% at 13mg/L
	7.9% at 57mg/L	2.7% at 61mg/L
Precision:between-run	6.5% at 11mg/L	10.8% at 13mg/L
	5.6% at 57mg/L	9.0% at 61mg/L

Table 27.3. Assay performance on The Binding Site Minineph.

a software key from the company's engineers. Once programmed, the FLC assays run in a similar manner to other protein tests. A single calibrator fluid is automatically diluted to form a calibration curve. The initial sample dilution is 1/100 with automatic dilution of samples that are outside the calibration range. *(Table 27.4)* The initial dilution of 1/100 has a good antigen excess capacity.

Assay trouble-shooting

If the assay is performing poorly the following issues should be considered and an engineer may be needed for assistance:-

1. Wash system (wash shoe, alignment and tubing). Problems with these components may lead to liquid remaining in the bottom of the cuvettes after cleaning. This may lead to carry-over problems in subsequent assays causing dilution errors and variable results. If fluid remains in the cuvettes after laundering, a service engineer should assess the wash system.

2. Syringes. Fluid leakage or excessive air in the syringes and buffer lines.

3. Programming. The assays require software programming with a service key (dongle). Check carefully for correct parameter programming before the engineer leaves.

	Kappa	Lambda
Range at 1/100	6-190mg/L	8-260mg/L
Sensitivity at 1/5	0.3mg/L	0.4mg/L
Assay time	18 min	18 min
Precision:within-run	3.1% at 14mg/L	8.4% at 15mg/L
	4.8% at 33mg/L	5.2% at 22mg/L
	4.2% at 51mg/L	4.8% at 72mg/L
Precision:between-run	6.3% at 12mg/L	8.1% at 18mg/L
	8.4% at 32mg/L	4.7% at 24mg/L
	7.4% at 55mg/L	7.5% at 72mg/L

Table 27.4. Assay performance on the Dade Behring BNII.

4. Leaking three-way valves. N-Reaction buffer used in many other BNII assays may leak across the three-way valve into the FLC assays. This leads to loss of curve reproducibility and poor assay precision (particularly at the low end of the curve). If this occurs the syringes should be primed with N-Diluent prior to running the assays. Avoid running assays that use N-Reaction buffer alongside the FLC assays until after the valve has been replaced.

References

1. **Bradwell AR, Carr-Smith HD, Mead GP, Tang LX, Showell PJ, Drayson MT, Drew R.** Highly sensitive automated immunoassay for immunoglobulin free light chains in serum and urine. Clin Chem 2001; **47**: 673-680.

2. **Katzmann JA, Clark RJ, Abraham RS, Bryant S, Lymp JF, Bradwell AR, Kyle RA.** Serum Reference Intervals and Diagnostic Ranges for Free Kappa and Free Lambda Immunoglobulin Light Chains: Relative Sensitivity for Detection of Monoclonal Light Chains. Clin Chem 2002; **48**: 1437-1444.

3. **Carr-Smith HD, Showell P, Bradwell AR**. Antigen excess assessment of free light chain assays on the Dade-Behring BNII nephelometer. Clin Chem 2002; **48 (**6): Suppl A-71: A23.

27.5. Dade Behring BN-ProSpec™

This instrument is available in some markets in an 'open-mode', or can be opened for serum FLC assays by the Dade Behring engineers with a software programme called 'Assay Builder'. The instrument is more precise than the BNII for a variety of reasons including the use of disposable cuvettes. The instrument uses the same format FLC kits as the BNII but with a different product code. Precision of the instrument is good, in part because of disposable cuvettes *(Table 27.5).*

Reference

1. **Tate JR, Gill D, Cobcroft R, Hickman PE.** Practical Considerations for the Measurement of Free Light Chains in Serum. Clin Chem 2003; **49**: 1252-1257.

2. **Showell PJ, Lynch EA, Overton J, Carr-Smith HD, Bradwell AR.** Evaluation of latex-enhanced nephelometric reagents for measuring free immunoglobulin light chains on the Dade Behring ProSpec. Clin Chem 2005; **51** (6): suppl. B-38.

	Kappa	Lambda
Range at 1/100	6-190mg/L	8-260mg/L
Sensitivity at 1/5	0.3mg/L	0.4mg/L
Assay time	18 min	18 min
Precision:within-run	4% at 16mg/L	2% at 25mg/L
	6% at 30mg/L	3% at 56mg/L
	4.2% at 51mg/L	4.8% at 72mg/L
Precision:between-run	4% at 25mg/L	2% at 22mg/L
	2% at 36mg/L	1% at 44mg/L
	4% at 80mg/L	1% at 141mg/L

Table 27.5. Assay performance on the BN ProSpec.

27.6. Olympus analysers (AU400, 640, 2700 and 5400)™

The Olympus chemistry analysers use turbidimetry for the measurement of plasma proteins. All have similar hardware and software but vary in their sample handling capacity. The instruments are open and can be programmed by the user. For the FLC assays, 6 pre-diluted standards are provided. The standard sample dilution is 1/10 which provides a good antigen excess capacity. Sample results outside this range are automatically re-measured at 1/100 or 1/5, while off-line dilutions are required for higher concentrations. Results correlate well with other FLC immunoassays and assay precision is particularly good.

At present, no specific technical issues have been encountered. Fogging of the glass cuvettes with the latex reagent is a potential problem. This can be prevented by adding a W2 wash with 1% Decon 90 before the normal weekly W2 wash programme.

	Kappa	Lambda
Range at 1/10	6-150mg/L	6-150mg/L
Sensitivity at 1/5	3mg/L	3mg/L
Assay time	8 min	8 min
Precision:within-run	2% at 22mg/L	1.6% at 31mg/L
	1.2% at 41mg/L	0.8% at 66mg/L
	1.9% at 153mg/L	6.8% at 183mg/L
Precision:between-run	5.8% at 22mg/L	5.4% at 27mg/L
	5.2% at 41mg/L	4.9% at 63mg/L
	6.0% at 135mg/L	4.5% at 178mg/L

Table 27.6. Assay performance on the Olympus analysers.

Reference

1. **Showell P, Matters D, Carr-Smith HD, Bradwell AR.** Evaluation of latex-enhanced turbidimetric reagents for measuring free immunoglobulin light-chains on the Olympus AU400. Clin Chem 2003; **49** (6): A105: D55.

27.7. Radim Delta™

This is a medium-sized, fully automated bench-top nephelometer, with similar characteristics and performance to the Dade-Behring BNII. The instrument produces calibration curves from a single calibration fluid. Samples with concentrations of FLCs outside the initial measuring range are automatically re-diluted by the instrument.

Reference

1. **Showell PJ, Lynch EA, Carr-Smith HD, Bradwell AR.** Evaluation of latex-enhanced nephelometric reagents for measuring free immunoglobulin light-chains on the Radim Delta. Clin Chem 2004; **50** (6): Suppl. A81: C40.

	Kappa	Lambda
Range at 1/100	6.0-190mg/L	8.0-260mg/L
Sensitivity at 1/5	0.3mg/L	0.4mg/L
Assay time	18 min	18 min
Precision:within-run	10.1% at 8.9mg/L	4.3% at 15.5mg/L
	5.7% at 31.7mg/L	2.0% at 75.2mg/L
	4.4% at 135.7mg/L	4.1% at 202.8mg/L
Precision:between-run	11.0% at 8.9mg/L	5.3% at 13.1mg/L
	7.6% at 32.9mg/L	5.2% at 47.6mg/L
	9.4% at 129.1mg/L	6.4% at 143.5mg/L

Table 27.7. Assay performance on the Radim Delta.

27.8. Roche Modular P™ analyser system and the Hitachi 911/912/917

These instruments measure serum proteins by turbidimetry. Most parameter channels are dedicated to Roche assays but a few can be used with other manufacturers' products. Single-vial calibrator fluids are used that are diluted automatically to generate the calibration curves. The starting sample dilutions are 1/5 for κ assays and 1/8 for λ assays. The instruments can be programmed to automatically re-dilute samples when results are outside the range of the calibration curve *(Table 27.8)*. Very high samples must be diluted off-line. There is good antigen excess capacity and results show a good correlation with the Dade Behring BNII.

Assay trouble-shooting

The following issues need to be considered with the Modular P.

1. Ensure correct settings for the parameters and technical limits. These change with each batch of kits.
2. Add an additional "joker-labelled" open channel reagent bottle with saline for diluent.
3. If the sodium hydroxide wash buffer bottle is empty, cuvettes become turbid and an "OVER" error message appears.

	Kappa	Lambda
Range	3.7-56mg/L(1/5)	7.0-93.3mg/L (1/8)
Sensitivity (neat)	0.8mg/L	1.0mg/L
Assay time	10-15 min	10-15 min
Precision:within-run	5.5% at 14.6mg/L	2.7% at 23.5mg/L
	4.7% at 25mg/L	.7% at 49 mg/L
	2.4% at 54mg/L	1.4% at 79mg/L
Precision:between-run	7.3% at 7mg/L	9.5% at 12mg/L
	9.5% at 15mg/L	6.1% at 24mg/L
	5.7 at 35mg/L	6.3% at 55mg/L

Table 27.8. Assay performance on the Roche Modular P.

4. If tolerance limits have been exceeded after the water wash, a "CELL" error message appears.
5. Wait until the calibrator rack has cleared the pipetting area before loading new controls. This ensures that the new curve information is allocated to the correct samples.

References

1. **Showell PJ, Long JM, Carr-Smith HD, Bradwell AR**. Evaluation of latex-enhanced turbidimetric reagents for measuring free immunoglobulin light-chains on the Hitachi 911/912. Clin Chem 2002; **48**: Suppl. A-66: A22.
2. **Overton J, Goodier D, Carr-Smith HD, Bradwell AR.** Evaluation of latex-enhanced turbidimetric reagents for measuring free immunoglobulin light-chains on the Roche Modular P. Clin Chem 2003; **49**: Suppl. A106: D60.

27.9. Tokyo Boeki Prestige 24i™ and Biolis

The Prestige 24i is a bench-top, random-access, chemistry and immunoassay instrument. It can perform 80 tests per hour. Up to 24 reagents can be used simultaneously and chemical reactions are temperature-controlled at 37°C. There is sufficient space to load 55 samples, 55 calibrators and controls. Urgent samples can also be added. Cuvettes are semi-disposable.

	Kappa	**Lambda**
Range at 1/10	6.5-196mg/L	3.8-128mg/L
Sensitivity at 1/1	0.65mg/L	0.38mg/L
Assay time	10 min	10 min
Precision:within-run	5.5% at 14.6mg/L	2.7% at 23.5mg/L
	4.7% at 25mg/L	1.7% at 49mg/L
Precision:between-run	8.8% at 14.3mg/L	2.2% at 22mg/L
	5.5% at 31mg/L	2.1% at 54mg/L

Table 27.9. Assay performance on the Tokyo Boeki Prestige 24i.

Trademarks

Advia ™ - Bayer Healthcare AG, Germany
BNII™ and BN ProSpec™ - Dade Behring GmbH., Marburg, Germany
FREELITE™ - The Binding Site Ltd., Birmingham, England
MININEPH™ - The Binding Site Ltd., Birmingham, England
IMMAGE™ - Beckman Coulter Inc., Brea, California, USA
Olympus™ and Olympus AU™ - Olympus Optical Company Ltd., Tokyo, Japan
Tokyo Boeki Prestige 24i™ - Tokyo Boeki Medical System Ltd., Japan

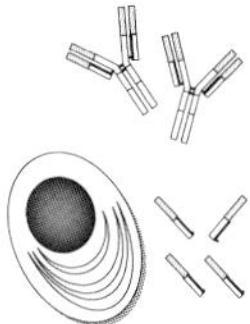

Chapter 28

Quality assurance for serum free light chain analysis

28.1. Introduction

It is essential that all laboratories participate in external quality control schemes when performing monoclonal protein analysis. Guidelines are described in many publications and are summarised in Chapter 25.

There are several national quality control (QA) schemes for assessing monoclonal immunoglobulins.[1-3] Typically, distributed samples comprise serum or urine and contain combinations of intact immunoglobulin monoclonal proteins and monoclonal FLCs. Results are generally satisfactory for serum samples but less good for urine, particularly when FLC concentrations are low.[4] The explanations for poor urine results are:- variations in electrophoretic techniques, the requirement to concentrate urine samples and difficulties with interpretation of the gels *(Chapter 25)*.

Many laboratories measuring monoclonal proteins could improve their results by the addition of FLC immunoassays. If the QA schemes encouraged the use of serum rather than urine tests, this might further improve clinical diagnostic accuracy. Wide availability of QA schemes for sFLC analysis should be encouraged.

28.2. The Binding Site QA scheme (QA003)

Because there are currently no international or national schemes, The Binding Site has developed its own sFLC QA programme. To date, there have been 27 distributions over nearly 5 years. Three of these contained both monoclonal intact immunoglobulins (IgG, IgA or IgM) and sFLCs. For the intact immunoglobulins in these samples, the diagnostic accuracy of the reporting laboratories was almost 100% by IFE and between 70-90% using SPE. In the same samples, sFLCs were correctly identified in only 5-35% of laboratories using electrophoretic tests.

Seven of the distributed samples contained monoclonal sFLCs alone. SPE was correct in only 1-5% of the laboratories while IFE was correct in 10-70% of laboratories. As expected, greater accuracy was obtained for samples containing high sFLC concentrations (values ranged from 50mg/L to 3,000mg/L - normal range <26.3mg/L).

In contrast, almost all laboratories using FLC immunoassays reported the FLCs correctly in the distributed samples. Figure 28.1 shows the results of analysis of one of these samples, from a patient with IIMM, that had a κ sFLC concentration of 420 mg/L.

The monoclonal band was undetectable by SPE and IFE.

Another of the distributed samples was from a patient with NSMM and contained no detectable monoclonal protein by all serum and urine electrophoretic tests *(Figure 28.2)*. This included uIFE on highly concentrated samples. sFLC immunoassays showed 250 mg/L of κ FLC and 11 mg/L of λ FLC. This was identified correctly only by those laboratories using sFLC immunoassays. It should be noted that weak, false-positive bands for FLCs may sometimes be seen by IFE. So-called 'free' light chain antisera used in IFE usually have some cross-reactivity with bound light chains in order to improve IFE sensitivity (see information leaflet in IFE kits).

28.3. College of American Pathologists (CAP) QA scheme

The College of American Pathologists (CAP) produces a serum paraprotein QA scheme with over 900 participants.[2] Reporting methods include SPE, IFE and monoclonal protein quantification. Most samples inevitably contain monoclonal FLCs. One of the distributed samples was particularly difficult to characterise, yet contained a monoclonal IgA λ of 6g/L (*Figure 28.3*). This was missed by 65% (593/916) of laboratories using SPE and 6% of laboratories using IFE but only 43% (398/916) of laboratories used the latter method.

sFLC measurements showed an elevated λ of 39mg/L (normal range 5.7-26.3mg/L) and an abnormal κ/λ ratio of 0.24 (normal range 0.26-1.65) indicating monoclonality (*Figure 28.3*). This abnormal FLC result would have alerted many laboratories to the presence of a monoclonal plasma cell disease.

28.4. French QA Scheme

La Agencé Francaise de Securité Sanitaire des Products de Santé (French quality control agency for health) have a quality control scheme for monoclonal

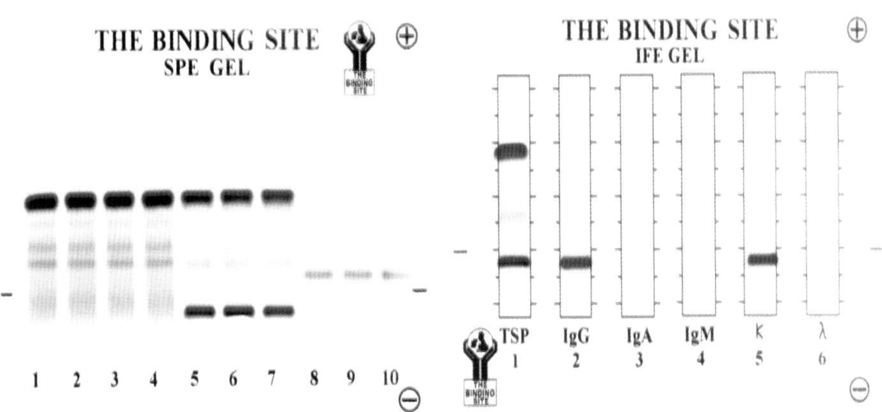

Figure 28.1. SPE and sIFE in a patient with IIMM. SPE comprised a normal sera (lanes 1-4) and the patient sample (IgGκ) applied 3 times (lanes 5-7) and a κ FLC positive urine sample (lanes 8-10). The κ sFLC concentration was 420 mg/L.

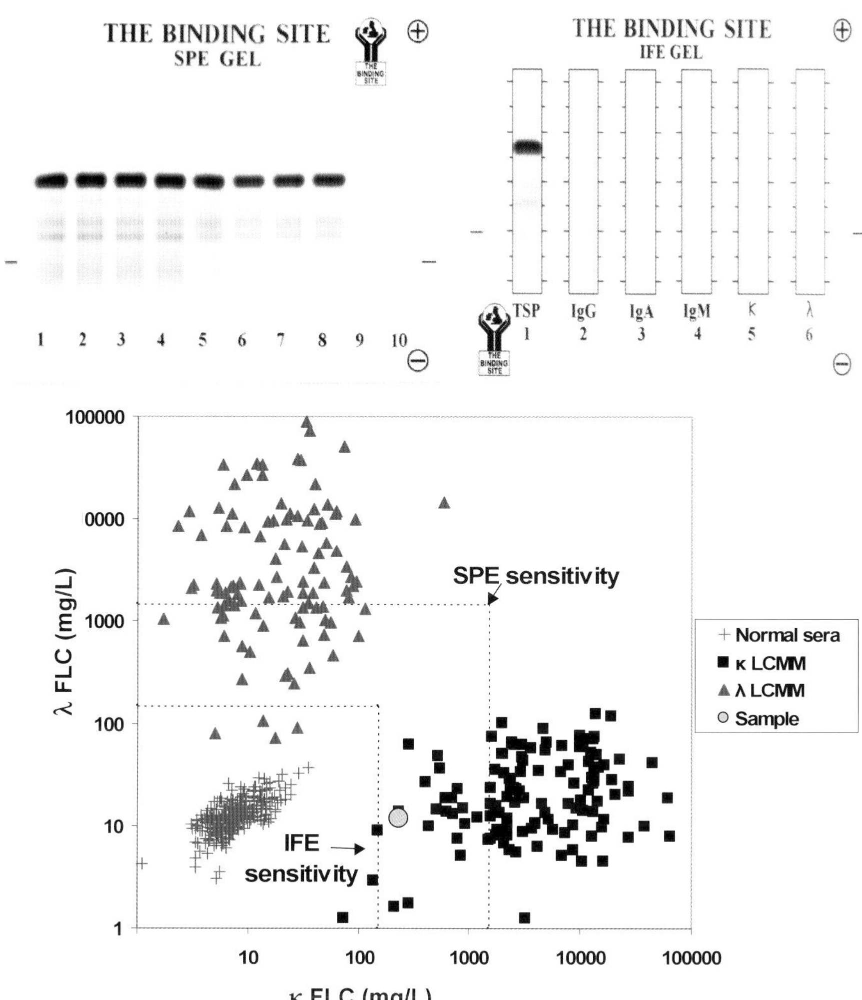

Figure 28.2. SPE, IFE and sFLC concentrations in a patient with NSMM. SPE comprised a normal sera (lanes 1-4) and the patient sample (lanes 5-8). sIFE was normal.

immunoglobulins.[3] One distributed serum sample was from a patient with IgD myeloma. Almost 95% of laboratories identified the IgDλ monoclonal immunoglobulin correctly, but only 17% of 1,118 laboratories reported the associated λ FLC. However, sFLC immunoassays showed a λ FLC concentration of 254mg/L and a κ/λ ratio of 0.0096 - the latter result being 30-fold outside the normal range (*Figure 28.4*).

28.5. UK NEQAS Monoclonal protein identification

The UK National External Quality Assessment Service for Immunology and

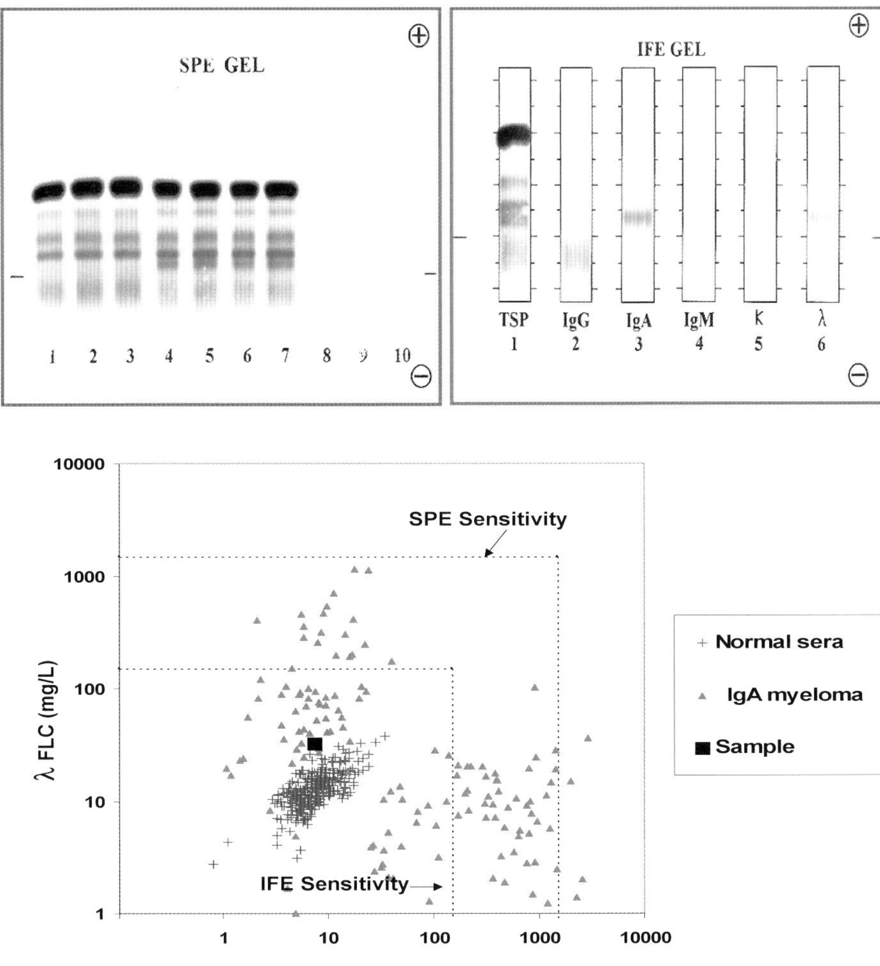

Figure 28.3. SPE, IFE and sFLC concentrations in a patient with IgAλ MM in relation to other patients with IgA MM (*Figure 10.2*). SPE comprised 3 normal sera (lanes 1-3) and the patient sample applied 4 times (lanes 4-7).

Immunochemistry (Sheffield, UK) provides a scheme for monoclonal proteins and FLCs. Approximately 30 laboratories currently participate in the FLC component and the usual quality assessment parameters are analysed.

28.6. Practical aspects of The Binding Site QA scheme QA003

There are 6 sets of samples issued per year and each contains unmatched serum and urine samples. The results that are returned to the laboratories include photocopies of the electrophoretic gels, comparisons with other laboratories' results and an 'expert

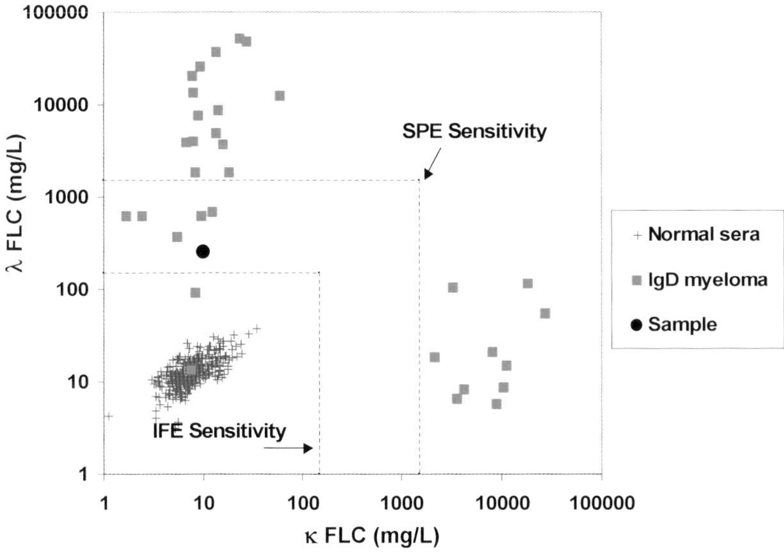

Figure 28.4. sFLC concentrations in a patient with IgDλ MM and results from other patients with IgD MM (*Figure 10.2*).

opinion' regarding the sample and results. Typical reports are shown in Figures 28.5 and 28.6.

The left hand side of the Figure 28.5 shows an SPE gel with normal sera for reference on the 4 left-hand lanes, then 3 lanes loaded with the unknown serum sample and on the right, 3 lanes loaded with the urine sample. In these samples the serum is negative but the urine positive by protein electrophoresis, while a λ band is visible by IFE. Figure 28.6 shows the λ results reported from all laboratories with the mean, standard deviation and the result from the reporting laboratory.

Laboratory and clinical reports accompanying results from The Binding Site QA003 distribution 64 *(Figures 28.5-28.7).*

Serum sample: IgG 7.9g/L, IgA 1.6g/L, IgM 0.77g/L, κFLC 13.7mg/L (NR 3.3-19.4), λ FLC 70mg/L (NR 5.7-26.3), κ/λ ratio 0.096 (NR 0.26-1.65) and β2 microglobulin 1.8mg/L. The sample appeared normal by SPE but a λ FLC band was detected by IFE.

Urine sample: κ FLC 4.2mg/L (NR 0.36-20.3mg/L), λ FLC 62mg/L (NR 0.81-17.3mg/L), κ/λ ratio 0.07. UPE showed a minor band on concentrated urine and IFE confirmed an abnormal λ FLC band.

Comment: The serum sample contained elevated λ FLCs of 70mg/L with no evidence of immunosuppression. The FLC band was not visible by SPE since the concentration was below the detection limit. By IFE, a λ monoclonal band was detected with no coincident heavy chains for IgG, A, M, D or E. sFLC assays showed an elevated

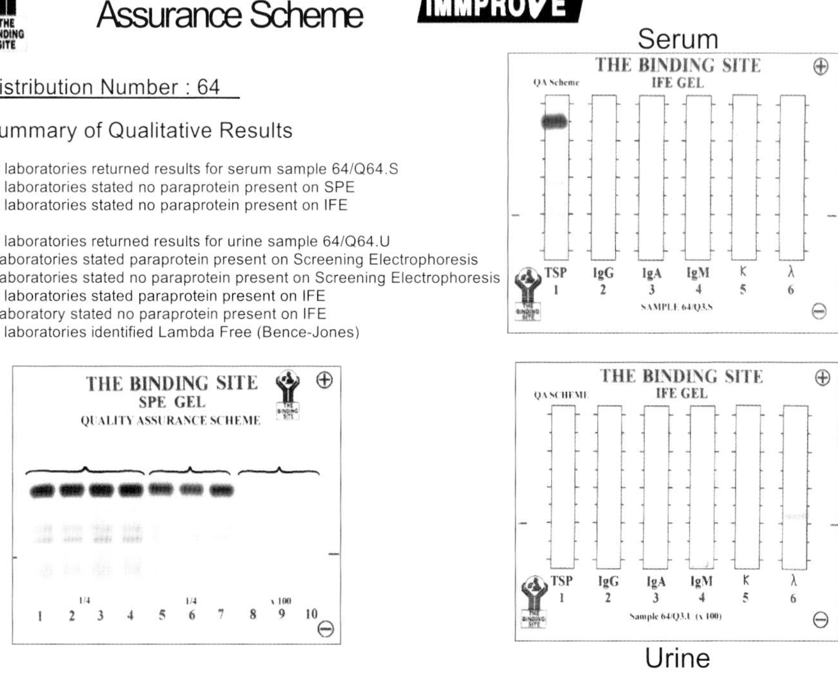

Figure 28.5. SPE and UPE tests on samples containing low concentrations of λ FLCs.

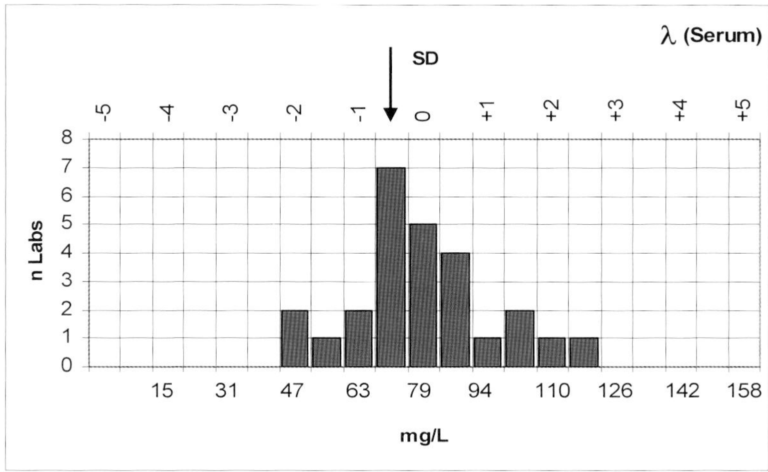

Figure 28.6. Frequency distribution of reported λ sFLC concentrations from QA003 Distribution No 64. The reporting laboratory's result is indicated by an arrow.

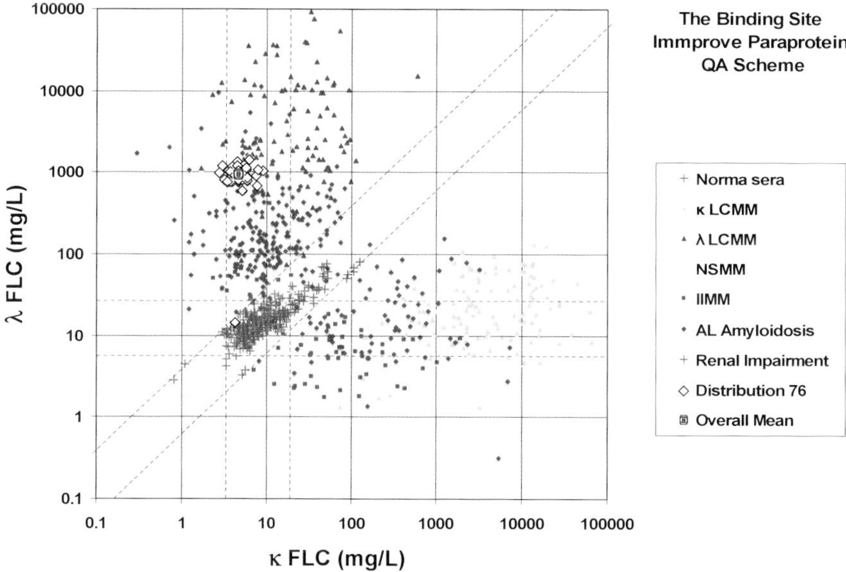

Figure 28.7. Combined results of The Binding Site Paraprotein Quality Assurance Scheme (QA003) from 94 laboratories.

λ concentration and a reduced κ/λ ratio. Tests on the urine sample showed similar results by electrophoretic tests and uFLC immunoassays. The latter can often be used to decypher urine electrophoretic test results that are difficult to interpret.

References

1. **UK NEQAS**, PO Box 401, Sheffield, S5 7YZ.

2. **College of American Pathologists, (CAP)** 324 Waukegan Road, Northfield, Illinois, 60093-2750, USA.

3. **La Agencé Francaise de Securité Sanitaire des Products de Santé,** 143-147 Boulevard Anatole, 93285 Saint Denis cedex, France.

4. **Ward AM, White PAE, Beetham R.** UK NEQAS Monoclonal Protein Identification Distribution 986. UK NEQAS Sheffield, 1998.

Section 6

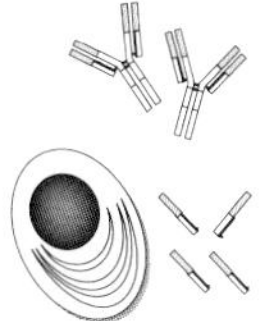

Appendices

Chapter 29

Classification of diseases with increased immunoglobulins

29.1. Monoclonal gammopathies

A. New classification

In May 2003, The International Myeloma Working Group published a review of the criteria for the diagnosis and classification of monoclonal gammopathies, MM and related disorders.[1] The aim was to standardise and simplify previous classification systems and provide easy definitions based on routinely available investigations. A uniform approach should facilitate comparisons of therapeutic trial data. The disease groups are as follows and their definitions are found in the respective chapters of this book.

1. MGUS. (*Chapter 19*)
2. Asymptomatic MM (smouldering MM or Durie and Salmon Stage I). (*Chapter 11*)
3. Symptomatic MM. (*Chapters 8 and 10*)
4. Nonsecretory MM. (*Chapter 9*)
5. Solitary plasmacytoma of bone. (*Chapter 18.1*)
6. Extramedullary plasmacytoma. (*Chapter 18.2*)
7. Multiple solitary plasmacytoma. (*Chapter 18.3*)
8. Plasma cell leukaemia. (*Chapter 18.4*)

B. Old classification

This classification includes the diseases indicated above and other types of monoclonal gammopathy.[2] Percentages refer to the frequency of a disease in relation to the total number of monoclonal gammopathies detected, although some variation occurs between different series of patients. The occurrence of monoclonal immunoglobulins with non-malignant conditions is uncommon but a proportion will contain chance associations with MGUS.

I. Malignant monoclonal gammopathies

a. Multiple myeloma (IgG, IgA, IgD, IgE, and FLC) 18%

1. Smouldering MM 4%
2. Plasma cell leukaemia
3. Nonsecretory MM 2%
4. Osteosclerotic MM (POEMS syndrome)
5. Plasmacytoma 3%

(a) Solitary plasmacytoma of bone

(b) Extramedullary (soft tissue) plasmacytoma

II. Waldenström's macroglobulinaemia 2%

III. Heavy-chain diseases (HCD) (rare)

a. Gamma-HCD (γ-HCD)

b. Alpha-HCD (α-HCD)

c. Mu-HCD (μ-HCD)

IV. AL amyloidosis (Primary) 10%

V. Monoclonal gammopathy of undetermined significance (MGUS) 50%

a. Single clone (IgG, IgA, IgD, IgM, and rarely, free light chains)

b. Biclonal and triclonal gammopathies

Lymphoma 5%
Chronic lymphocytic leukaemia 2%
Chronic myelomonocytic leukaemia
Chronic neutrophilic leukaemia
Refractory anaemia with or without blast cells
Lymphoproliferative diseases 14%
Gaucher's disease
Myelin associated glycoprotein (MAG) and polyneuropathy

Non-malignant disorders associated rarely with monoclonal proteins (usually MGUS)

1. **Dermatological diseases**
   Lichen myxoedematosus (IgGl), scleroderma, pyoderma gangrenosum, necrobiotic xanthogranuloma, discoid lupus erythematosus, psoriasis, cutaneous lymphoma
2. **Immunosuppression**
   AIDS and HIV infection, renal transplantation, bone marrow transplantation
3. **Liver diseases**
   Chronic hepatitis, cirrhosis, primary biliary cirrhosis
4. **Miscellaneous**
   Rheumatoid arthritis, inflammatory seronegative polyarthritis, polymyositis (IgGκ), polymyalgia rheumatica, myasthenia gravis, angioneurotic oedema (C1 inactivator deficiency)

29.2. Polyclonal gammopathies

Chronic infections, autoimmune diseases and many tumours cause increases in polyclonal immunoglobulins and presumably polyclonal FLC concentrations. Skin, pulmonary and gut diseases are more likely to cause increases in IgA concentrations while systemic infections will increase all immunoglobulins but particularly IgG. The percentages indicate the frequency of the various disorders from a study at The Mayo Clinic.[3] Clearly, results will vary in different parts of the world.

1. Connective tissue diseases (22%)

Sjögren's syndrome, Rheumatoid arthritis, Systemic lupus erythematosus, Mixed connective tissue disease, Overlap syndrome, Juvenile rheumatoid arthritis, Progressive systemic sclerosis, Ankylosing spondylitis, Fibrosing alveolitis,
CREST syndrome, Temporal arteritis, Raynaud's phenomenon, Cutaneous vasculitis, Familial Mediterranean fever, Eosinophilic fasciitis, Inclusion body myositis

2. Liver diseases (61%)

Autoimmune hepatitis, Viral hepatitis, Primary biliary cirrhosis, Primary sclerosing cholangitis, Cryptogenic cirrhosis
Primary hemochromatosis, Ethanol-induced liver injury, $\alpha 1$-antitrypsin deficiency

3. Chronic Infections (6%)

Subacute bacterial endocarditis, Renal abscess, Cystic fibrosis, Whipple's disease
Brucellosis, Lyme disease
Malaria, Worm infestations, Tropical splenomegaly syndrome
Mycobacterium Tuberculosis, Mycobacterium leprae, Leishmania organisms, Trypanosoma cruzi, Toxocara canis
HIV-1, Varicella, Vaccinia

4. Lymphoproliferative disorders (5%)

Pseudolymphoma, Kikuchi disease, Malignant lymphoma, Castleman disease
Angioimmunoblastic lymphadenopathy with dysproteinemia
Large granular lymphocytic leukaemia, Chronic lymphocytic leukaemia, Hairy cell leukemia, Plasma cell leukaemia
Histiocytosis X, Sinus histiocytosis with massive lymphadenopathy
Cutaneous eruptive histiocytoma
Intracranial plasma cell granulomata
Systemic cutaneous plasmacytosis
Proteinaceous lymphadenopathy with hypergammaglobulinemia
Chronic active EBV infection syndrome
Severe autoimmune lymphoproliferative syndrome

5. Other haematological conditions

Myelodysplastic syndromes

Idiopathic neutropenia, Idiopathic thrombocytopenic purpura
Severe hemophilia A, Thalassemia major, Sickle cell anemia
Benign hypergammaglobulinemic purpura of Waldenström, Cryoglobulinemia
Fanconi anemia

6. Non-hematological malignancies (3%)
Gastric carcinoma, Lung cancer, Hepatocellular carcinoma, Renal cell carcinoma, Ovarian cancer, Chondrosarcoma

7. Neurological conditions
Acquired chronic dysimmune demyelinating polyneuropathy
HTLV-1-associated myelopathy
Chronic progressive sensory ataxic neuropathy
Pure motor neuron disease and plasma cell dyscrasia
Microangiopathy of vasa nervorum in dysglobulinemic neuropathy

8. Diseases with associated immune system abnormalities
Graves' disease, Chronic ulcerative colitis, Chronic autoimmune pancreatitis
Sarcoidosis
Syndrome of IgG2 subclass deficiency, Hyper IgE syndrome
Hyperimmunoglobulinemia D and Periodic fever syndrome

9. Drugs
Aminophenazone, asparaginase, ethotoin, hydralazine hydrochloride, mephenytoin, methadone, oral contraceptives, phenylbutazone, phenytoin.

10. Miscellaneous conditions
Gaucher's disease, Meniere's disease, Cardiac myxoma, Asbestos exposure
Cryptogenic organising pneumonitis, Lymphoid interstitial pneumonia
Distal renal tubular acidosis
Hyperimmunisation

References

1. **Kyle RA, Child JA, Durie BGM, Blade J, Boccadoro M, Ludwig H et al.** Criteria for the classification of monoclonal gammopathies, multiple myeloma, and related disorders: a report of the International Myeloma Working Group. Br J Haem 2003; **121**: 749-757.

2. **Monoclonal Gammopathies of Undetermined Significance in: Myeloma**: Eds. Mehta J, Singhal S. 2002: Martin Dunnitz Ltd. United Kingdom. p419.

3. **Dispenzieri A, Gertz MA, Therneau TM, Kyle RA.** Retrospective Cohort Study of 148 Patients With Polyclonal Hypergammaglobulinaemia. Mayo Clin Proc 2001; **76**: 476-487.

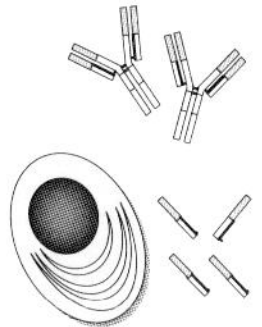

Chapter 30

Questions and answers about free light chains

30.1 Questions about urine testing for free light chains

1. Why are existing assays for urine FLCs poor?

There are several reasons. UPE with scanning of the bands is inaccurate if there is accompanying proteinuria. Urine IFE is non-quantitative but is more sensitive than UPE. Dye uptake tests, dipsticks and many other widely used tests for proteinuria are unreliable as they largely fail to measure small, cationic proteins such as free κ and λ. 24-hour urine collections are frequently not collected reliably so measurements of FLC excretion may be inaccurate.

2. Can I replace existing UPE and IFE tests with uFLC assays?

No. FLC assays will produce direct, quantitative results for uFLCs but are not always more sensitive than UPE tests. It is preferable to measure serum rather than uFLC concentrations because the removal of FLCs by the renal tubules has a huge effect on the amount of FLCs entering the urine. Also, FLC κ/λ ratios in urine are much more variable than in serum because of renal tubular absorption.

3. Why might patients show a poor correlation between uFLC M-spike concentrations measured by UPE and uFLCs measured by immunoassays?

UPE involves scanning gels for FLC bands but these can be obscured or confused by other proteins present in urine. In contrast, FLC assays are specific but will also measure polyclonal FLCs in urine. Polymerisation or fragmentation of FLC molecules will affect measurements by either assay, but to different extents.

4. How does proteinuria affect FLC measurements?

Moderate to heavy proteinuria makes interpretation of UPE difficult particularly when obscuring immunoglobulins are present. FLC assays are affected only by increased monoclonal and polyclonal FLC excretion and not by other proteins.

5. How are assays for monoclonal uFLCs affected by polyclonal uFLCs?

FLC assays measure both polyclonal and monoclonal FLCs. Renal impairment will lead to increases in both polyclonal κ and λ urine FLC concentrations and may produce abnormal urine κ/λ ratios. Large amounts of polyclonal FLCs may be excreted in diseases such as SLE and may prevent low concentrations of monoclonal FLCs from being detected as abnormal κ/λ ratios.

6. In urine, how do FLC assays and IFE compare?

Urinary FLC assays are sometimes, but not always, more sensitive than urine IFE and are quantitative. Clonality is judged by κ/λ ratios for FLCs and visually by IFE. There is a poor correlation between FLC concentrations and the intensity of staining on IFE because of the IFE antibody.

7. Will ladder banding be a problem using FLC tests?

Ladder banding is the term used to describe repeating bands of κ and/or λ seen in concentrated urine samples on IFE gels. It is due to minor differences in charge on polyclonal FLC molecules. The pattern may be confused with, and potentially obscure, genuine monoclonal FLC bands. Ladder banding does not indicate the presence of monoclonal FLCs. uFLC immunoassays are not affected by ladder banding but the presence of polyclonal FLCs will affect measurements of monoclonal FLCs.

8. How do urine and sFLC tests compare?

There is a poor correlation between serum and uFLC concentrations in individual patients. This is because the kidney metabolises large amounts of FLC molecules, preventing them from entering the urine. There is a much better correlation between changes in serum and uFLC concentrations.

30.2 Clinical questions about serum testing for free light chains

9. What diseases cause elevation of monoclonal FLC levels in serum?

Monoclonal elevations of free κ and λ occur in the same diseases that produce monoclonal gammopathies with intact immunoglobulins. The number of diseases is extensive but clearly MM and AL amyloidosis are important. A list of diseases associated with monoclonal gammopathies is given in Chapter 29.

10. Why are serum tests preferable to urine tests?

Since the kidney can metabolise between 10 and 30g of FLCs per day in the proximal tubules, urinary FLC results do not accurately reflect FLC production by the tumour. This results in a poor correlation between serum and uFLC concentrations and makes urine testing unreliable.

11. How many more MM patients will be detected if sFLC assays are run alongside SPE?

LCMM comprises between 15-18% of all MM. Approximately, half to two thirds of these patients will have abnormalities by SPE. This especially applies to patients who are producing large quantities of FLCs, are in renal failure or have associated hypogammaglobulinaemia. The remaining LCMM patients with normal SPE (5-7%) and 70% of those with NSMM (2%) will be detected by sFLC assays. Most patients with AL amyloidosis and other rare monoclonal gammopathies will also be detected. In addition, normal individuals with FLC MGUS will be identified. Intact immunoglobulin MGUS occurs in approximately 3% of people aged over 70 and more frequently with increasing age. Therefore, at least 10-15% additional patients with monoclonal gammopathies will be detected using sFLC. The study by Bakshi et al., (Chapter 23) detected an additional 50% of patients and included B-CLL and other plasma cell dyscrasias.

12. I currently screen for MM using IFE. Will sFLC assays be of additional benefit?
Yes, for two reasons. sFLC analysis will detect monoclonal gammopathies that are missed by IFE. Also, quantification of sFLCs, at the time of clinical presentation provides a base line result for subsequent disease monitoring.

13. How many more MM patients will be detected if I perform sFLC assays together with SPE and IFE?
FLC serum assays are more sensitive for FLC detection than both SPE and IFE so approximately 5% extra patients with low concentration monoclonal FLCs will be detected. Some of these patients will have LCMM, NSMM or AL amyloidosis. Many of these patients also have FLCs in the urine but some do not. If monoclonal FLCs are detected in the serum then there is little value in performing additional urine tests. However, there are rare patients that have normal sFLC concentrations but have detectable FLCs in concentrated urine by IFE. These include patients with AL amyloidosis but not patients with LCMM.

14. How many more MGUS patients will be detected using sFLC assays?
MGUS have historically comprised intact immunoglobulins and these are detected using SPE. FLC only MGUS have been observed in the urine but only rarely. FLC MGUS have recently been detected in serum using FLC immunoassays at a frequency of approximately 20% of intact immunoglobulin MGUS (3% of samples from individuals over 70 years of age). Since MGUS comprises 60-80% of monoclonal gammopathies, many new FLC MGUS patients will be detected. These may be the precursor of LCMM and AL amyloidosis and are a focus of considerable clinical interest.

15. Can sFLC assays be used to follow-up patients with LCMM?
Yes, serum is preferable to urine for monitoring patients for several reasons. Serum samples are easier to collect than 24-hour urine samples and serum is a more reliable fluid for assessing changes in production of FLCs. Also, normal serum concentrations of FLCs are less variable than urine concentrations so abnormal results are more easily assessed. Since serum is more sensitive for detection of FLCs than urine, sFLCs are more effective for assessing minimal residual disease.

16. How will sFLC tests benefit patients with NSMM?
By definition, these patients have no detectable monoclonal proteins in their serum and urine by conventional electrophoresis tests and have to be monitored by marrow biopsies or bone scans. sFLC tests are clearly useful in these patients and more accurate

than bone marrow biopsies that can miss patchy tumour deposits. sFLC concentrations assess FLC production by the whole bone marrow (and extramedullary sites) so are probably a better reflection of overall tumour activity than isolated bone marrow aspirations. sFLC tests will lead to a reduced number of bone marrow biopsies in most of these patients. However, as for all tumours, a tissue diagnosis, obtained by biopsy, is essential to establish the initial diagnosis, even if the FLC test results are grossly abnormal.

17. Are sFLC measurements helpful in patients with AL amyloidosis?

AL amyloidosis is a difficult disease to diagnose because existing serum and urine tests are not sufficiently sensitive to identify all patients. sFLC measurements not only identify more patients than electrophoresis tests of serum and urine but also they are important for monitoring disease progress. The short serum half-life of FLCs makes them a mandatory test for evaluating responses to treatment and identifying relapse.

18. What are the normal values for serum and urine FLCs?

Publications from Birmingham University and The Mayo Clinic have shown similar results. The data from The Mayo Clinic contains results from older people and indicates that sFLC concentrations increase in normal individuals aged >70 years due to deteriorating glomerular filtration. Results from patients should be compared with the age-matched, normal range data. However, all laboratories should make some assessment of normal ranges in their own laboratories since there will be minor variations resulting from differences in race, age, exposure to infections, the use of different instruments, etc.

Normal ranges are usually established by reference to standards (comprising purified proteins) that have been agreed by international committees. Since there is no international agreement, at present, and because of the novelty of the FLC tests, no definitive statement on the accuracy of the normal ranges can be made. In time, agreed reference materials will be manufactured and international agreement established. Existing normal ranges will then be adjusted to take into account any recommendations.

19. Is the absolute value of the FLCs or the free κ/λ ratio more important?

sFLC abnormalities should be assessed from the concentrations of the clonal FLC, the alternate FLC and the κ/λ ratio. This is optimally performed using a κ/λ log plot for each patient's result (see Figure on page iv) which is compared with normal range and disease group data. This elegantly distinguishes monoclonal FLC diseases from polyclonal FLC abnormalities and individuals that are in the normal range. Since renal function is frequently affected in MM patients, the alternate FLC concentrations are often elevated but the κ/λ ratio usually remains highly abnormal.

If the patient has bone marrow suppression, the individual FLC concentrations might be low, in which case the κ/λ ratio may be more helpful. This is typical of patients undergoing chemotherapy and in those patients with NSMM and AL amyloidosis with bone marrow suppression. Clinical judgement should be used in these cases. If either the FLC concentrations or the κ/λ ratios are outside the normal range then the cause should be investigated. Consideration should be given to assessment of renal function and causes of increased immunoglobulin production such as autoimmune diseases, chronic infections and some malignant tumours.

20. If MM patients are in complete remission, how useful is the sFLC result?

FLC results are more useful than existing SPE or IFE because they are more sensitive and, therefore, more likely to detect residual disease. Also, sFLC concentrations are more likely to be elevated than uFLC levels when patients are in remission. Thus, some patients apparently in full remission by existing tests might have abnormal FLC concentrations and their clinical status will need to be revised. Some patients who relapse between monitoring periods may be more easily identified using sFLC assays rather than SPE or IFE.

21. What happens to monoclonal FLC concentrations when patients develop renal impairment?

As patients develop renal impairment the concentrations of κ and λ polyclonal serum FLCs increase. This is associated with an increase in the monoclonal FLC but the κ/λ ratio will also increase slightly because of the relative reduction in clearance of κ molecules *(Chapter 11.2)*. However, changes in the κ/λ ratio are a better guide to changes in clinical status when glomerular filtration rates are changing than the concentrations of the monoclonal FLC. Changes in the concentrations of creatinine or cystatin C should be assessed, under these circumstances, in order to provide an independent assessment of renal function and a correction factor for the κ/λ ratios.

22. Does bone marrow suppression affect FLC concentrations?

Bone marrow suppression, either because of bone marrow replacement by tumour or resulting from chemotherapy, leads to a reduction in the concentrations of polyclonal FLCs. Typically, at the time of diagnosis, the alternate FLC is suppressed and there is a grossly distorted κ/λ ratio. κ/λ ratios play an important role in assessing changing FLC concentrations in these patients and may even be useful when the concentrations of the monoclonal FLCs are below normal levels.

23. Will sFLC concentrations help in understanding tumour kinetics?

This is an important issue. At present, intact monoclonal immunoglobulins in serum or FLCs in urine are used to monitor the progress of patients. The half-life of IgG is 3-4 weeks, so reductions in tumour mass with chemotherapy may not be reflected in serum monoclonal protein changes for several weeks.

The half-life of FLCs is only a few hours - extending to 2-3 days when renal function is impaired. Thus, reductions in tumour mass with chemotherapy can be identified earlier when the patients are being monitored using sFLC tests. Indeed, changes in tumour mass might be assessed between each cycle of chemotherapy allowing subsequent treatments to be specifically tailored to individual patients. Changes in urine and serum levels of FLCs broadly correspond but renal tubular reabsorption prevents accurate assessment of tumour responses from urine measurements.

Approximately 95% of patients with MM, excreting intact immunoglobulins have abnormal sFLCs. It is likely, because of the short half-life of FLCs, discussed above, that disease monitoring in many of these patients will be better using sFLC levels rather than intact immunoglobulin concentrations.

24. Can sFLC assays be used for transplantation monitoring?

Yes, sFLC assays are useful for monitoring post transplantation progress in AL amyloidosis and MM and may indicate early relapse and early responses.

25. What diseases cause elevated serum polyclonal FLC concentrations?

Serum polyclonal FLC concentrations increase if there is increased production or reduced glomerular filtration of κ and λ proteins. Increased production results from any disease that stimulates B-cell proliferation such as infections, autoimmune diseases, various tumours etc. For example, in active SLE, total immunoglobulin production increases 3-4 fold with a corresponding increase in sFLC concentrations.

Reduced glomerular filtration of FLCs occurs in renal damage because almost all FLC removal is via the glomerular pores and the proximal renal tubules. In renal failure, sFLC concentrations may rise 10-20 fold but in all cases both free κ and λ are elevated, so the free κ/λ ratio remains normal. In many diseases, particularly SLE, increases in polyclonal FLC concentrations are due to a combination of increased FLC production and reduced renal filtration.

In situations of increased polyclonal FLC production or reduced filtration, there may be moderate distortions of κ/λ ratios (e.g., 3-4 standard deviations from the normal range). These patients are borderline abnormal and should be investigated appropriately.

30.3 Laboratory questions about serum testing for free light chains

26. Should sFLC tests be used as a screen for monoclonal gammopathies instead of SPE?

No. SPE detects intact immunoglobulin monoclonal proteins and some FLC monoclonal proteins. In contrast, sFLC assays detect FLC monoclonal gammopathies, either alone, or in association with intact monoclonal immunoglobulins. Approximately 95% of patients with intact monoclonal immunoglobulins have abnormal sFLCs, but not all, particularly those patients with low concentration MGUS.

27. Will any monoclonal proteins detected by SPE and/or IFE be missed by sFLC tests?

Yes. Monoclonal proteins can be intact immunoglobulins or FLCs. Since sFLC assays are >100 times more sensitive than electrophoretic tests it is most unlikely that FLCs will be detected in serum by SPE or IFE yet be normal by FLC assays. However, intact immunoglobulin monoclonal immunoglobulins by tradition (especially MGUS) are detected by IFE and SPE, but may have normal FLC concentrations. Studies indicate that all LCMM and ~95% of AL amyloidosis patients are correctly identified by sFLC assays.

28. If the sFLC concentration is many thousands of mg/L why is there no band on SPE?

The sensitivity of SPE for monoclonal bands depends upon the width of the band and its position in the gel in relation to other plasma proteins. Narrow monoclonal bands in the gamma region in association with hypogammaglobulinaemia will be visible at 200-400mg/L. The same band in a beta position, perhaps superimposed on transferrin, will be invisible. The monoclonal protein may need to be over 2,000mg/L to be visible in this area of the gel. In addition, monoclonal FLCs may be polymerised to different extents and then they migrate on electrophoresis gels as diffuse bands. This is frequently found in NSMM and is well-documented in LCMM. In these patients, even 5,000mg/L of monoclonal protein may be difficult to detect above the background of the other plasma proteins.

29. Many sera tested by SPE have bands that are barely visible. I worry that I might be missing MM patients. At present I ask for IFE on these samples. Can sFLC testing help?

Yes, the sFLC assays will detect all patients with LCMM and most patients with NSMM and AL amyloidosis. IFE will not detect many of these patients. Since sFLC immunoassays are 100-fold more sensitive than serum IFE, sFLC abnormalities, visible by IFE, will be exceptionally rare if the sFLC tests are normal. Urine IFE or uFLC measurements may be helpful in these rare cases.

30. Serum albumin levels are reduced in patients with nephrotic syndrome and gross proteinuria. Are sFLC levels also reduced in these patients with proteinuria and will FLC monoclonal gammopathies be missed?

No. Renal damage never increases the glomerular filtration rate of small molecules such as FLCs or creatinine since they normally pass relatively unhindered through the glomerular pores. Molecules as large as albumin are not normally filtered by the kidney but they are cleared in nephrotic syndrome as the glomerular pores become damaged. The extra protein leakage overwhelms the proximal tubular reabsorption mechanisms allowing many different proteins to appear in the urine. The protein leakage damages the tubules in the process which become sclerotic. Renal clearance of all small proteins is then reduced. This leads to an increase in sFLC levels (and creatinine). In the early stages of the process, FLCs are increased in the urine because of increased competition with albumin for reabsorption by the proximal tubules.

Renal impairment leads to increases in both κ and λ FLCs in the serum. Therefore, when both are elevated the likely cause is a reduction in glomerular filtration. There is a correlation between changes in the concentrations of serum creatinine, cystatin C and FLCs during changes in renal function.

31. How can clonality be judged using FLC assays?

Using electrophoresis methods, clonality is judged by the appearance of a narrow protein band. Using FLC assays, clonality is judged by the numerical ratio of free κ to free λ concentrations. In a similar manner, B-cell clonality in leukaemia is assessed by cellular κ/λ ratios using flow cytometry. Arguably, numerical FLC ratios are more accurate than visual assessments of stained bands on electrophoresis gels. Furthermore, in NSMM, clonality may not be apparent by any electrophoretic procedure but is usually identified by serum κ/λ ratios. In the situation of biclonal gammopathies, with increased synthesis of both free κ and λ molecules, free κ/λ ratios may be normal but the concentrations of both FLCs will be raised.

32. How do we report borderline results?

All tests have borderline results. For FLCs, clinical results should be judged against normal and disease state sera from the laboratory, and from national and international reference ranges. The normal range recommended for the free κ/λ ratios is greater than that used for most tests in order to provide a large safety margin for normal individuals.

Since FLC results are quantitative, less experience is required compared with protein electrophoresis. This leads to less subjective interpretation of results.

33. What is the frequency of false positive and false negative results, and how are they dealt with?

All tests produce false positive and false negative results and these need to be assessed for clinical significance. Reference ranges have been developed in collaboration with The Mayo Clinic and include individuals up to 90 years of age. Some of these individuals have minor degrees of renal impairment. This increases the concentrations of the FLCs, and the κ/λ ratios, and is apparent on a κ/λ log plot. The difference between the normal and abnormalsamples is then selected using standard deviations from the mean. If all of the 282 normal samples in the Mayo Clinic study are used, this represents four standard deviations from the mean and is greater than normally chosen cut off levels. Therefore, test samples outside this range will most likely indicate patients with monoclonal gammopathies.

Negative sFLC results occur in a few patients with NSMM, AL amyloidosis and LCDD. Also, rare patients have monoclonal proteins in the urine detected only by IFE. The molecular form of these FLC molecules is unknown but they may be abnormal in shape or size and this may prevent their detection by the FLC antibodies.

34. Why is the free κ/λ ratio different from the total κ/λ ratio in normal subjects?

Approximately twice as many κ molecules are produced as λ. Since free λ is mostly in dimeric form it has a half-life (determined by glomerular filtration) that is approximately three times that of monomeric κ FLCs. This causes free λ molecules to accumulate in the serum more than free κ molecules and alters the free κ/λ ratio from 1.8 to 0.6. When the light chains are bound to immunoglobulins they are metabolised as the whole immunoglobulin, which is independent of light chain type, so total κ/λ ratio is 1.8:1.

35. Why should I change from using a total light chain measurement to a more expensive FLC assay?

Normal sFLC concentrations are <30mg/L, which is much lower than total light chain concentrations of 1,000-3,000 mg/L. Patients who have levels of monoclonal FLCs between these two ranges cannot be assessed using total light chain assays. Since this applies to most patients with AL amyloidosis, NSMM and many LCMMs, sFLC assays have considerable benefit in these diseases.

36. How does the sensitivity of sFLC tests compare with CZE?

CZE of serum is more sensitive than SPE but less sensitive than IFE for detecting monoclonal proteins. In a recent study, it was shown that sFLC assays detected all monoclonal FLCs from patients with LCMM that were missed by CZE but detected by IFE. If CZE is used for initial detection of monoclonal proteins, sFLC assays will detect additional patients.

37. Since the FLC reagents use polyclonal antibodies, how is batch to batch variation minimised?

The FLC antisera are produced by immunisation with many different monoclonal FLC proteins. These are not representative of all monoclonal FLCs but the antibody target is the constant region of the molecule that has little structural variation. However, tumour produced monoclonal FLCs may be truncated, have amino acid substitutions or additions and may be abnormally polymerised. Therefore, occasional patient's monoclonal FLCs may not be detected reliably by the immunoassays or may be detected differently with different antiserum batches. It is, therefore, ideal laboratory practice to assay current and previous samples alongside each other. This is no different from the situation when measuring IgG with different antiserum batches.

To minimise batch-to-batch variation, antisera pools are large, are prepared from multiple immunisations and are carefully controlled to maintain consistency. Many monoclonal proteins are tested when new batches are prepared but there is a limit to the number of different monoclonal proteins that can be used.

Monoclonal antibodies have been assessed in some studies to measure FLCs but they have proved to be unreliable. Polyclonal antisera are superior since they detect more monoclonal FLC molecules and they detect them more reliably.

38. If I am going to use sFLC tests how do they fit into my laboratory protocols?

The preferred option is to measure FLCs alongside SPE at the time of the presentation blood sample. SPE will identify IIMM patients while FLC assays will identify LCMMs, most NSMMs and other FLC diseases such as AL amyloidosis. Low concentration, intact immunoglobulin MGUS sera (less than 2-5g/L) will not be detected using these two procedures. A strategy of performing SPE and IFE as a screen for FLC monoclonal proteins and not FLC immunoassays will result in some patients with LCMM, NSMM and AL amyloidosis being missed. FLC assays, performed on a patient's presentation sample, are also important for providing a baseline for subsequent disease monitoring.

For easy interpretation, results should be reported using a logarithmic κ/λ plot, alongside existing clinical data.

When monitoring patients with FLC diseases, results should be reported alongside other analyses. IFE may add little to the combined use of SPEand FLC tests apart from identifying some low level intact immunoglobulin MGUS samples.

39. Does antigen excess occur with FLC assays?

Yes, for two reasons. The range of monoclonal sFLCs is huge, from a few mg/L to many g/L. Hence, assay conditions causing antigen excess occur on a regular basis. In addition, the small size of FLC molecules and the variety of different shapes and sizes may produce antigen excess conditions at relatively low concentrations for some samples. For accurate results, care must be taken to dilute high concentration samples into the appropriate assay range. If in doubt, samples should be re-analysed at higher dilutions.

40. Which instrument should I use for measuring FLCs?

Nephelometers and turbidimeters have a similar level of sensitivity and precision for measuring sFLCs. Instruments vary in their ability for sample handling, in providing clean cuvettes for each test, for evaluating antigen excess, etc. Generally, the large clinical chemistry analysers are the best platforms for measuring sFLCs.

41. How accurate are the quantitative FLC results?

Quantification of monoclonal FLCs by immunoassay is less accurate than scanning bands on SPE gels. This is the same situation as using nephelometry for measuring intact immunoglobulin monoclonal proteins. Studies have shown that purified monoclonal FLCs assessed by accurate quantitative protein tests may give quite different results compared with immunoassays for FLCs. The explanation is that the antibody assays cannot be expected to produce consistent results for all molecular shapes and polymeric forms of FLCs.

Since the exact amount of serum or uFLCs, at the time of diagnosis, bears little relationship to disease outcome, accurate quantification is relatively unimportant. Of greater concern is the reproducibility of the assay results in individual patients during treatment. It is apparent that FLC measurements produce consistent results during chemotherapy and this provides the basis for their value in managing patients with the various monoclonal diseases. Indeed, sFLC tests are much more reproducible than electrophoresis tests.

42. The patient has high serum and urine polyclonal FLCs with an abnormal urine κ/λ ratio. What does this mean?

High concentrations of both FLCs in the urine and serum indicate a degree of renal impairment. If the kidney becomes further damaged then both serum and urine concentrations may rise further. This is because with increasing renal damage, glomerular filtration falls and sFLC concentrations increase. This leads to the circulating FLCs being filtered by the remaining nephrons. As their proximal tubules become overwhelmed by the increase in filtered FLCs there is more leakage into the urine. Improving renal function is characterised by reductions in both serum and uFLC concentrations.

The mechanism of abnormal uFLC κ/λ ratios seen in some of these patients can be explained by the renal handling of the molecules. In patients with renal damage, the glomerular pores become altered in size so that monomeric and dimeric FLCs may be filtered differently. In addition, the proximal tubular reabsorption mechanism is partly dependent upon molecular charge, which is different for each FLC type. Thus, there may be differential clearance and adsorption of κ or λ molecules. This may lead to small distortions of serum and urine κ/λ ratios in patients with renal impairment.

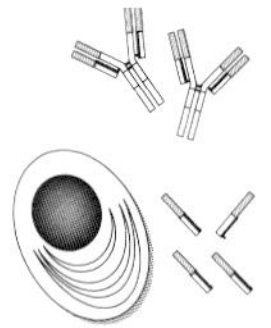

Chapter 31

Serum free light chain publications

Abstracts in black, papers and book chapters in blue.

1999

1. **Bradwell AR, Drew R, Showell PJ, Carr-Smith HD, Mead GP**. Clinical potential of free immunoglobulin light-chain measurements. Clin Chem 1999; **45**: 6, pA54. No181.
2. **Tang LX, Showell PJ, Mead GP, Carr-Smith HD, Drew R, Bradwell AR**. An automated nephelometric immunoassay for quantification of free light-chains in human serum and urine. Clin Chem 1999; **45**: 6, pA54, No179.

2000

1. **Bradwell AR, Tang LX, Drayson MT, Drew RL**. Immunoassays for detection of free light chains in sera of patients with nonsecretory myeloma. Blood 2000; **96**:16, p271b, 4906.
2. **Carr-Smith HD, Edwards J, Showell P, Drew R, Tang LX, Bradwell AR.** Preparation of an immunoglobulin free light-chain reference material. Clin Chem 2000; **46**: 6: pA180, No. 699.
3. **Harris J, Tang LX, Showell PJ, Carr-Smith HD, Drew R, Bradwell AR.** Assays for immunoglobulin free light chains in serum on the Beckman IMMAGE™. Clin Chem 2000; **46**: 6: pA180, No 701.
4. **Tang LX, Showell P, Carr-Smith HD, Mead GP, Drew R, Bradwell AR.** Evaluation of F(ab)2-based latex enhanced nephelometric reagents for free immunoglobulin light-chains on the Behring Nephelometer II. Clin Chem 2000; **46**: 6: pA181, No 705.

2001

1. **Abraham RS, Katzmann JA, Clark RJ, Lymp JF, Dispenzieri A, Lust JA, Bradwell AR.** Light chain myeloma: Correlation of serum nephelometric analysis for the quantitation of immunoglobulin free light chain with urine Bence Jones protein. Clin Chem 2001; **47**: 6 A33, No. 108.
2. **Abraham RS, Katzmann JA, Clark RJ, Dispenzieri A, Lust JA, Bradwell AR.** Detection of serum immunoglobulin free light chains in primary amyloidosis and light chain deposition disease by nephelometry. Clin Chem 2001; **47**:6 A32, No.107.
3. **Bradwell AR, Mead GP, Carr-Smith HD, Drayson MT**. Detection of Bence Jones Myeloma and Monitoring of Myeloma Chemotherapy Using Serum Immunoassays Specific for Free Immunoglobulin Light Chains. Blood 2001; **98**; 11:p157a No 663.
4. **Bradwell AR, Carr-Smith HD, Mead GP, Tang LX, Showell PJ, Drayson MT, Drew RL.** Highly sensitive, automated immunoassay for immunoglobulin free light chains in serum and urine. Clin Chem 2001; **47**: 4: 673-680.
5. **Bradwell AR, Drayson MT, Mead GP**. Measurement of free light chains in urine. Clin Chem 2001; **47**:11, p2069-2070.
6. **Bradwell AR, Smith L, Drayson MT, Mead GP, Carr-Smith HD.** Serum Free Light Chain measurements for identifying and monitoring patients with nonsecretory multiple myeloma. Clin Chem Lab Med 2001; **39** pS167, PO-F038.
7. **Bradwell AR, Carr-Smith HD, Smith L, Mead GP**. Detection and monitoring of nonsecretory myeloma using an assay for free light chains in serum. Clin Chem 2001; **47**:6, pA43, No 142.
8. **Carr-Smith HD, Smith L, Showell P, Mead GP, Drayson MT, Bradwell AR.** Development of Serum Free Light Chain Immunoassays for the detection and monitoring of patients with Bence Jones Myeloma. Hematol J. 2001; **1** p29, No 070.
9. **Carr-Smith HD, Smith L, Showell P, Mead GP, Drayson MT, Bradwell AR.** Detection and Monitoring of Nonsecretory Myeloma using assay for Free Light Chains in Serum. Hematol J. 2001; **1** p30, No 071.

10. Clark RJ, Katzmann JA, Abraham RS, Lymp JF, Kyle RA, Bradwell AR. Detection of monoclonal free light chains by nephelometry: Normal ranges and relative sensitivity. Clin Chem 2001;**47**:6 A27, No. 90.

11. Drayson MT, Tang LX, Drew R, Mead GP, Carr-Smith HD, Bradwell AR. Serum free light-chain measurements for identifying and monitoring patients with nonsecretory multiple myeloma. Blood 2001; **97**: 9: 2900-2902.

12. Hansson L-O, Dijlai-Merzog R, Danielsson O, Bradwell AR. Quantitation of the Free Light Chain Kappa and Lambda Serum, Urine and Cerebrospinal Fluid (CSF) using The Binding Site (F)ab2-based nephelometric method on the IMMAGE® system. Clin Chem 2001; **47**:6 pA32, No 106.

13. Katzmann JA, Clarke RJ, Abraham RS, Lymp JF, Carr-Smith HD, Kyle RA, Bradwell AR. Detection of monoclonal Free Light Chains in serum by nephelometry: Normal ranges and relative sensitivity. Proceedings of the Monoclonal Gammopathies & the Kidney, Poitiers France 2001: P2.

14. Mead GP, Carr-Smith HD, Drayson MT, Hawkins PN, Bradwell AR. Serum Free Light Chain Immunoassays As An Aid In The Diagnosis And Monitoring Of Light Chain Monoclonal Gammopathies: J Bone & Mineral Metab. 2001;**19**:Suppl. p64: No.44.

15. Smith L, Mead GP, Carr-Smith HD, Drayson MT, Bradwell AR. Detection and Monitoring of Bence Jones Myeloma using Serum Free Light Chain Measurements. Clin Chem Lab Med 2001; **39**, PO-F039, pS68.

16. Smith L, Mead GP, Carr-Smith HD, Drayson MT, Bradwell AR. Development of serum free light chain immunoassays for the detection and monitoring of patients with Bence Jones myeloma. Clin Chem 2001; **47**:6, pA33, No141.

2002

1. Abraham RS, Clark RJ, Bryant SC, Lymp JF, Larson T, Kyle RA, Katzmann JA. Correlation of serum immunoglobulin free light chain quantitation with urine Bence Jones protein in Light Chain Myeloma. Clin Chem 2002; **48**, 655-657.

2. Bradwell AR, Carr-Smith HD, Mead GP, Drayson MT. Serum free light chain immunoassays and their clinical application. Clin Appl Imm Rev 2002; **3**: 17-33.

3. Bradwell AR, Carr-Smith HD, Mead GP, Harvey TC, Drayson MT. Management of patients with light chain myeloma using serum free light chain immunoassays. Clin Chem 2002; **48**:6 Suppl. pA17, No A-51.

4. Bradwell AR, Mead GP, Drayson MT, Carr-Smith HD. Serum immunoglobulin free light chain measurement in intact immunoglobulin multiple myeloma. Blood 2002; **100**:11 No 5054, p373b.

5. Bradwell AR, Drayson MT, Mead GP, Galvin G. Serum Free Light Chain Immunoassays for Monitoring Patients with Light Chain producing and Nonsecretory Multiple Myeloma. Blood 2002; **100:**11 No 5091.

6. Carr-Smith HD, Showell P, Bradwell AR. Antigen excess assessment of free light chain assays on the Dade-Behring BNII nephelometer. Clin Chem 2002; **48**:6; A-71 p A23.

7. Carr-Smith HD, Mead GP, Drayson MT, Hawkins PN, Bradwell AR. Detection and monitoring of light chain monoclonal gammopathies using serum free light chain immunoassays. Clin Chem Lab Med 2002; No.042: pS205.

8. Carr-Smith HD, Showell PJ, Long JM, Bradwell AR. Development and evaluation of turbidimetric reagents for measuring free immunoglobulin light-chains on the Hitachi 911/912. Clin Chem Lab Med 2002; No.043: pS205.

9. Carr-Smith HD, Showell PJ, Matters DJ, Long JM, Bradwell AR. Development and evaluation of nephelometric reagents for measuring free immunoglobulin light-chains on a modified Mininephᵀᴹ. Clin Chem Lab Med 2002; No.044: pS205.

10. Hermsen D, Bradwell AR, Reinaauer H. Evaluation of an Automated Nephelometric Immunoassay for Quantification of Free Light Chains in Serum. J Lab Med 2002; **26** (9/10):No. Q18:p536.

11. Hofmann W, Guder WG, Bradwell AR, Garbrecht M. Kappa and Lambda Light Chain in Serum and Urine in Patients with Monoclonal Gammopathy. J Lab Med 2002; **26** (9/10):No.019, p513.

12. Hofmann W, Guder WG, Bradwell AR, Garbrecht M. Detection of free Kappa and Lambda light chain in serum and urine in patients with monoclonal gammopathy. Onkologie: Int J Canc Res & Treatment;

2002; **25**: No. 752: p212.

13. Katzmann JA, Clark RJ, Abraham RS, Bryant S, Lymp JF, Bradwell AR, Kyle RA. Serum Reference Intervals and Diagnostic Ranges for Free κ and Free λ Immunoglobulin Light Chains: Relative Sensitivity for Detection of Monoclonal Light Chains. Clin Chem 2002; **48**: 1437-1444.

14. Lachmann HJ, Gallimore R, Gillmore JD, Smith L, Bradwell AR, Hawkins PN. Detection of monoclonal free light chains by nephelometry in systemic AL amyloidosis. Clin Chem 2002; **48**: A164: pE45.

15. Lachmann HJ, Gallimore R, Gillmore JD, Smith L, Bradwell AR, Hawkins PN. Correlation of changes in nephelometric quantification of serum monoclonal free light chains following chemotherapy and outcome in systemic AL amyloidosis. Clin Chem 2002; **48**: A165: pE46.

16. Lachmann HJ, Gallimore R, Gillmore JD, Carr-Smith HD, Bradwell AR, Hawkins PN. Changes in the concentration of circulating Free Immunoglobulin Chains and outcome in Systemic AL Amyloidosis. Blood 2002; **100**:11. No 5090.

17. Le Bricon T, Bengoufa D, Benlakehal M, Bousquet B, Erlich D. Urinary free light chain analysis by the Freelite[R] immunoassay: a preliminary study in multiple myeloma. Clin Biochem 2002; **35**: 565-567.

18. Marien G, Bradwell AR, Blanckaert N, Bossuyt X. Detection of monoclonal proteins in sera by capillary zone electrophoresis and free light-chain measurements. Clin Chem 2002; **48**:6, No E-52, pA167.

19. Marien G, Oris E, Bradwell AR, Blanckaert N, Bossuyt X. Detection of monoclonal proteins in sera by capillary zone electrophoresis and free light chain measurements. Clin Chem 2002; **48**: 1600-1601.

20. Mead GP, Carr-Smith HD, Drayson MT, Bradwell AR. Detection of Bence Jones myeloma and monitoring of myeloma chemotherapy using immunoassays specific for free immunoglobulin light chains. Br J Haematol 2002; **117**: Suppl 1: No 195,p69.

21. Mead GP, Stubbs PD, Carr-Smith HD, Drew R, Drayson MT, Bradwell AR. Nephelometric measurement of serum free light chains in nonsecretory myeloma. Clin Chem 2002; **48**:6 Suppl, pA23, No A-70.

22. Showell PJ, Long JM, Carr-Smith HD, Bradwell AR. Evaluation of latex-enhanced turbidimetric reagents for measuring free immunoglobulin light-chains on the Hitachi 911/912. Clin Chem 2002; **48**: 6 Suppl, No A-66, pA22.

23. Showell PJ, Matters DJ, Long JM, Carr-Smith HD, Bradwell AR. Evaluation of latex-enhanced nephelometric reagents for measuring free immunoglobulin light-chains on a modified Minineph™. Clin Chem 2002; **48:** 6 Suppl; A-67, pA17.

24. Sirohi B, Powles R, Kulkarni S, Carr-Smith HD, Sankpal S, Patel G, Singhal S, Iqbal J, Bradwell AR. Serum Free Light Chain Assessment in Myeloma Patients who are in Complete Remission by Immunofixation. Blood 2002; **100**:11: No 5095.

25. Tate JR, Grimmett K, Mead GP, Cobcroft R, Gill D. Free light chain ratios in the serum of myeloma patients in complete remission following autologous peripheral blood stem cell transplantation. Clin Chem. 2002; **48**:6 Suppl No. E-50, p A166.

2003

1. Abraham RS, Katzmann JA, Clark RC, Bradwell AR, Kyle RA, Gertz MA. Quantitative analysis of serum free light chains. A new marker for the diagnostic evaluation of primary systemic amyloidosis. Am J Clin Pathol 2003; **119**: (2): 274-278.

2. Alyanakian M-A, Abbas A, Delarue R, Arnulf B, Bradwell AR, Aucouturier P. Free immunoglobulin light chains serum levels in the follow-up of patients with monoclonal gammopathies: correlation with the 24H urinary light-chain excretion. Clin Chem 2003; **49**: pA105, D-54.

3. Arneth B, Fischer C, Birklein F, Lackner KJ. The suitability of Kappa Free Light Chains in Cerebrospinal Fluid. Clin Chem Lab Med. 2003; **41** (10) No.P7.85, pA107.

4. Bradwell AR, Clinical applications of serum free light chain immunoassays. Clin Lab Imm 2003; **27**: 7: 8-12

5. Bradwell AR, Carr-Smith HD, Mead GP. Clinical utility of serum free light chain assays. Clin Chem Lab Med 2003; **41**: S72.

6. Bradwell AR, Carr-Smith HD, Mead GP, Harvey TC, Drayson MT. Serum test for assessment of patients with Bence Jones myeloma. Lancet 2003; **361**: 489-491.

7. Bradwell AR, Galvin GP, Mead GP, Carr-Smith HD. Practical use of serial measurements of serum free light chains to monitor response to treatment of multiple myeloma. Blood 2003; **102** (11), A5234.

8. Bradwell AR, Mead G, Carr-Smith H, Galvin G, Pratt G. Efficacy of high dose myeloma treatment and response to individual chemotherapy agents in myeloma is indicated by changes in serum free light chain concentrations. Blood 2003; **102** (11), A2547.

9. Bradwell AR, Mead GP, Drayson MT, Kyle RA, Katzmann JA. Role of serum free light chain measurements in disease diagnosis and monitoring. The Hematology Journal 2003; **4,** P7.4: pS46.

10. Carr-Smith HD, Bradwell AR. Serum free light chain assay development - specificity, sensitivity, standardisation and protocols. Clin Chem Lab Med 2003; **41**: S72.

11. Carr-Smith HD, Mead GP, Smith L, Drayson MT, Bradwell AR. Serum free light chain levels in patients with intact immunoglobulin myeloma. Br J Haematol 2003; **121**: 198, p66.

12. Cohen AD, Zhou P, Xiao Q, Fleisher M, Kalakonda N, Akhurst T, Chitale DA, Moskowitz C, Dhodapkar MV, Teruya-Feldstein J, Filippa DA, Comenzo RL. Systemic AL amyloidosis due to Non-Hodgkin's Lymphoma: An unusual clinicopathologic association. Blood 2003; **102** (11), A4838.

13. Graziani M, Merlini G, Petrini C, IFCC Committee on Plasma Proteins; SIBioC Study Group on Proteins. Guidelines for the analysis of Bence Jones proteins. Clin Chem Lab Med. 2003 **41**(3): 338-346.

14. Helmke KH, Oppermann MO, Teuber WT, Michels HM, Ventur YV, Welcker MW, v.Landenberg PL. Freie Immunglobulin-Leichtketten im Serum bei rheumatischen Erkrankungen.Z Rheumatol 2003; **62**, Suppl.1: No. PFr-40, p105

15. Hermsen D, Bradwell AR. Nephelometric detection of free kappa and lambda light chains in serum in patients with suspected monoclonal gammopathy. Onkologie 2003; **26**: P697, p125

16. Herzog W, Hofmann W. Detection of free kappa and lambda light chains in serum and urine in patients with monoclonal gammopathy. Blood 2003; **102** (11), A5190.

17. Hofmann W, Herzog W. Detection of free kappa and lambda light chain in serum and urine in patients with monoclonal gammopathy. Onkologie 2003; **26**: P694, p124

18. Hunter HM, Peggs K, Powles R, Apperley J, Mahendra P, Canenagh J, Littlewood T, Potter M, Hunter A, Pagliuca, Williams C, Cook G, Towlson K, Marks D, Russell NH. A comparison of outcome for patients undergoing non-myeloablative stem cell transplantation compared to conventional conditioning for multiple myeloma. Blood 2003; **102** (11), A2705.

19. Katzmann JA, Clark RJ, Rajkumar VS, Kyle RA. Monoclonal free light chains in sera from healthy individuals: FLC MGUS. Clin Chem 2003; **49**: pA24, No. A-74

20. Keren DF, Techniques to measure free kappa and free lambda chains in serum and/or urine. In: Protein Electrophoresis in Clinical Diagnosis 2003. Pub: Arnold, London.

21. Lachmann HJ, Gallimore R, Gillmore JD, Carr-Smith HD, Bradwell AR, Pepys MB, Hawkins PN. Outcome in systemic AL amyloidosis in relation to changes in concentration of circulating free immunoglobulin light chains following chemotherapy. Brit J Haematol 2003; **122**: 78-84

22. Martin W, Clark RJ, Shanafelt T, Katzmann JA, Bradwell AR, Abraham R, Kay NE, Witzig TE. Detection of serum free light chains in patients with B-cell non-Hodgkin lymphoma (NHL) and chronic lymphocytic leukemia (CLL). Blood 2003; **102** (11), A4827.

23. Mead GP, Carr-Smith H, Drayson M, Bradwell AR. Serum free light chain concentrations and their use for disease monitoring in multiple myeloma patients with intact immunoglobulin monoclonal proteins. The Hematology Journal 2003; 170, pS163.

24. Mead GP, Carr-Smith HD, Drayson MT, Bradwell AR. Elevated serum free light chain concentrations in multiple myeloma patients with intact immunoglobulin monoclonal proteins; their use for disease monitoring. The Hematology Journal 2003; **4** (2), No.0407, pS125.

25. Mead GP, Carr-Smith HD, Drayson MT, Bradwell AR. Diagnosis and monitoring of multiple myeloma using serum free light chain concentrations. Onkologie 2003; **26**: P695, p124

26. Mead GP, Carr-Smith HD, Drayson MT, Bradwell AR. Serum free light chain assays provide improved monitoring of myeloma therapy. Br J Haem 2003; **121**, Suppl. 1: p69: No. 205.

27. Mead GP, Carr-Smith HD, Drayson MT, Bradwell AR. Serum free light chain levels in patients with intact immunoglobulin myeloma. Clin Chem 2003; **49**: D-61, pA107.

28. Mead GP, Drayson MT, Carr-Smith HD, Bradwell AR. Measurement of Immunoglobulin Free

Light Chains in Serum. Clin Chem 2003; **49**(11): 1957-1958 *(letter reply).*

29. Mead G, Pratt G, Bradwell AR. Frequent measurement of total immunoglobulin and serum free light chains in myeloma patients during peripheral blood stem cell transplantation. The Hematology Journal 2003; **171**, pS163.

30. Myers B, Lachmann H, Russell NH. Novel combination chemotherapy for primary (AL) amyloidosis myeloma: clinical, laboratory and serum amyloid-P protein scan improvement. Br J Haem; 2003: **121**: 815-819.

31. Myers B, Russell NH, McMillan AK. Use of a novel combination chemotherapy for AL-Amyloidosis: cyclophosphamide, thalidomide and dexamethasone - serum free light chain (SFLC) and serum amyloid protein P (SAP) scan results. Blood 2003; **102** (11), A5249.

32. Nowrousian MR, Brandhorst D, Daniels R, Sammet C, Schuett P, Ebeling P, Buttkereit U, Opalka B, Flasshove M, Moritz T, Seeber S. Free light-chain measurement in serum compared with immunofixation of urine in patients with multiple myeloma. Blood 2003; **102** (11), A5197.

33. Nowrousian MR, Brandhorst D, Daniels R, Sammet C, Schuett P, Ebeling P, Seeber S. Comparison between free light chain measurement in serum and immunofixation of urine in patients with multiple myeloma. Onkologie 2003; **26**: P696, p124

34. Ong S, Sethi S. Assessment of free light chains assays in serum on the Beckman IMMAGE. Clin Chem 2003; **49**: No. D-59, pA106.

35. Overton J, Goodier D, Carr-Smith HD, Bradwell AR. Evaluation of latex-enhanced turbidimetric reagents for measuring free immunoglobulin light-chains on the Roche Modular P. Clin Chem 2003; **49**, D-60, pA106

36. Patten PE, Ahsan G, Kazmi M, Fields PA, Chick GW, Jones RR, Bradwell AR, Schey SA. The early use of the serum free light chain assay in patients with relapsed refractory myeloma receiving treatment with thalidomide analogue (CC-4047). Blood 2003; **102** (11), A1640.

37. Rajkumar SV, Kyle RA, Therneau TM, Bradwell AR, Melton J, Katzmann JA. Presence of monoclonal free light chains in serum predicts risk of progression in monoclonal gammopathy of undetermined significance (MGUS). Blood 2003; **102** (11), A3481.

38. Showell P, Matters D, Bradwell AR. Evaluation of latex-enhanced turbidimetric reagents for measuring free immunoglobulin light-chains on the Olympus AU400™. Proceedings of ACB National Meeting, 2003; No.**13**, p52.

39. Showell P, Matters D, Carr-Smith HD, Bradwell AR. Evaluation of latex-enhanced turbidimetric reagents for measuring free immunoglobulin light-chains on the Olympus AU400™. Clin Chem 2003; **49**: (6): pA105, D-55.

40 Sirohi B, Powles R, Kulkarni S, Carr-Smith HD, Patel G, Das M, Iqbal J, Bradwell AR, Dearden C, Mehta J. Serum free light chain assessment in myeloma patients who are in complete remission (CR) by immunofixation predicts early relapse. Blood 2003; **102** (11), A5195.

41. Smith L, Showell P, Matters D, Carr-Smith HD, Bradwell AR. Evaluation of latex-enhanced turbidimetric reagents for measuring free immunoglobulin light-chains on the Olympus AU400™. Clin Chem & Lab Med. 2003; **W-497**; pS 520.

42. Smith LJ, Long J, Matters DJ, Carr-Smith HD, Bradwell AR. Sample storage and stability for free light chain assays. Proceedings of ACB National Meeting, 2003; **No.2**, p47.

43. Smith LJ, Long J, Matters DJ, Carr-Smith HD, Bradwell AR. Sample storage and stability for free light chain assays. Clin Chem 2003; **49**: (6): D-57, pA105.

44. Smith LJ, Long J, Carr-Smith HD, Bradwell AR. Measurement of immunoglobulin free light chains by automated homogeneous immunoassay in serum and plasma samples. Clin Chem 2003; **49:** (6): D-58, pA106.

45. Smith LJ, Mead GP, Bradwell AR. Comparative sensitivity of serum and urine assays for free light chains. Clin Chem Lab Med 2003; **41**: pS72.

46. Tate RJ, Gill D, Cobcroft R, Hickman PE. Practical considerations for the Measurement of Free Light Chains in Serum. Clin Chem 2003; **49**: 8: 1252-1257

47. Tate RJ, Mollee P, Gill D. Measurement of Immunoglobulin Free Light Chains in Serum. Clin Chem 2003; **49** (11): 1958 *(Letter)*

48. Terpos E, Politou M, Szydio R, Nadal E, Avery S, Olavarria E, Kanfer E, Goldman JM, Apperley JF, Rahemtulla A. Autologous stem cell transplantation normalises abnormal bone resorption through the reduction of RANK/OPG ratio in multiple myeloma. Blood 2003; **102** (11), A3658.

49. Wands C, Powell MP. The development of serum free light chain immunoassay on the Bayer Advia 1650. Proc ACB National Meeting. 2003; **No.3**, p47.

2004

1. Alyanakian MA, Abbas A, Delarue R, Arnulf B, Aucouturier P. Free Immunoglobulin Light-chain Serum Levels in the Follow-up of Patients With Monoclonal Gammopathies: Correlation with 24-hr Urinary Light-chain Excretion. Am J Hemat 2004; **75**: 246-248.

2. Augustson BM, Reid SD, Mead GP, Drayson MT, Child JA, Bradwell AR. Serum Free Light Chain Levels In Asymptomatic Myeloma. Blood 2004; **104**: 11: No. 4880.

3. Berard A, Bouabdallah K. Chaines legeres libres: interet pour le diagnostic et le suivi des gammapathies monoclonales. Infos Biologiste Tribune 2004; **8**: 12-13.

4. Bergen III HR, Abraham RS, Johnson KL, Bradwell AR, Naylor S. Characterisation of amyloidogenic immunoglobulin light chains directly from serum by on-line immunoaffinity isolation. Biomedical Chromatography 2004; **18**: 191-201.

5. Bird JM, Cavenagh J, Samson D, Mehta A, Hawkins P, Lachmann H. Guidelines on the diagnosis and management of AL amyloidosis. Br J Haematol 2004; **125**: 681-700.

6. Bradwell AR, Garbincius J, Holmes EW. The Free Kappa to Free Lambda Ratio (SFKLR) as an Adjunct to Serum Protein Electrophoresis for the Detection of Monoclonal Proteins in the Serum. Blood 2004: **104**: 11: No. 4856.

7. Carr-Smith HD, Harland B, Anderson J, Overton J, Wieringa G, Bradwell AR. The effect on laboratory organisation of introducing serum free light chain assays. Clin Chem 2004; **50** (6): Suppl, pA76; C-22.

8. Carr-Smith HD, Harland B, Anderson J, Overton J, Wieringa G, Bradwell AR. Evaluation of latex-enhanced turbidimetric reagents for measuring free immunoglobulin light chains on the Bayer Advia 1650. Clin Chem 2004; **50** (6): Suppl, pA82; C-44.

9. Chou PP, Praither JD, Grainger A, Knight R. Serum free light chain assays. Clin Chem 2004; **50** (6): Suppl, pA76; C-24.

10. Cohen AD, Zhou P, Reich L, Quinn A, Fircanis S, Drake L, Hedvat C, Teruya-Feldstein J, Filippa DA, Fleisher M, Comenzo RL. Risk-adapted intravenous melphalan followed by adjuvant dexamethazone (D) and Thalidomide (T) for newly diagnosed patients with systemic AL amyloidosis (AL): Interim results of a phase II study. Blood 2004: **104**: 11: No.542.

11. Engelhardt M, Rapple D, Weis A, Bisse E, Thorst G. Serum Free Light Chain (FLC) Measurement in Multiple Myeloma (MM) Patients (pts) Correlate with Known Monoclonal Paraprotein, Disease Stage and Therapy Response. Blood 2004; **104**: 11: No. 4907.

12. Fischer CB, Arneth B, Koehler J, Lotz J, Lackner KJ. Kappa Free Light Chains in cerebrospinal fluid as Markers of Intrathecal Immunoglobulin Synthesis. Clin Chem 2004; **50**: 1809-1813.

13. Fischer CB, Arneth B, Koehler J, Lackner K. The suitability of kappa free light chains in cerebrospinal fluid diagnostics. Clin Chem 2004; **50** (6): Suppl, pA49; B-47.

14. Gertz MA. Freelite™ Immunoglobulin Free Light Chain Assay. Diagnostic Serum Test Enables Identification and monitoring of MM. Myeloma Today; 2004; **6** (2):5-6.

15. Gertz M, Comenzo R, Falk RH, Fermand J-P, Hazenberg BP, Hawkins PN, Merlini G, Moreau P, Ronco P, Sanchorawala V, Sezer O, Solomon A, Grateau G. Definition of organ involvement and treatment response in primary systemic amyloidosis (AL): A consensus opinion from the 10th International Symposium on amyloid and amyloidosis. Blood 2004; **104**: 11: No. 754.

16. Gertz M, Lacy M, Dispenzieri A. Therapy for immunoglobulin light chain amyloidosis: The new and the old. Blood Reviews 2004; **18** (1) 17-37.

17. Goodman HJB, Lachmann HJ, Bradwell AR, Hawkins PN. Intermediate Dose Intravenous Melphalan and Dexamethasone Treatment in 144 patients with Systemic AL Amyloidosis. Blood 2004; **104**: 11: No. 755.

18. Guis L, Diemert MC, Ghillani P ,Choquet S, Leblond V, Vernant JP, Musset L. The quantitation of serum free light chains: Three case reports. Clin Chem 2004; **50** (6): Suppl, pA183; F-38.

19. Hermsen D, Herzog W. Nephelometric detection of serum free kappa and lambda light chains in patients with suspected monoclonal free light chain gammopathies. Clin Chem 2004; **50** (6): Suppl, pA75; C-19.

20. Herzog W, Hofmann W. Detection of free Kappa and Lambda light chain in serum and urine in patients with monoclonal gammopathy. Clin Chem 2004; **50** (6): Suppl, pA182; F-34.

21. Herzum I, Bruder-Burzlaff B, Heinz R, Wahl HG. Reliability of the New FREELITE Assay for Quantification of Free Light Chains in Urine. Clin Chem 2004; **50** (6): Suppl, pA80; C-36.

22. Hoffman W, Garbrecht M, Bradwell AR, Guder WG. A New Concept for Detection of Bence Jones Proteinuria in Patients with Monoclonal Gammopathy. Clin Lab 2004; **50**: 181-185.

23. Jaccard A, Moreau P, Aucouturier P, Ronco P, Fermand J-P, Hermine O. Amylose immunoglobulinique. Hematologie 2003; **9**: 6 485-95.

24. Katzmann J, Dispenzieri A, Abraham R, Kyle R. Performance of Free Light Chain Assays in Clinical Practice. Blood 2004; **104**: 11:No.757.

25. Mead G, Bradwell AR, Lovell R, Pratt G. Changes in Serum Free Light Chain Concentrations after High-Dose Melphalan and Autologous Stem Cell Transplant in Myeloma Patients. Bone Marrow Transplant 2004; **33**: Suppl 1:S1-380.

26. Mead GP, Carr-Smith HD, Drayson MT, Morgan GT, Child JA, Bradwell AR. Serum free light chains for monitoring multiple myeloma. Br J Haem 2004; **126**: 348-354.

27. Mead GP, Carr-Smith HD, Galvin G, Pratt G, Bradwell AR. Efficacy of High Dose Treatment and Response to Individual Chemotherapy Agents in Myeloma is Indicated by Changes in Serum Free Light Chain Concentrations. Clin Chem 2004; **50** (6): Suppl, pA75; C-20.

28. Mead GP, Reid S, Augustson B, Drayson MT, Bradwell AR, Child JA. Correlation of Serum Free Light Chains and Bone Marrow Plasma Cell Infiltration in Multiple Myeloma. Blood 2004; **104**: 11: No. 4865.

29. Merlini G. Editorial: Sharpening Therapeutic Strategy in AL Amyloidosis. Blood 2004; **104**: 6: 1593-1594.

30. Merlini G, Palladini G, Bosoni, Lavatelli F, D'Eril GM, Bradwell AR, Moratti R. Circulating free light chain concentration correlates with degree of cardiac dysfunction in AL amyloidosis. Clin Chem 2004; **50** (6): Suppl, pA69; B113.

31. Nakano T, Nagata A, Takahashi H. Ratio of urinary free immunoglobulin light chain kappa to lambda in the diagnosis of Bence Jones proteinuria. Clin Chem Lab Med 2004; **42** (4): 429-434.

32. Rajkumar SV, Kyle RA, Therneau TM, Clark RJ, Bradwell AR, Melton LJ III, Larson DR, Plevak MF, Katzmann JA. Presence of monoclonal free light chains in the serum predicts risk of progression in monoclonal gammopathy of undetermined significance. Br J Haem 2004; **127**: 308-310.

33. Rajkumar SV, Kyle RA, Therneau TM, Melton LJ III, Bradwell AR, Clark RJ, Larson DR, Plevak MF, Dispenzieri A, Katzmann JA. Presence of an Abnormal Serum Free Light Chain Ratio is an Independent Risk Factor for Progression in Monoclonal Gammopathy of Undetermined Significance (MGUS). Blood 2004; **104**: 11: No. 3647.

34. Räpple D, Weis A, Deschler B, Bisse E, Englehardt M. Lambda (λ) - and Kappa (κ) - Free Light Chains in Multiple Myeloma (MM) Patients Correlate with Known Monoclonal Paraprotein, Disease Stage and Therapy Response. Onkologie 2004; **27** (suppl 3): 183.

35. Reid SD, Drayson MT, Mead GP, Augustson B, Bradwell AR. Serum free light chains are a more sensitive marker of serological remission in multiple myeloma patients. Clin Chem 2004; **50** (6): Suppl, pA79; C-34.

36. Reid S, Mead GP, Drayson MT, Bradwell AR. Comparison of immunofixation electrophoresis with serum free light chain measurement for determining complete remission in Light Chain Multiple Myeloma. Bone Marrow Transplant 2004; **33:** Suppl 1:S1-380.

37. Sanchorawala V, Seldin DC, Wright DG, Skinner M, Finn KT, Falk RH. Pulsed Low Dose Intravenous Melphalan in Patients with AL Amyloidosis, Ineligible for Aggressive Treatment with High-Dose Melphalan and Stem Cell Transplantation. Blood 2004; **104**: 11:No. 2393.

38. Sanchorawala V, Wright DG, Magnani B, Skinner M, Finn KT, Seldin DC. Serum Free Light

Chain Responses after High-Dose Intravenous Melphalan and Autologous Stem Cell Transplantation for AL (Primary) Amyloidosis. Blood 2004; **104**: 11:No. 942.

39. Showell PJ, Lynch EA, Carr-Smith HD, Bradwell AR. Evaluation of latex-enhanced nephelometric reagents for measuring free immunoglobulin light-chains on the Radim Delta. Clin Chem 2004; **50** (6): Suppl, pA81; C-40.

40. Sirohi B, Powles R, Kulkarni S, Carr-Smith HD, Patel G, Das M, Iqbal J, Bradwell AR, Dearden C, Mehta J. Serum free light chain ratio is predictive of early relapse in patients who are in complete remission by immunofixation. Bone Marrow Transplant 2004; **33:** Suppl 1:S1-380.

41. Tate JR, Mollee P, Gill D. Serum free light chain ratios do not detect relapse in some patients with intact immunoglobulin myeloma post autologous peripheral blood stem cell transplantation. Clin Chem 2004; **50** (6): Suppl, pA51; B-54.

42. Thompson EJ. Editorial. Quality versus Quantity: Which is better for cerebrospinal fluid IgG. Clin Chem 2004; **50**: 1721-1722.

43. Urban S, Oppermann M, Reucher SW, Schmolke M, Hoffmann U, Hiefinger-Schindlbeck R, Helmke K. Free light chains (FLC) of immunoglobulins as parameter resembling disease activity in autoimmune rheumatic diseases. Proceedings of EULAR, 9-12 June, 2004 (www. EULAR.ORG).

2005

1. Abdalla S, Goodman HJB, Hawkins PN. Thalidomide alone and in combination with other agents in the treatment of patients with AL amyloidosis. Haematologica 2005; **90** (s1): PO.1411.

2. Abdalla S. The use of Serum free light chain assay in clinical practice. Haematologica 2005; **90** (s1): PO.405: p107.

3. Akar H, Seldin DC, Magnani B, O'Hara C, Berk JL, Schoonmaker C, Cabral H, Dember LM, Sanchorawala V, Connors LH, Falk RH, Skinner M. Quantitative serum free light-chain assay in the diagnostic evaluation of AL amyloidosis. In: Amyloid and Amyloidosis; Eds Grateau G, Kyle RA, Skinner M: CRC Press: 2005; 90-92.

4. Akar H, Seldin DC, Magnani B, O'Hara C, Berk JL, Schoonmaker C, Cabral H, Dember LM, Sanchorwala V, Connors LH, Falk RH, Skinner M. Quantitative serum free light chain assay in the diagnostic evaluation of AL amyloidosis. Amyloid 2005; **12** (4): 210-215.

5. Augustson BM, Katsavara H, Reid SD, Mead GP, Shirfield M, Bradwell AR. Monoclonal gammopathy screening: Improved sensitivity using the serum free light chain assay. Haematologica 2005; **90** (s1): 195: PO1302.

6. Augustson BM, Reid SD, Cohen D, Hawkins K, Mead G, Drayson M, Child JA, Bradwell AR. Normalisation Of Serum Free Light Chains and Negative Immunofixation Electrophoresis May Be Predictive Of Progression Free Survival And Overall Survival Following High Dose Melphalan. Haematologica 2005; **90**(s1): 107: PO403.

7. Augustson BM, Reid SD, Mead GP, Drayson MT, Child JA, Bradwell AR. Serum Free Light Chain Levels In Asymptomatic Myeloma. Haematologica 2005; **90** (s1): 195: PO1303.

8. Bakshi NA, Guilbranson R, Garstka D, Bradwell AR, Keren DF. Serum Free Light Chain (FLC) Measurement Can Aid Capillary Zone Electrophoresis (CZE) In Detecting Subtle FLC M-Proteins. Am J Clin Path 2005; **124**: 214-218.

9. Bergon E, Miravalles E, Bergon E, Miranda I, Bergon M. The predictive power of serum Kappa/Lambda ratios for discrimination between monoclonal gammopathy of undetermined significance and Multiple Myeloma. Clin Chem Lab Med 2005; **43** (3): 349.

10. Bradwell AR. Serum free light chain assays move to centre stage. Editorial Clin Chem 2005; **51** (5): 805-807.

11. Bradwell AR, Evans ND, Chappell MJ, Cockwell P, Reid SD, Harrison J, Hutchison C, Mead GP. Rapid Removal of Free Light Chains from Serum by Hemodialysis for Patients with Myeloma Kidney. Blood 2005; **106** (11): 3482, p972a.

12. Bradwell AR, Mead GP, Chappell MJ, Evans ND. Model for assessing free light chain kinetics when monitoring patients with multiple myeloma. Haematologica 2005; **90** (1): p110, No.PO411.

13. Brockhurst I, Harris KPG, Chapman CS. Diagnosis and monitoring a case of light-chain deposition disease in the kidney using a new, sensitive immunoassay. Nephrol Dial Transplant 2005; **20**: 1251-1253.

14. Carr-Smith HD, Abraham R, Mead GP, Goodman H, Hawkins P, Bradwell AR. Measurement of serum free light chains in AL amyloidosis. In: Amyloid and Amyloidosis; Eds Grateau G, Kyle RA, Skinner M: CRC Press: 2005; 154-156.

15. Carr-Smith H, Mead G, Bradwell AR. Serum Free Light Chain Assays as a Replacement for Urine Electrophoresis. Haematologica 2005; **90**(s1): p107, PO404.

16. Cavallo F, Rasmussen E, Zangari M, Tricot G, Fender B, Fox M, Burns M, Bart Barlogie B. Serum Free-Lite Chain (sFLC) Assay in Multiple Myeloma (MM): Clinical Correlates and Prognostic Implications in Newly Diagnosed MM Patients Treated with Total Therapy 2 or 3 (TT2/3). Blood 2005; **106** (11): 3490: P974a.

17. Chapuis-Cellier C, Foray V, Chazaud A, Troncy J. Contribution of the quantification of free light chains in 273 patients presenting with a newly discovered monoclonal gammapathy. Haematologica 2005; **90** (s1): PO408: p109.

18. Chapuis-Cellier C, Foray V, Chazaud A, Troncy J. Apparent discrepancies in the Quantitation of Free light chains in serum of patients presenting with a monoclonal gammopathy. Haematologica 2005; **90** (s1): PO409: p109.

19. Cohen AD, Zhou P, Reich L, Ford A, Hedvat C, Teruya-Feldstein J, Filippa DA, Fleisher M, Comenzo RL. Interim analysis of a Phase II study of risk-adapted intravenous melphalan followed by adjuvant dexmethasone (D) and thalidomide (T) for newly diagnosed patients with systemic AL amyloidosis (AL).Haematologica 2005; **90** (s1): PO1407.

20. Comenzo RL. Light chains ahoy: Pirating Thal/Dex for AL too. Editorial, Blood 2005; **105** (7): 2625.

21. Commenzo RL, Zhou P, Reich L, Costello S, Quinn A, Fircanis S, Drake L, Hedvat C, Teruya-Feldstein J, Filippa D, Fleisher M. Risk-adapted intravenous melphalan with adjuvant Thalidomide and Dexamethazone for newly diagnosed untreated patients with systemic AL amyloidosis: interim report of a phase II trial. In: Amyloid and Amyloidosis; Eds Grateau G, Kyle RA, Skinner M: CRC Press: 2005; 112-115.

22. Commenzo RL, Zhou P, Reich L Costello S, Quinn A, Fircanis S, Drake L, Hedvat C, Teruya-Feldstein J, Filippa D, Fleisher M. Prospective evaluation of the utility of the serum free light chain assay (FLC), Clonal Ig V_LR gene identification and troponin 1 levels in a phase II trial of risk-adapted intravenous melphalan with adjuvant Thalidomide and Dexamethasone for newly diagnosed untreated patients with systemic AL amyloidosis. In: Amyloid and Amyloidosis; Eds Grateau G, Kyle RA, Skinner M: CRC Press: 2005; 167-169.

23. Comenzo RL, Zhou P, Wang L, Nimer SD, Olshen AB. Plasma Cell Gene-Expression Profiles in Patients with Systemic AL Amyloidosis: Responses to Melphalan and Stem Cell Transplant Are Associated with Differential Expression of Genes Involved in Translation, Protein Degradation and Detoxification. Blood 2005; **106** (11): 3405: p951a.

24. Das M, Mead GP, Sreekanth V, Anderson J, Blair S, Howe T, Cavet J, Liakopoulou E. Serum Free Light Chain (SFLC) Concentration Kinetics in Patients Receiving Bortezomib: Temporary Inhibition of Protein Synthesis and Early Biomarker for Disease Response. Blood 2005; **106** (11): 5094: p355b.

25. Dellerba MP, James M, Butler SJ, Kelsey PR. Serum Free Light Chain Measurement in Patients with Multiple Myeloma and Amyloidosis AL. Clin Chim Acta 2005; **355**: Supp S: s137.

26. Desplat-Jego S, Feuillet L, Pelletier J, Bernard D, Cherif AA, Boucrout J. Quantification of Immunoglobulin Free Light Chains in CerebroSpinal Fluid by Nephelometry. J Clin Imm 2005; **25** (4): 338-345.

27. Dingli D, Kyle RA, Rajkumar VS, Nowakowski GS, Larson DR, Bida JP, Gertz MA, Dispenzieri A, Melton III LJ, Therneau TM, Katzmann JA. Immunoglobulin Free Light Chains at Diagnosis: Predictors of Progression and Survival in Solitary Plasmacytoma of Bone. Blood 2005; **106** (11): 5080; p352b.

28. Dispenzieri A, Lacy MQ, Katzmann JA, Rajkumar VS, Abraham RS, Hayman SR, Kumar SK, Clark R, Kyle RA, Litzow MR, Inwards DJ, Elliott MA, Micallef IM, Ansell SM, Porrata LF, Johnston P, Zeldenrust SR, Witzig TE, Greipp PR, Lust JA, Russell SR, Gertz MA. Absolute Values of Serum Immunoglobulin Free Light Chains Predict for Survival in Patients with Primary Systemic Amyloidosis Undergoing Peripheral Blood Stem Cell Transplant. Blood 2005; **106** (11): 422: p127a.

29. Foray V, Chapuis-Cellier C. Contribution of serum free light chain immunoassays in diagnosis and monitoring of free light chain monoclonal gammopathies. Immuno-analyse et Biologie Specialisee 2005; **20**: 385-393.

30. Forsyth JM, G. Hill PG, Rai BS, Mayne S, Mead GP. Serum Free Light Chain Measurement Can Replace Urine Electrophoresis in the Detection of B Cell Proliferative Disorders. Blood 2005; **106** (11): 5081: 352b.

31. Forsyth JM, Hill PG, Rai BS, Mayne S, Mead G. Serum free light chains in screening for B cell proliferative disorders. Clin Chim Acta 2005; **355**: WP18.30: pS437-S438.

32. Gertz MA, Comenzo R, Falk RH, Fermand JP, Hazenberg BP, Hawkins PN, Merlini G, Moreau P, Roncon P, Sanchorawala V, Sezer O, Solomon A, Grateau G. Definition of organ involvement and treatment response in primary systemic amyloidosis (AL): A concensus opinion from the 10th International Symposium on Amyloid and Amyloidosis. Haematologica 2005; **90** (s1), PO1405

33. Gertz MA, Comenzo R, Falk RH, Fermand JP, Hazenberg BP, Hawkins PN, Merlini G, Moreau P, Ronco P, Sanchorawala V, Sezer O, Solomon Al, Grateau G. Definition of Organ Involvement and Treatment Response in Immunoglobulin Light Chain Amyloidosis (AL): A Consensus Opinion From the 10th International Symposium on Amyloid and Amyloidosis. Am J Hem 2005; **79**: 319-328.

34. Gertz MA, Lacy MQ, Dispenzieri A, Hayman SR, Kumar SK, Ansell SM, Elliott MA, Gastineau DA, Inwards DJ, Johnston PB, Micallef IN, Porrata LF, Litzow MR. Role of Second Stem Cell Transplant in Patients with Amyloidosis Who Are Refractory or Relapsing. Blood 2005; **106** (11): 5469: p455b.

35. Giarin MM, Di Bello C, Battaglio S, Falco P, Giaccone L, Boccadoro M. Serum free light chains: a new tool for diagnosis and management of multiple myeloma. Haematologica 2005; **90**: Supl 3: P235: p179.

36. Gillmore JD, Wechalekar AD, Goodman HJB, Lachmann HJ, Offer M, Joshi J, Hawkins PN. Cardiac Followed by Autologous Stem Cell Transplantation for Systemic AL Amyloidosis. Blood 2005; **106** (11): 1158: p338a.

37. Goodman HJB, Wechalekar, Lachmann HJ, Bradwell AR, Hawkins PN. Clonal disease response and clinical outcome in 229 patients with AL amyloidosis treated with VAD-like chemotherapy. Haematologica 2005; **90** (s1): PO1408: p201.

38. Gupta S, Comenzo RL, Hoffman BR, Fleisher M. National Academy of Clinical Biochemistry Guidelines for the use of Tumor Markers in Monoclonal Gammopathies. 2005 nacb.org.

39. Hammer F, Rolinski B, Scherberich JE. Impact of chronic renal failure on serum concentrations of free polyclonal immunoglobulin light chains. Nephro-News, Proceedings of Congress of Nephrology 2005; **10**: P05: p66.

40. Hassoun H, Reich L, Klimek VM, Dhodapkar M, Cohen A, Kewalramani T, Riedel ER, Hedvat CV, Teruya-Feldstein J, Filippa DA, Fleisher M, Nimer SD, Comenzo RL. The Serum Free Light Chain Ratio after One or Two Cycles of Treatment Is Highly Predictive of the Magnitude of Final Response in Patients Undergoing Initial Treatment for Multiple Myeloma. Blood 2005; **106** (11): 3481: p972a.

41. Hassoun H, Reich L, Klimek VM, Dhodapkar M, Cohen A, Kewalramani T, Zimman R, Drake L, Riedel ER, Hedvat CV, Teruya-Feldstein J, Filippa DA, Fleisher M, Nimer SD, Comenzo RL. Doxorubicin and dexamethosone followed by thalidomide and dexamethasone is an effective well tolerated initial therapy for multiple myeloma. Br J Haem 2005; **132**: 155-161.

42. Hazenberg BPC, Bijzet J, de Wit H, van Steijn J, Vellenga E, van Rijswijk MH. Diagnostic value of free kappa and lambda light chains in fat tissue of patients with systemic AL Amyloidosis. In: Amyloid and Amyloidosis; Eds Grateau G, Kyle RA, Skinner M: CRC Press: 2005; 107-108.

43. Henon KT, Dispenzieri A, Katzmann JA, Lacy MQ, Ramirez-Alvarado M, Gertz MA, Kyle RA, Abraham RS. Circulating soluble light chain oligomers in sera of patients with light chain amyloidosis. Haematologica 2005; **90** (s1): PO1406: p200.

44. Herzog W, Mead GP, Drayson MT, Bradwell AR. Serum free light chain immunoassays in the diagnosis of monoclonal Gammopathies. Nephro-News, Proceedings of Congress of Nephrology Sept 2005, P12.04; p102.

45. Herzog W, Mead GP, Reid SD, Hewins P, Cockwell P, Bradwell AR. The effect of renal impairment and dialysis on serum free light chain measurement. Nephro-News, Proceedings of Congress of Nephrology Sept 2005; P08.03; p81.

46. Hill P, Forsyth J, Mayne S, Mead G. Comparison of serum free light chain measurement and urine electrophoresis for detection of B cell proliferative disorders. Haematologica 2005; **90** (s1): p108: PO406.

47. Hill PG, Forsyth JM, Rai BS, Mayne S, Mead GP. Serum free light chain measurement can replace urine electrophoresis for detecting B cell proliferative disorders. Clin Chem 2005; **51** (6):B-6.

48. Ihenetu KU, Abudu N, Miller J, Elin RJ. Free light chain assay shows greater clinical sensitivity than electrophoresis for detecting plasma cell dyscrasias. Clin Chem 2005; **51** (6): B-157.

49. Kang SY, Suh JT, Lee HJ, Yoon HJ, Lee WI. Clinical usefulness of free light chain concentration as a tumor marker in Multiple Myeloma. Ann Hematol 2005; **84**: 588-593.

50. Katsavara H, Reid SD, Augustson BM, Mead GP, Shirfield M, Drayson MT, Bradwell AR, Narayanan M. Screening for monoclonal gammopathy: Improved sensitivity using serum free light chain assays. Clin Chim Acta 2005; **355**: Suppl S285.

51. Katzmann JA. Quantitative free light chain assays for the diagnosis and monitoring of monoclonal gammopathies. J of Ligand Chemistry 2005; **27** (4): 246-255.

52. Katzmann J, Abraham RS, Dispenzieri A, Lust JA, Kyle RA. Diagnostic performance of Quantitative Kappa and Lambda Free Light Chain Assays in Clinical Practice. Clin Chem 2005; **51** (5); p878-881.

53. Katzmann JA, Dispenzieri A, Abraham RS, Lust JA, Kyle RA. Diagnostic Performance of Free Light Chain Assays in Clinical Practice. Clin Chem 2005; **51** (6): Suppl: D-16.

54. Keren DF. Serum protein electrophoresis evaluation of monoclonal gammopathies (M-proteins). J of Ligand Chemistry 2005: **27** (4): 218-226.

55. Kühnemund A, Liebisch P, Bauchmüller K, Haas P, Kleber M, Bisse E, Schmitt-Graff A, Engelhardt M. Secondary light chain multiple myeloma with decreasing IgA paraprotein levels correlating with renal insufficiency and progressive disease: Clinical course of two patients and review of the literature. Onkologie 2005; **28** (suppl 3): 165.

56. Kumar S, Gertz MA, Hayman SR, Lacy MQ, Dispenzieri A, Zeldenrust SR, Lust JA, Greipp PR, Kyle RA, Fonseca R, S. Rajkumar VS. Use of the Serum Free Light Chain Assay in Assessment of Response to Therapy in Multiple Myeloma: Validation of Recently Proposed Response Criteria in a Prospective Clinical Trial of Lenalidomide Plus Dexamethasone for Newly Diagnosed Multiple Myeloma. Blood 2005; **106** (11): 3479: p971a.

57. Kyrtsonis M-C, Sachanas S, Vassilakopoulos TP, Kafassi N, Tzenou T, Papadogiannis A, Kalpadakis C, Antoniadis AG, Dimopoulou MN, Angelopoulou MK, Siakantaris MP, Dimitriadou EM, Kokoris SI, Plata E, Tsaftaridis P, Panayiotidis P, Pangalis GA. Bortezomib in Patients with Relapsed-Refractory Multiple Myeloma (MM). Clinical Observations. Blood 2005; **106** (11): 5193: p382b.

58. Leleu X, Moreau A-S, Coiteux V, Guieze R, Hennache B, Facon T, Parker P, Reid SD, Mead GP, Bradwell AR. Serum Free Light Chain Assays in Solitary Bone Plasmacytoma. Clin Chim Acta 2005; **355**: Suppl S285.

59. Leleu X, Moreau A-S, Coiteux V, Guieze R, Hennache B, Facon T, Parker P, Reid SD, Mead GP, Bradwell AR. Serum Free Light Chain Assays in Solitary Bone Plasmacytoma. Br J Haem 2005; **129**; 59-60: 186: Suppl 1.

60. Leleu X, Moreau AS, Hennache B, Dupire S, Faucompret JL, Facon T, Bradwell AR, Reid S, Mead G. Serum Free Light Chain Immunoassays Measurement for Monitoring Solitary Bone Plasmacytoma. Haematologica 2005; **90** (1): 110: PO410.

61. Lorenz EC, Gertz MA, Fervenza FC. Long-term renal outcome of autologous stem cell transplantation in light chain deposition disease. Blood 2005; **106** (11): 5518.

62. Matsuda M, Yamada T, Gono T, Shimojima Y, Ishii W, Fushimi T, Sakashita K, Koike K, Ikeda S. Serum levels of free light chain before and after chemotherapy in primary systemic AL Amyloidosis. Internal Medicine 2005; **44** (5): 428-433.

63. Mead GP, Carr-Smith HD, Drayson MT, Morgan GT, Child JA. Response to: Serum free light chains for monitoring multiple myeloma. Br J Haem 2004; **128**: 406-408. (*Reply to letter by Tate et al).*

64. Mead GP, Reid S, Augustson B, Drayson MT, Bradwell AR, Child JA. Comparison of serum and urine free light chain measurements with bone marrow assessments in multiple myeloma. Haematologica 2005; **90** (s1): 108: PO407.

65. Mead GP, Reid SD, Cockwell P, Hewins P, Bradwell AR. The Effect of Renal Impairment and

Dialysis on Serum Free Light Chain measurement. Haematologica 2005; **90** (s2): 0237: p95.

66. Merkel S, Peest D, Witte T, Haller H, Schwarz A. Rekurrenz einer Leichtkettennephropathie im Transplantat - Therapiemöglichkeiten. Nephro-News, Proceedings of Congress of Nephrology Sept 2005, P03.08; p50.

67. Moesbauer U, Schieder H, Renges H, Ayuk F, Zander A, Kröger N. Serum Free Light Chain [FLC] Assay in Multiple Myeloma Patients who Achieved Negative Immunofixation after Allogeneic Stem Cell Transplantation. Blood 2005; **106** (11): 2023: 572a.

68. Mollee P, Tate J, Dimeski G, Gill D. Falsely Low Serum Free Light Chain Concentration in Patients with Monoclonal Light Chain Diseases. Blood 2005; **106** (11): 5077: 351b.

69. Munshi NC. Determining the undetermined. Editorial: Blood 2005; **106**: 3: 767-768.

70. Myers B. Cardiac amyloidosis. Clin Med 2005; **6**: 2-3. *Letter.*

71. Nowrousian MR, Brandhorst D, Sammet C, Kellert M, Daniels R, Schuett P, Poser M, Mueller S, Ebeling P, Welt A, Bradwell AR, Buttkereit U, Opalka B, Flasshove M, Moritz T, Seeber S. Serum Free Light Chain Analysis and Urine Immunofixation Electrophoresis in Patients with Multiple Myeloma. Clin Cancer Res 2005; **11** (24): 8706-8714.

72. Nowrousian MR, Brandhorst D, Sammet C, Kellert M, Daniels R, Schuett P, Poser M, Mueller S, Ebeling P, Welt A, Buttkereit U, Opalka B, Flasshove M, Seeber S, Moritz T. Relationship between Serum Concentrations and Urinary Excretions of Monoclonal Free Light Chains (mFLC) Detectable as Bence Jones Proteins (BJP) by Immunofixation Electrophoresis (IFE) in Patients with Multiple Myeloma (MM). Blood 2005; **106** (11): 5060: 347b.

73. Offer M, Wechalekar AD, Goodman HJB, Gillmore JD, Lachmann HJ, Bradwell AR, Hawkins PN. Standard Oral Melphalan Chemotherapy for AL Amyloidosis Revisited Using the Serum Free Light Chain Assay. Blood 2005; **106** (11): 3495: 976a.

74. Palladini G, Perfetti V, Perlini S, Obici L, Lavatelli F, Caccialanza R, Invernizzi R, Comotti B, Merlini G. The combination of thalidomide and intermediate-dose dexamethasone is an effective but toxic treatment for patients with primary amyloidosis (AL). Blood 2005; **105** (7): 2949-2951.

75. Palladini G, Perlini S, Vezzoli M, Perfetti V, Lavatelli F, Ferrero I, Obici L, Caccialanza R, Bradwell AR, Merlini G. The reduction of the serum concentration of the amyloidogenic light-chain in cardiac AL results in prompt improvement of myocardial function and prolonged survival despite unaltered amount of myocardial amyloid deposits. In: Amyloid and Amyloidosis; Eds Grateau G, Kyle RA, Skinner M: CRC Press: 2005; 73-75.

76. Peterson MR, Sumabat F, Nesbet L, Mullaney S, Smith D, Herold DA. Analysis of serum immunoglobulin free light chains in chronic hemodialysis patients. Am J Clin Path 2005; **124**: 23: p459.

77. Pietrantuono A. Que sont les tests Freelite™. Bulletin des Syndicat National des Biologistes des Hopitaux 2005; **11**: 2.

78. Pratt G, Mead GP, Bradwell AR. Changes in Serum Free Light Chain Concentrations as a marker of chemosensitivity after High-Dose Melphalan and Autologous Stem Cell Transplant in Myeloma Patients. Haematologica 2005; **90** (s1): PO413: 111.

79. Rajkumar VS. MGUS and Smoldering Multiple Myemloma: Update on Pathogenesis, Natural History, and Management. Hematology (Am Soc Hematol Educ Program). 2005; p340-345.

80. Rajkumar SV, Kyle RA, Therneau TM, Melton III JL, Bradwell AR, Clark RJ, Larson DR, Plevak MF, Katzmann JA. Abnormal serum free light chain ratio is an independent risk factor for progression in monoclonal gammopathy of undetermined significance (MGUS). Haematologica 2005; **90**(s1): 194: PO1301.

81. Rajkumar SV, Kyle RA, Therneau TM, Melton JL III, Bradwell AR Clark RJ, Larson DR, Plevak MF, Dispenzieri A, Katzmann JA. Serum free light chain ratio is an independent risk factor for progression in monoclonal gammopathy of undetermined significance. Blood 2005; **106**: 812-817.

82. Ramasamy I. Free immunoglobulin light chain serum levels in B cell dyscrasias. Clin Chem 2005; **51** (6): B-122.

83. Reid SD, Augustson BM, Katsavara H, Drayson MT, Mead GP, Shirfield M, Bradwell AR, Narayanan M. Monoclonal Gammopathy Screening: Improved Sensitivity Using Serum Free Light Chain Assays. Clin Chem 2005; **51** (6): suppl: B20.

84. Reid SD, Augustson BM, Katsavara H, Mead GP, Shirfield M, Drayson MT, Bradwell AR, Narayanan M. Screening for Monoclonal Gammopathy: Improved Sensitivity Using Serum Free Light Chain Assays. Br J Haem 2005; **129**: 81: Suppl 1.

85. Reid SD, Leleu X, Moreau AS, Coiteux V, Guieze R, Hennache B, Facon T, Parker P, Mead GP, Bradwell AR. Serum Free Light Chain Assays in Solitary Bone Plasmacytoma. Clin Chem 2005; **51** (6) suppl: D-13.

86. Reid SD, Cockwell P, Hewins P, Millard JL, Mead GP, Bradwell AR. Haemodialysis removes free light chains from serum. Clin Chem 2005; **51** (6): suppl: D-12.

87 Reid SD, Cockwell P, Hewins P, Mead GP, Bradwell AR. Efficient Removal of Serum Free Light Chains by Haemodialysis. Haematologica 2005; **90** (s1): 117: PO512.

88. Reid SD, Hewins P, Cockwell P, Millard JL, Mead GP, Bradwell AR. Haemodialysis removes free light chains from serum. Clin Chim Acta 2005; **355**: suppl: S188.

89. Romeril KR, White G, Ritchie D. Thalidomide therapy in relapsed/refractory light chain myeloma. Haematologica 2005; **90** (s1): PO708.

90. Sanchorawala V, Seldin DC, Magnani B, Skinner M, Wright DG. Serum free light chain responses after high-dose intravenous melphalan and autologous stem cell transplantation for AL (primary) amyloidosis. Bone Marrow Transplantation 2005; **36**: 597-600.

91. Sanchorawala V, Wright DG, Quillen K, Fisher C, Skinner M, Sedlin DC. Early Serum Free Light Chain Responses Following High-Dose Melphalan and Stem Cell Transplantation for AL Amyloidosis Predict Treatment Outcomes. Blood 2005; **106** (11): 1160, p339a.

92. Shimojima Y, Matsuda M, Gono T, Ishii W, Fushimi T, Hoshii Y, Yomada T, Ikeda S. Correlation between serum levels of free light chain and phenotype of plasma cells in bone marrow in primary AL amyloidosis. Amyloid 2005; **12** (1):33-40.

93. Showell PJ, Lynch EA, Overton J, Carr-Smith HD, Bradwell AR. Evaluation of latex-enhanced nephelometric reagents for measuring free immunoglobulin light chains on the Dade Behring ProSpec. Clin Chem 2005; **51** (6) suppl: B-38.

94. Smith DE, Abadie J, Bankson D, Mead GP. Assessment of Serum Free Light Chain Assay for Screening for Plasma Cell Disorders. Blood 2005; **106** (11): 2563, p720a.

95. van Steijn J, Bijzet J, de Wit H, Hazenberg BPC, van Gameren II, van de Belt K, Vellenga E. Serum levels of free kappa and lambda light chains in patients with systemic AL, AA and ATTR Amyloidosis. In: Amyloid and Amyloidosis; Eds Grateau G, Kyle RA, Skinner M: CRC Press: 2005; 105-106.

96. Tate JR, Mollee P, Dimeski G, Gill D. Falsely low serum free light chain concentrations in patients with monoclonal light chain diseases. Clin Chem 2005; **51** (6) suppl: B-31.

97. Tate JR, Mollee P, Gill D. Serum free light chains for monitoring multiple myeloma. Br J Haem 2005; **128**: 405-406. *(letter).*

98. Tate J, Mollee P, Gill D. Utility of serum free light chains for monitoring myeloma post autologous stem cell transplantation. Haematologica 2005; **90** (s1): PO.412.

99. Walker R, Rasmussen E, Cavallo F, Jones-Jackson L, Anaissie E, Alpe T, Epstein J, an Rhee F, Zangari M, Tricot G, Shaughnessy J, Barlogie B. Correlation of Suppression of FDG PET Uptake with Serum Free Light Chain Levels - Both FDG PET-CT and Serum Clonal Free Light Chain Response Precede and Predict the Likelihood of Subsequent Complete Remission in Newly Diagnosed Multiple Myeloma. Blood 2005; **106** (11): 3493, p975a.

100. Walker SA, Roddie PH, Ashby JP. Evaluation of serum free light chain (FLC) measurements as an alternative to urine Bence Jones (BJP) analysis in a routine laboratory setting. Clin Chim Acta 2005; **355**: Suppl S: S438.

101. Wechalekar AD, Goodman HJB, Gillmore JD, Lachmann HJ, Offer M, Bradwell AR, Hawkins PN. Efficacy of Risk-Adapted Cyclophosphamide, Thalidomide and Dexamethasone in Systemic AL Amyloidosis. Blood 2005; **106** (11): 3496, p976a.

102. Wechalekar AD, Goodman HJB, Gillmore JD, Lachmann HJ, Offer M, Bradwell AR, Hawkins PN. Clinical Profile and Treatment Outcome in 92 Patients with AL Amyloidosis Associated with IgM Paraproteinaemia. Blood 2005; **106** (11): 3498, p977a.

103. Wechalekar AD, Lachman HJ, Goodman HJB, Bradwell AR, Hawkins PN. Role of serum free light chains in diagnosis and monitoring response to treatment in light chain deposition disease. Haematologica 2005; **90** (s1): PO1414.

104. Yagmur E, Mertens PR, Gressner AM, Kiefer P. Free Light Chain κ/λ - ratios are also of diagnostic value for patients with renal insufficiency. Nephro-News. Proceedings of Congress of Nephrology Sept 2005; P12.04: 102-103.

2006

1. **Campbell P, Murdock C.** Cardiac amyloidosis - sustained clinical and free light chain response to low dose thalidomide and corticosteroids. Int Med J 2006; **36:** 137-139. *Letter*

2. **Pratt G, Mead GP, Godfrey KR, Ying H, Evans ND, Chappell MJ, Lovell R, Bradwell AR.** The tumour kinetics of multiple myeloma following autologous stem cell transplantation as assessed by measuring serum free light chains. Leukaemia and Lymphoma 2006; **47** (1): 21-28.

3. **Smith A, Wisloff F, Samson D on behalf of the UK Myeloma Forum, Nordic Myeloma Study Group and the British Committee for Standards in Haematology.** Guidelines on the diagnosis and management of Multiple Myeloma 2005. Br J Haem 2006; **132**: 410-451.

4. **Van Der Heijden M, Kraneveld A, Redegeld F.** Free immunoglobulin light chains as target in the treatment of chronic inflammatory diseases. Eur J Pharmacol 2006; **533** (1-3): 319-326. (Epub)

In press or submitted

1. **Abdalla S, Lachmann H, Hawkins P.** The use of serum free light chain assay in clinical practice. *Submitted.*

2. **Bradwell AR, Evans ND, Chappell MJ, Cockwell P, Reid SD, Harrison J, Hutchison C, Mead GP.** Rapid removal of free light chains from serum by hemodialysis for patients with myeloma kidney. *In Press.*

3. **Dispenzieri A, Lacy MQ, Katzmann JA, Rajkumar VS, Abraham RS, Hayman SR, Kumar SK, Clark R, Kyle RA, Litzow MR, Inwards DJ, Ansell SM, Micallef IM, Porrata LF, Elliott MA, Johnston P, Greipp PR, Witzig TE, Zeldenrust SR, Russell SR, Gastineau D, Gertz MA.** Absolute Values of Serum Immunoglobulin Free Light Chains Predict for Survival in Patients with Primary Systemic Amyloidosis Undergoing Peripheral Blood Stem Cell Transplant. Blood 2006; *In Press.*

4. **Evans ND, Hattersley J, Hutchison C, Hu Y, Godfrey KR, Bradwell AR, Mead GP, Chappell MJ.** Modelling of haemodialysis in limiting serum free light chains in patients with renal failure. *Submitted*

5. **Hill PG, Forsyth JM, Rai BS, Mayne S, Mead GP**. Serum free light chain measurement can replace urine electrophoresis for detecting B cell proliferative disorders. *Submitted.*

6. **Hutchison CA, Bradwell AR, Reid SD, Cockwell P, Mead GP, Barnett AH.** Free light chain abnormalities in diabetic patients with and without microalbuminuria. *Submitted*

7. **Hutchison CA, Cockwell P, Reid SD, Chandler K, Millard J, Mead GP, Evans N, Chappell MJ, Bradwell AR.** Removal of serum free light chains by hemodialysis in patients with multiple myeloma. *In Press.*

8. **Katzmann JA.** The Quantitation of Serum Free Light Chains: Clinical Utility. Clin Lab News 2006; *In Press.*

9. **Palladini G, Lavatelli F, Rosso P, Perlini S, Perfetti V, Vezzoli M, Bosoni T, Obici L, Bradwell AR, Melzi D'Eril G, Fogari R, Moratti R, Merlini G.** Circulating amyloidogenic free light chains and serum N-terminal natruiretic peptide type B decrease simultaneously in association with improvement of survival in AL amyloidosis. Blood 2006; *In Press.*

10. **Reid SD, Cockwell P, Millard J, Chandler K, Hutchison CA, Mead GP, Bradwell AR.** MGUS incidence in a chronic kidney disease population. *In Press.*

11. **Showell PJ, Scurvin ML, Chinyimba AL, Carr-Smith HD, Bradwell AR.** Evaluation of latex-enhanced turbidimetric reagents for measurement of free immunoglobulin light-chains on The Binding Site automated analyser. *In Press.*

Index

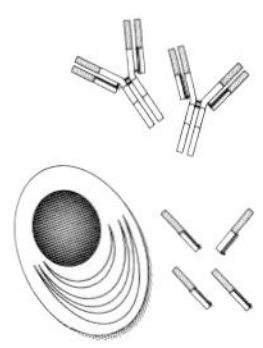

Important pages marked in bold
Figures and clinical case histories are high-lighted in blue
Questions and answers are high-lighted in red - p249-59
Chapter summaries are high-lighted in red

A

N

O

P

Q